HEART DISEASE

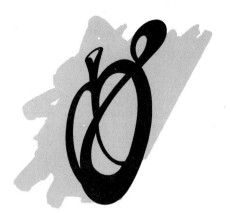

Review and Assessment

A Question and Answer Book with Explanations and References

MICHAEL E. MENDELSOHN, M.D.

Instructor in Medicine, Harvard Medical School;
Associate Physician, Brigham and Women's Hospital, Boston

BRADFORD C. BERK, M.D., Ph.D.

Assistant Professor of Medicine, Harvard Medical School;
Associate Physician, Brigham and Women's Hospital, Boston

Edited by

EUGENE BRAUNWALD, A.B., M.D., M.S. (hon.), M.D. (hon.)

Hersey Professor of the Theory and Practice of Physic;
Herrman Ludwig Blumgart Professor of Medicine, Harvard Medical School;
Chairman, Department of Medicine,
Brigham and Women's and Beth Israel Hospitals, Boston

1989

W. B. SAUNDERS COMPANY

Harcourt Brace Jovanovich, Inc.

Philadelphia, London, Toronto, Montreal, Sydney, Tokyo

W. B. SAUNDERS COMPANY

Harcourt Brace Jovanovich, Inc.

The Curtis Center
Independence Square West
Philadelphia, PA 19106

Library of Congress Cataloging-in-Publication Data

Mendelsohn, Michael E.

Heart disease: review and assessment: a question and answer book
with explanations and references / Michael E. Mendelsohn,
Bradford C. Berk; edited by Eugene Braunwald.

p.   cm.

Includes bibliographies.

Study guide to: Heart disease: a textbook of cardiovascular
medicine / edited by Eugene Braunwald. 3rd ed. 1988.

1. Heart—Diseases—Examinations, questions, etc.
2. Cardiovascular system—Diseases—Examinations,
questions, etc.   I. Berk, Bradford C.   II. Braunwald,
Eugene, 1929–   III. Title. [DNLM: 1. Heart
Diseases—examination questions.   WG 200 H4364 1988
Suppl.]

RC681.H362 1988 Suppl.   616.1′2—dc19   88–39826

ISBN 0–7216–2242–9

Manuscript Editor: Edna Dick

Production Manager: Frank Polizzano

HEART DISEASE: Review and Assessment   ISBN   0–7216–2242–9

Last digit is the print number: 9   8   7   6   5   4   3   2

PREFACE

Heart Disease: Review and Assessment consists of 623 multiple-choice questions designed to provide a comprehensive and useful review of the broad field of cardiology. It is a companion study guide representative of the major areas covered in *Heart Disease: A Textbook of Cardiovascular Medicine*. *Heart Disease: Review and Assessment* is designed to aid in the education of cardiology fellows and cardiologists as well as residents in internal medicine, internists, and other physicians who wish to attain a high level of expertise in cardiology as well as the ability to solve clinical problems. It should be especially helpful to cardiology fellows and others preparing for the Subspecialty Examination in Cardiovascular Disease of the American Board of Internal Medicine.

The basic question types are in the format of the aforementioned examination. Each question is followed by an answer, sometimes quite detailed, and is referenced to specific pages in *Heart Disease, 3rd edition*, as well as to other pertinent references. By allowing two and a half minutes to answer each question, the time constraints of the board examination may be simulated.

This is the first edition of *Heart Disease: Review and Assessment* and was prepared in response to a number of requests. We hope that it will be useful. The authors, the editor, and W. B. Saunders invite comments and suggestions from the reader.

Ms. Kathryn Saxon and Ms. Patricia DeLosh rendered invaluable assistance in the preparation of the manuscript. We are grateful to Marion Laboratories, Inc. for an educational grant that aided the development of this book.

MICHAEL E. MENDELSOHN, M.D.

BRADFORD C. BERK, M.D., PH.D.

EUGENE BRAUNWALD, M.D.

ABBREVIATIONS

A_2	=	second aortic sound	LBBB	=	left bundle branch block
AF	=	atrial fibrillation	LPHB	=	left posterior hemiblock
APC	=	atrial premature contraction	LV	=	left ventricle
ASD	=	atrial septal defect	LVH	=	left ventricular hypertrophy
AV	=	atrio-ventricular	LVOT	=	left ventricular outflow tract
BP	=	blood pressure	MI	=	myocardial infarction
CHF	=	congestive heart failure	MRI	=	magnetic resonance imaging
CT	=	computerized tomography	P_2	=	second pulmonic sound
CVP	=	central venous pressure	PVC	=	premature ventricular contractions
CXR	=	chest x-ray	RA	=	right atrium
EKG	=	electrocardiogram	RBBB	=	right bundle branch block
ETT	=	exercise tolerance testing	RV	=	right ventricle
HOCM	=	hypertrophic obstructive cardiomyopathy	S_1	=	first heart sound
HR	=	heart rate	S_2	=	second heart sound
JVP	=	jugular venous pressure	S_3	=	third heart sound
LA	=	left atrium	S_4	=	fourth heart sound
LAHB	=	left anterior hemiblock	VSD	=	ventricular septal defect

CONTENTS

PART I: EXAMINATION OF THE PATIENT

CHAPTERS 1 THROUGH 12

DIRECTIONS: Each question below contains five suggested responses. Select the ONE BEST response to each question.

1. Each of the following statements concerning the history in congenital heart disease is true EXCEPT:

   A. Murmurs due to aortic or pulmonic stenosis are often apparent within the first 48 hours of life
   B. A large left-to-right shunt may lead to frequent episodes of pneumonia in early infancy
   C. Rubella in the first 2 months of pregnancy is associated with several cardiac malformations, including patent ductus arteriosus and supravalvular aortic stenosis
   D. A history of squatting is most frequently associated with valvular pulmonic or aortic stenosis
   E. A maternal viral illness in the third trimester may lead to neonatal myocarditis

2. All of the following statements about pulsus paradoxus are true EXCEPT:

   A. A reduction in the systolic arterial pressure of up to 8 mm Hg during inspiration is within normal limits and reflects a small reduction in LV stroke volume and a transmission of negative intrathoracic pressure to the aorta
   B. Pulsus paradoxus is observed frequently in cardiac tamponade
   C. Pulsus paradoxus is observed in patients with pulmonary disease associated with wide swings in intrathoracic pressure
   D. In the presence of aortic regurgitation, pulsus paradoxus is less likely to develop, despite the presence of tamponade
   E. Pulsus paradoxus may occur in hypertrophic obstructive cardiomyopathy (HOCM)

3. Each of the following comments about the phonocardiograms displayed *below* is correct EXCEPT:

   A. A long, late-peaking crescendo-decrescendo murmur is noted during systole
   B. The second heart sound is soft and single
   C. A prominent third heart sound recorded at the apex is synchronized with an accentuated *a* wave in the apex cardiogram
   D. The carotid pulse tracing shows a relatively slow rate of rise
   E. The first heart sound has two components, the second of which is loudest and coincides with the carotid pulse, consistent with an ejection sound

4. The diagnosis most consistent with the phonocardiograms displayed is

   A. hypertrophic obstructive cardiomyopathy (HOCM)
   B. AS, supravalvular
   C. AS, calcific, valvular, mild
   D. AS, calcific, valvular, severe
   E. ventricular septal defect

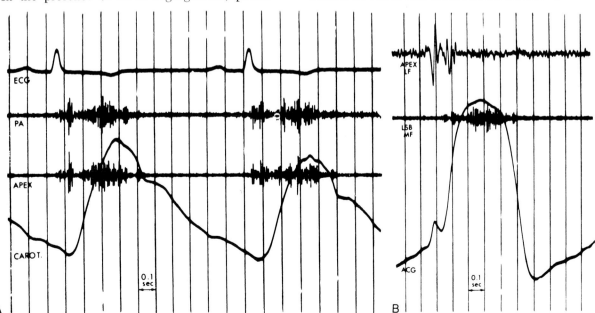

From Tavel, M.E.: Clinical Phonocardiography and External Pulse Recording. 3rd ed. Chicago, Year Book Medical Publishers, 1978, p. 327.

5. Each of the following statements about the measurement of cardiac output is true EXCEPT:

   A. The Fick principle states that the total uptake or release of a substance by an organ is the product of blood flow to the organ and the arteriovenous difference of the substance measured
   B. The normal range of cardiac index is 2.6 to 4.2 liters/min/m^2
   C. Angiographic measurement of LV end-diastolic and end-systolic volumes permits calculation of stroke volume, which may be used with heart rate to calculate cardiac output
   D. In patients with low cardiac output, the thermodilution method provides a more accurate measurement of cardiac output than the Fick O$_2$ method
   E. Provided that no intracardiac shunt is present, measurement of pulmonary blood flow and the difference between systemic and pulmonary arterial O$_2$ content allows calculation of the systemic blood flow

6. Each of the following statements concerning cyanosis is true EXCEPT:

   A. The bluish discoloration of cyanosis results from either an increased amount of reduced hemoglobin or the presence of abnormal hemoglobin pigments
   B. Central cyanosis is characterized by decreased arterial oxygen saturation
   C. Patients with marked polycythemia become cyanotic at higher levels of arterial oxygen saturation than patients with normal hematocrit
   D. Peripheral cyanosis most commonly results from impaired pulmonary function
   E. Localization of peripheral cyanosis to a single extremity may suggest arterial or venous obstruction

7. All of the following statements about the ECG depicted *below* are correct EXCEPT:

   A. The basic rhythm is atrial fibrillation
   B. The abnormal beat is an example of the Ashman phenomenon
   C. As opposed to early excitation, the abnormal conduction of the Ashman beat is a function of an altered duration of the refractory period rather than of changing prematurity of stimulation
   D. RBBB morphology is more commonly associated with this type of aberrancy
   E. Because the bundle of His has the longest refractory period, it is the likely anatomic location of the conduction delay

8. Each of the following statements about cardiac catheterization is true EXCEPT:

   A. Patients with ball-cage prosthetic aortic valves can safely undergo retrograde left ventricular catheterization
   B. Transseptal left-heart catheterization should not be attempted in patients with suspected severe mitral valve obstruction
   C. Catheterization of outpatients has been demonstrated to be a safe and cost-effective alternative in appropriately selected patients
   D. A percutaneous brachial arterial approach may be used in adults provided that the catheters used are of small size
   E. Porcine heterograft valves in the aortic position can safely be crossed in the course of performing a retrograde left ventricular catheterization

9. All of the following statements with reference to digital cardiac angiography are true EXCEPT:

   A. Less contrast media is needed than with conventional imaging because dye intensity needs to be only slightly above background
   B. The spatial resolution of digital arteriography on a 256 × 256 matrix is adequate for high-quality coronary angiography and analyses of arteries smaller than 0.4 mm
   C. Use of time-of-contrast-arrival maps before and after induced hyperpnea allows study of flow reserve
   D. There is close agreement between measurements of left ventricular volume obtained digitally and with standard-dose cineangiograms but a higher incidence of ventricular arrhythmias with the latter technique
   E. Digital *intravenous* ventriculography, in comparison with radionuclide rest-exercise studies, provides better spatial resolution and improved wall motion analysis

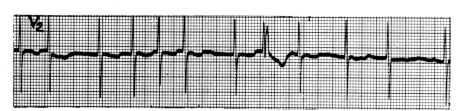

From Marriott, H.J.L.: Rhythm Quizlets: Self Assessment. Philadelphia, Lea & Febiger, 1987, p. 14.

10. A patient with a long history of pulmonary emboli undergoes noninvasive assessment of cardiac status by Doppler echocardiography. Assuming the following values:

    RA pressure = 4 mm Hg
    Peak Doppler flow signal across the tricuspid valve = 4 meters/second

    The patient's right ventricular systolic pressure is:

    A. 64 mm Hg
    B. 68 mm Hg
    C. 50 mm Hg
    D. 20 mm Hg
    E. Insufficient information to determine the value

11. Findings easily shown on *both* two-dimensional and M-mode echocardiography in mitral stenosis include all the following EXCEPT:

    A. Doming of the mitral valve leaflets
    B. Inadequate separation of the anterior and posterior leaflets of the valve during diastole
    C. Increased thickness of the valve leaflets
    D. The presence of fibrosis and calcifications as revealed by an increase in the number of echoes
    E. An increase in left atrial size due to left atrial hypertension

12. The electrocardiogram depicted is consistent with

    A. reversal of the limb leads
    B. left posterior hemiblock

    C. right ventricular hypertrophy
    D. counterclockwise rotation and left anterior hemiblock
    E. none of the above

13. Exercise tolerance testing (ETT) of asymptomatic subjects may be of clinical value because:

    A. the risk ratio for individuals who manifest an ischemic response has been found to average more than 5 in several major studies
    B. less than 1 per cent of patients tested will have false-negative results
    C. among patients who develop ST-segment elevation during an ETT, approximately 10 per cent have left main coronary disease
    D. although the mortality rate for ETT is about 10/10,000 tests, this is less than the number of lives saved as a result of diagnosis
    E. of those with positive tests, more than 70 per cent subsequently develop coronary artery disease

14. All of the following statements with regard to radionuclide angiocardiography are true EXCEPT:

    A. The correlation between ejection fractions derived by radionuclide and contrast ventriculography is excellent (r > 0.9)
    B. Assessment of systolic function and regional wall motion is possible

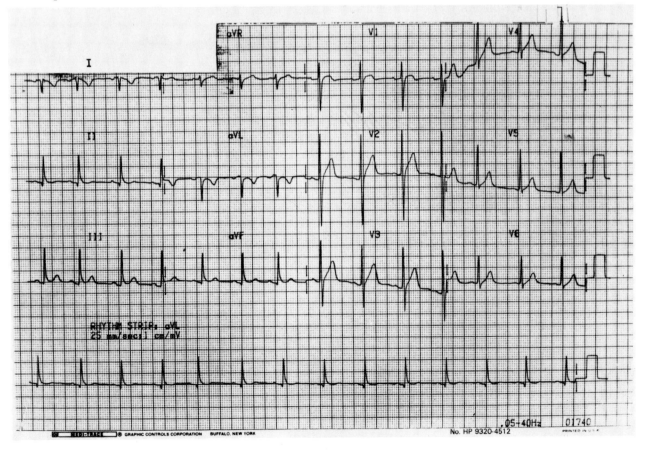

C. Spatial resolution, especially of the ventricular edges, is poor

D. Despite background subtraction algorithms, the geometry of the left ventricle relative to the detector critically affects determination of the left ventricular ejection fraction

E. LV ejection fraction = $\dfrac{EDC - ESC}{EDC - BC}$

    Where EDC = end diastolic counts
           ESC = end systolic counts
           BC = background counts

15. All of the following statements are correct with regard to thallium-201 perfusion scintigraphy EXCEPT:

A. Thallium-201 is a K^+ analog

B. Extraction of thallium by the myocardium is not affected by inhibition of the Na^+,K^+-ATPase by digoxin

C. Coronary blood flow increases uniformly throughout the ventricle in normal subjects during exercise; coronary artery stenosis results in reduced thallium extraction during exercise by myocardium in the distribution of the obstructed coronary vessel

D. Like microspheres, thallium stays trapped in the myocardium for 16 to 24 hours

E. Prior administration of dipyridamole results in a doubling of the dose of thallium, which is concentrated in the myocardium

DIRECTIONS: Each question below contains five suggested answers. For EACH of the FIVE alternatives listed you are to respond either YES (Y) or NO (N). In a given item ALL, SOME, OR NONE OF THE ALTERNATIVES MAY BE CORRECT.

16. With reference to intracardiac shunts, which of the following statements are true?

A. In normal subjects, O_2 content in different portions of the right atrium may vary by as much as 2 volumes per cent (20 ml O_2/liter), reflecting that streaming of blood received from the superior vena cava, the inferior vena cava, and the coronary sinus occurs in the right atrium

B. Atrial septal defect, anomalous pulmonary venous drainage, and ruptured sinus of Valsalva may all lead to significant step-up in O_2 saturation values between the venae cavae and the right atrium

C. Because of the normal variability in O_2 saturation, shunts with pulmonary-to-systemic flow ratios (Qp/Qs) ≤ 1.3 at the level of the pulmonary artery or right ventricle may escape detection by oximetry run analyses

D. When a shunt is unidirectional (e.g., left-to-right only), its magnitude is calculated as the difference between the pulmonary and systemic blood flows as determined using the appropriate variations of the Fick equation

E. In patients with a pure right-to-left shunt, such as in tetralogy of Fallot, the calculated left-to-right shunt will be a negative value

17. With reference to the magnetic resonance image (MRI) shown in the figure *below*, true statements

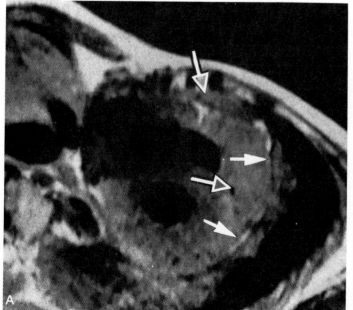

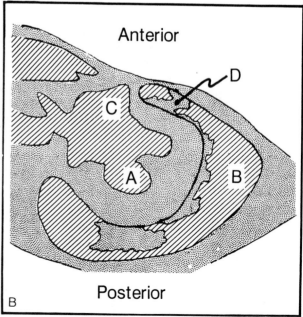

From Levine, H.J., and Southern, J.F.: A 58-year-old woman with progressive pericardial disease. N. Engl. J. Med. *316*:1402, 1987.

include which of the following? (Please note that the solid arrows delineate the epicardial fat line.)

A. The structure labeled "A" is the main pulmonary artery
B. The structure labeled "B" is the pericardial space
C. The structure labeled "C" is the right ventricle
D. The structure anterior to "D" is a paracardiac mass
E. The contents of the structure labeled "B" could be blood or transudate

18. Correct statements regarding the utility of echocardiography in myocardial ischemia and myocardial infarction include which of the following?

A. During systole, the left ventricle normally increases in thickness
B. At one year following a transmural myocardial infarction, ventricular wall thickness remains normal in diastole, but systolic thickening is abolished, indicative of infarction
C. The presence of a ventricular aneurysm is suggested echocardiographically by identification of a thrombus in the left ventricular inferior wall surrounded by a pericardial sac
D. LV mural thrombi occur most commonly with anterior myocardial infarctions
E. M-mode echocardiography is a sensitive way to detect a ventricular septal defect during acute MI

19. Each of the following are true statements about coronary artery anatomy EXCEPT:

A. The left coronary artery is dominant in 10 to 23 per cent of humans
B. The interventricular septum is the most densely vascularized area of the heart
C. Over 90 per cent of patients have between one and three diagonal vessels branching off the left anterior descending artery
D. A ramus medianus branch arising between the left anterior descending coronary (LAD) and circumflex arteries is present in approximately 10 per cent of patients
E. The position of the coronary sinus identifies the position of the circumflex artery, which runs in or near the atrioventricular groove

20. With reference to the electrocardiographic diagnosis of myocardial infarction, which of the following are true?

A. Less than 75 per cent of patients have a diagnostic ECG initially
B. Serial ECGs will increase the diagnostic sensitivity to greater than 80 per cent
C. About 30 per cent of patients with old Q wave myocardial infarction will eventually "lose" their Q wave
D. Patients with inferior myocardial infarctions and

reciprocal ST depressions in leads V_1 to V_4 usually have associated circumflex artery disease
E. Right ventricular infarction can be diagnosed with high sensitivity (> 75 per cent) by ST segment elevation in V_4R.

21. With reference to the jugular venous pulse (JVP), true statements include which of the following?

A. Two principal observations made from examination of the neck veins include the level of venous pressure and the type of venous wave pattern
B. Tricuspid regurgitation and right ventricular failure respond to the abdominojugular reflex test with a sustained rise in jugular venous pressure
C. The v wave results from right atrial pressure rise in response to blood flow into the right atrium during ventricular systole when the tricuspid valve is shut
D. Cannon (giant) a waves are observed when the right atrium contracts against a closed tricuspid valve, as in atrioventricular dissociation
E. Kussmaul's sign is a paradoxical fall in the height of the jugular venous pulse during inspiration which occurs frequently in patients with chronic constrictive pericarditis

22. With reference to complications of cardiac catheterization, which of the following statements are true?

A. The likelihood of death occurring from cardiac catheterization is less than 0.5 per cent
B. The likelihood of acute MI occurring from cardiac catheterization is less than 0.5 per cent
C. The incidence of death from cardiac catheterization is greater in patients under 1 year of age
D. Mortality from catheterization of patients with significant left main coronary artery disease is less than 0.5 per cent
E. The presence of valvular disease is associated with a higher risk of death at cardiac catheterization

23. Correct statements regarding the clinical interpretation of exercise stress testing include which of the following?

A. A finding of 0.1 mV of ST-segment depression *after* exercise is more specific than 0.1 mV ST-segment depression *during* exercise
B. A patient with a 50 per cent stenosis in the right coronary artery will probably develop ischemic ECG changes in leads II, III, and aV_f at a peak-pressure product of $\leq 15,000$ mm Hg $\times$ beats/min
C. In most exercise protocols the systolic blood pressure rises about 8 to 10 mm Hg per stage
D. Maximal predicted exercise heart rate is approximately $220 - $ (the patient's age)
E. In normal exercise there may be ≥ 0.1 mV J-point depression

24. Which of the following statements comparing first-pass and equilibrium angiocardiography are true?

    A. Both techniques yield accurate measurements of global left ventricular ejection fraction
    B. Regional wall motion abnormalities are assessed with equal accuracy
    C. Physiological or pharmacological interventions are better assessed by the equilibrium technique
    D. The number of studies is more limited by first-pass technique
    E. Interventions that result in rapid changes in heart rate are assessed better by equilibrium technique

25. With reference to technetium-99m-pyrophosphate (^{99m}Tc-PYP) imaging, true statements include which of the following?

    A. Uptake begins to increase within 1 hour of permanent coronary artery occlusion
    B. Intensity of radiopharmaceutical uptake reaches a peak by 48 hours
    C. The concentration ratio of ^{99m}Tc-PYP in infarct to normal myocardium is frequently greater than 10:1
    D. Approximately 50 per cent of the injected dose is actually extracted by bone
    E. The highest concentration ratio occurs in the central zones of necrosis where there is no blood flow

DIRECTIONS: Each question below contains four suggested responses of which ONE OR MORE ARE CORRECT. Select

    A   if 1, 2, and 3 are correct
    B   if 1 and 3 are correct
    C   if 2 and 4 are correct
    D   if 4 is correct
    E   if 1, 2, 3, and 4 are correct

26. Transient perfusion defects on thallium-201 scintigraphy are seen in which of the following settings?

    1. Patients with muscular myocardial bridges
    2. Patients with diffuse myocardial disease
    3. Patients with severe aortic valve stenosis
    4. Patients with mitral valve prolapse

27. Abnormalities that may enter into the differential diagnosis of chest pain or discomfort include:

    1. pulmonary hypertension
    2. Mallory-Weiss syndrome
    3. scalenus anticus syndrome
    4. congenital absence of the pericardium

28. True statements concerning ejection sounds include:

    1. Ejection sounds of aortic origin are most prominent in association with a deformed aortic valve, such as a bicuspid valve, or in congenital or rheumatic AS
    2. While aortic ejection sounds due to a dilated aortic root may be less prominent than those associated with valvular disease, they have a similar timing early in systole
    3. A decrease in intensity of the pulmonic ejection sound with inspiration is heard in pulmonic valve stenosis
    4. It can be shown by echophonocardiography that high-frequency ejection sounds start before the aortic or pulmonic valve is completely open

29. The cardiac catheterization tracing illustrated *below* could be associated with which of the following features?

    1. A large systolic pressure gradient between left ventricle and aorta

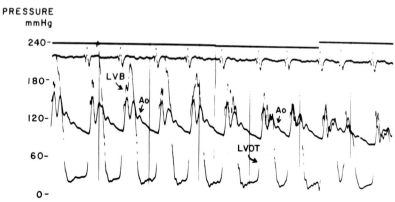

PRESSURE
mmHg

240 —
180 — LVB
           Ao
120 —
                        Ao
60 —   LVOT
0 —

From Levinson, G.E.: Aortic stenosis. *In* Dalen, J.E., and Alpert, J.S. (eds.): Valvular Heart Disease. 2nd ed. Boston, Little, Brown & Company, 1987, p. 257.

2. A bifid aortic pulse contour
3. Increased ventricular stiffness resulting in prominent *a* waves and an elevated left ventricular end-diastolic pressure
4. A slow and delayed rise in the aortic pressure as compared with that of the left ventricle

---

30. Rotation of the heart within the chest cavity results in which of the following changes in the ECG?

    1. A "horizontal" heart leads to a QRS complex in aVL that resembles leads V_5 and V_6
    2. "Clockwise rotation" causes the "rS" portions of the QRS complex to be present in leads V_2 to V_5
    3. A "vertical" heart leads to a QRS complex in lead aVF that resembles leads V_5 and V_6
    4. "Counterclockwise rotation" can mimic right ventricular hypertrophy

---

31. Infarct scintigraphy with ^{99m}Tc-pyrophosphate may be positive in diagnosis of which of the following clinical situations?

    1. Myocardial contusion
    2. Transmural infarction 2 days old
    3. Transmural infarction 2 months old
    4. Right ventricular infarction

---

32. Which of the following statements concerning catheterization laboratory evaluation of valve orifice areas are true?

    A. Valve area in cm² is calculated as
    Flow (in ml/sec) ÷ K × (mean pressure gradient in mm Hg)$^{1/2}$ where K is an empirical constant for the valve in question
    B. The presence of valvular regurgitation will result in a falsely low calculated valve area because the actual flow is greater than the flow calculated from the systemic cardiac output
    C. Calculation of mitral valve area often relies on substitution of a confirmed pulmonary capillary wedge pressure for left atrial pressure
    D. Stenotic valve areas calculated in patients with coexisting regurgitation should be considered to be the upper limits of the true valve area

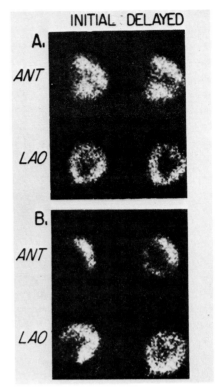

INITIAL DELAYED

From Okada, R.D., Boucher, C.A., Strauss, H.W., and Pohost, G.M.: Exercise radionuclide imaging approaches to coronary artery disease. Am. J. Cardiol. *46*:1188, 1980.

33. The myocardial scintigrams in *A* are from a normal patient. The scintigrams in *B* demonstrate the following features:

    1. a perfusion defect that is partly reversible
    2. an inferior perfusion defect
    3. an irreversible perfusion defect
    4. an increase in lung uptake of the radioisotope on the initial image

---

34. Computed tomography of the pericardium can delineate or differentiate the following features:

    A. loculated pericardial effusions and hemopericardium from transudative fluid
    B. congenital absence of the pericardium
    C. constrictive pericarditis with thickened pericardium from restrictive cardiomyopathy
    D. mucoid-secreting pericardial cysts from solid tumors

DIRECTIONS: The group of questions below consists of lettered headings followed by a set of numbered items. For each numbered item select the ONE lettered heading with which it is MOST closely associated. Each lettered heading may be used ONCE, MORE THAN ONCE, OR NOT AT ALL.

For each of the chest roentgenograms (A–D), match the most appropriate cardiac diagnosis:

35. mitral stenosis

36. aortic regurgitation

37. atrial septal defect

38. pericardial effusion

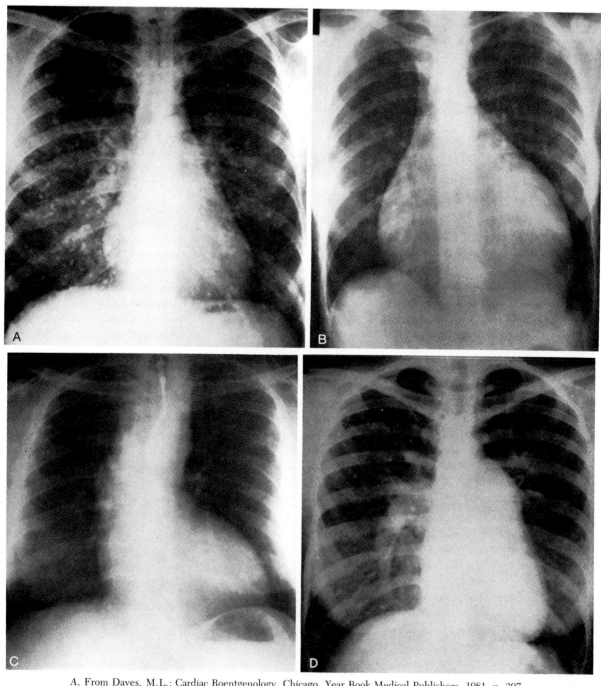

A, From Daves, M.L.: Cardiac Roentgenology. Chicago, Year Book Medical Publishers, 1981, p. 397.
B, From Daves, M.L.: Cardiac Roentgenology. Chicago, Year Book Medical Publishers, 1981, p. 470.
C, From Daves, M.L.: Cardiac Roentgenology. Chicago, Year Book Medical Publishers, 1981, p. 413.
D. From Daves, M.L.: Cardiac Roentgenology. Chicago, Year Book Medical Publishers, 1981, p. 271.

For each statement or definition, match the appropriate sign on physical examination:

    A. Hill's sign
    B. de Musset's sign
    C. Duroziez's sign
    D. Quincke's sign
    E. Traube's sign

39. "Pistol shot" sounds heard over the femoral artery when a stethoscope is placed on it

40. Systolic blood pressure in the popliteal artery exceeds that in the brachial artery by more than 20 mm Hg

41. Bobbing of the head in synchrony with each heart-beat.

42. A systolic murmur heard upon gradual compression of the proximal femoral artery, with a diastolic murmur heard upon compression of the artery distally

---

For each arteriogram or set of arteriograms on the following 2 pages (A–E), match the appropriate descriptive phrase.

43. RAO projection; LAD artery, demonstrating myocardial bridging with narrowing in systole and near-normal caliber in diastole

44. LAO projection; right coronary arteriogram demonstrating anomalous origin of the left circumflex artery from the proximal RCA

45. LAO projection; collateral vessels arising from the distal right coronary artery and supplying an occluded LAD artery

46. RAO projection; catheter-induced coronary spasm and restoration of normal caliber with introduction of nitroglycerin

47. LAO projection; showing early filling of a markedly dilated left circumflex artery and subsequent coronary sinus opacification due to a congenital fistula

---

The figure (top right) illustrates the Doppler flow signal obtained while interpolating the blood flow across the aortic valve of a patient from the supra-sternal notch.

    A. 40 mm Hg
    B. 32 mm Hg
    C. Increased
    D. Decreased
    E. No change

48. The transvalvular pressure gradient in mm Hg

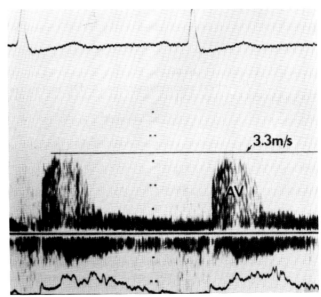

From Nishimura, R.A., et al.: Doppler echocardiography: Theory, instrumentation, technique and application. Mayo Clin. Proc. 60:331, 1985.

49. The effect of inappropriate angulation between the Doppler beam and the blood jet on the peak flow signal in the continuous wave mode

50. The aortic valve gradient (mm Hg) obtained by the Doppler measurement versus that obtained during cardiac catheterization

---

For each disease listed, match the appropriate descriptive phrase

    A. Ellis–van Creveld syndrome
    B. Down syndrome
    C. Werner syndrome
    D. Kearns-Sayre syndrome
    E. Holt-Oram syndrome

51. Prominent medial epicanthus, hypoplastic mandible, low-set ears, and endocardial cushion defect

52. Congenital heart disease accompanying dwarfism, polydactyly, hypoplastic fingernails, and ectodermal dysplasia

53. Proptosis, premature graying of the hair, frontal baldness, cataract formation, and premature coronary atherosclerosis

54. Ptosis, retinopathy, and external ophthalmoplegia in association with complete heart block

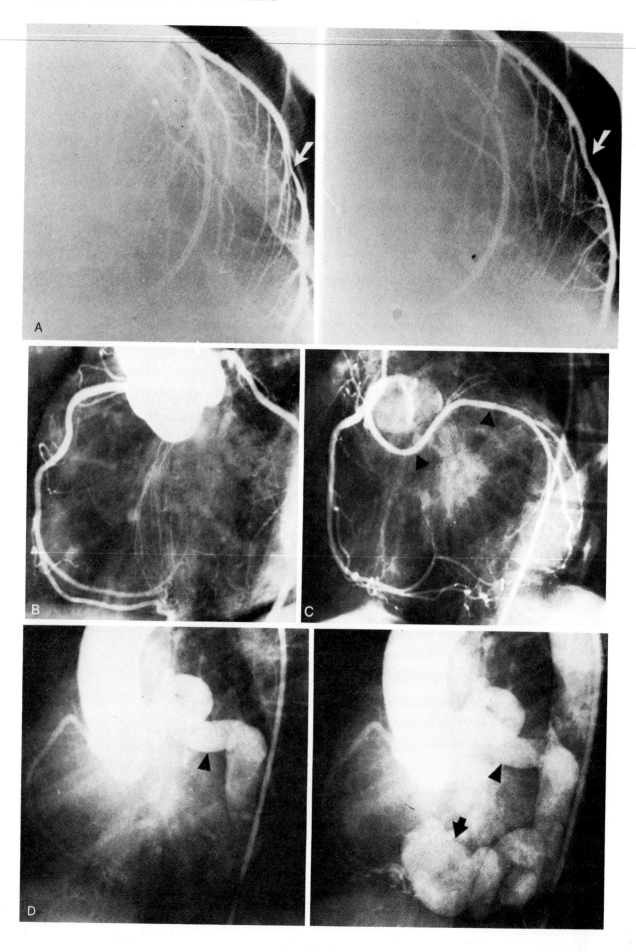

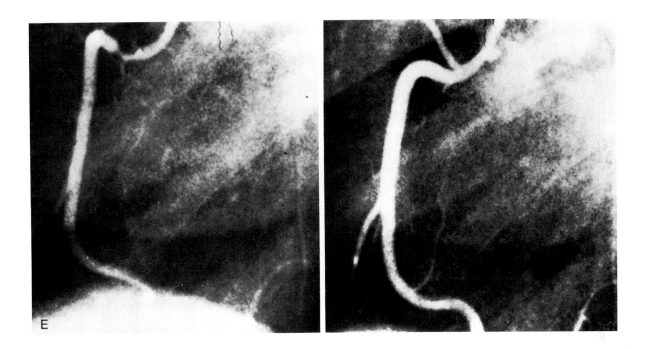

A, From Levin, D.C.: Pitfalls in coronary arteriography. *In* Abrams, H.L. (ed.): Coronary Arteriography: A Practical Approach. Boston, Little, Brown & Company, 1983, p. 251.

B, From Paulin, S.: Interarterial coronary anastomoses in relation to arterial obstruction demonstrated in coronary arteriography. Invest. Radiol. 2:147, 1967.

C, From Levin, D.C.: Anomalies and anatomic variations of the coronary arteries. *In* Abrams, H.L. (ed.): Coronary Arteriography: A Practical Approach. Boston, Little, Brown & Company, 1983, p. 290.

D, From Levin, D.C., Fellows, K.E., and Abrams, H.L.: Hemodynamically significant primary anomalies of the coronary arteries. Angiographic aspects. Circulation 58:25, 1978. Reprinted by permission of the American Heart Association, Inc.

E, From Abrams, H.L.: Angiography in coronary disease. *In* Abrams, H.L. (ed.): Coronary Arteriography: A Practical Approach. Boston, Little, Brown & Company, 1983, p. 225.

For each electrocardiogram, match the appropriate interpretation.

55. left posterior hemiblock

56. Wolff-Parkinson-White syndrome

57. right bundle branch block and left anterior hemiblock

58. right ventricular hypertrophy

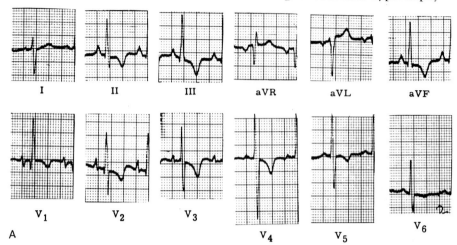

A, From Goldman, M.J.: Principles of Clinical Electrocardiograpahy. 11th ed. Los Altos, CA, Lange Medical Publications, 1982, p. 363.

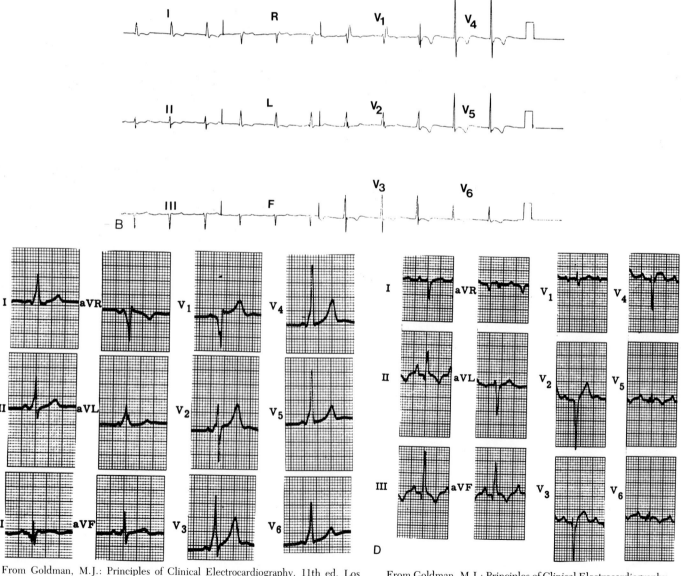

From Goldman, M.J.: Principles of Clinical Electrocardiography. 11th ed. Los Altos, CA, Lange Medical Publications, 1982, p. 277.

From Goldman, M.J.: Principles of Clinical Electrocardiography. 11th ed. Los Altos, CA, Lange Medical Publications, 1982, p. 133.

ELECTROCARDIOGRAMS

DIRECTIONS: Each of the 12-lead ECGs below is introduced by a brief descriptive phrase. For each electrocardiogram, perform a systematic reading. Begin with noting any atrial, AV junctional, or ventricular rhythms present and point out whether any AV conduction abnormalities or atrial-ventricular interactions exist. Determine whether criteria are met for abnormal voltage, ventricular hypertrophy, or intraventricular conduction disturbances. Continue by noting abnormal ST- and/or T-wave changes as well as any Q wave MI that may be apparent. Conclude by citing any suggested clinical abnormality compatible with each tracing.

59. An elderly man seen in a nursing home with a complaint of occasional dizziness

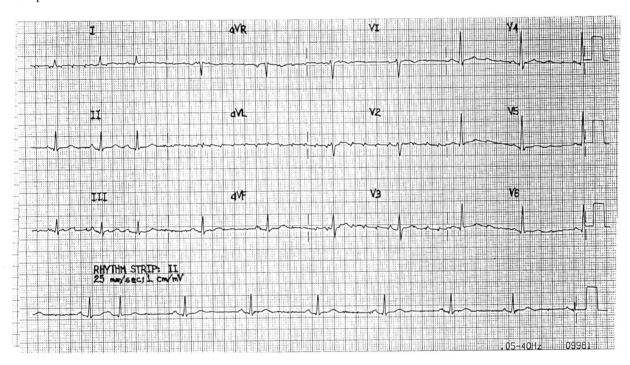

60. An elderly woman with severe dyspnea on exertion

61. A 54-year-old woman with weight loss

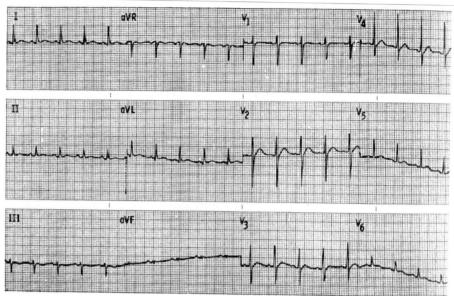

Chung, E.K.: Electrocardiography: Practical Applications with Vectorial Principles. 3rd ed. Boston, Appleton-Century-Crofts, 1985, p. 532.

62. An exercise tolerance test tracing from a 46-year-old man

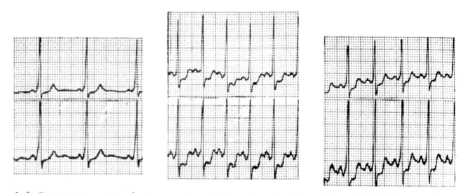

Left, Preexercise; *center*, during exercise; *right*, postexercise. From Chung, E.K. Electrocardiography: Practical Applications with Vectorial Principles. 3rd ed. Boston, Appleton-Century-Crofts, 1985, p. 456.

63. A 68-year-old woman with dyspnea and edema

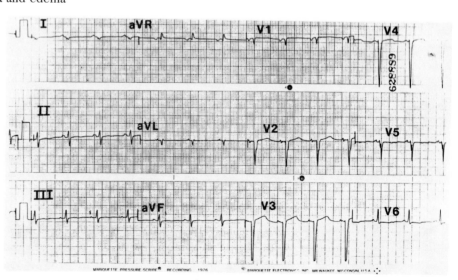

64. A 60-year-old man with history of chest pain

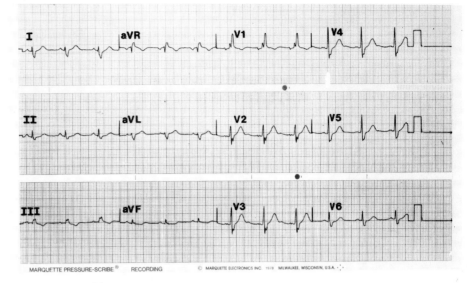

65. An 18-year-old woman in the emergency room with chest pain

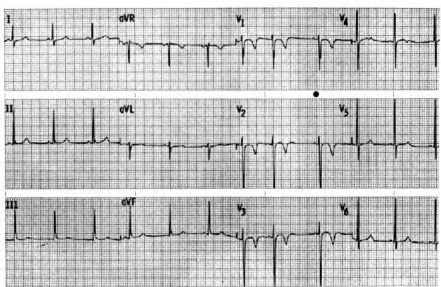

Chung, E.K.: Electrocardiography: Practical Applications with Vectorial Principles. 3rd ed. Boston, Appleton-Century-Crofts, 1985, p. 692.

66. A 20-year-old man with a heart murmur

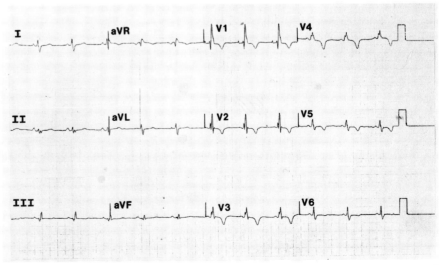

67. A 54-year-old woman with atypical chest pain

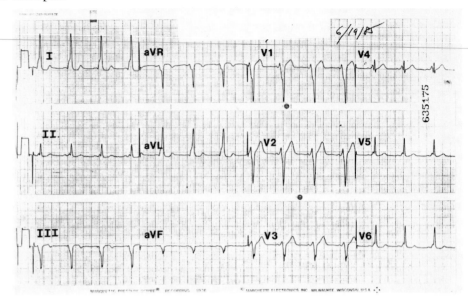

68. A 56-year-old diabetic woman in the coronary care
unit

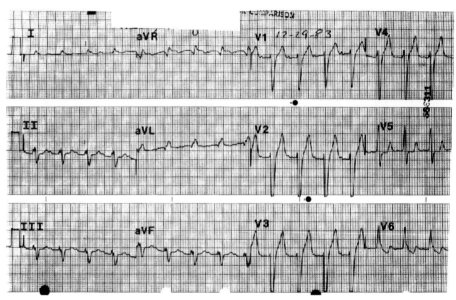

69. A 48-year-old man in the emergency room with
nausea

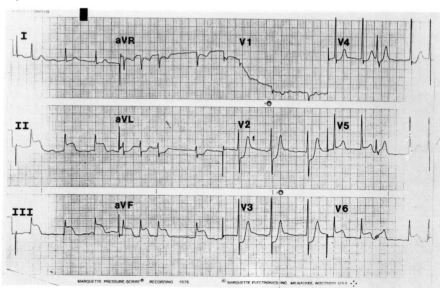

70. A 48-year-old man in the coronary care unit

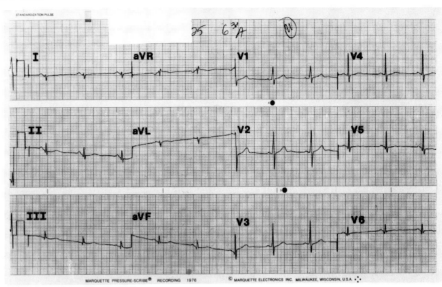

71. A 58-year-old man in the cardiology clinic

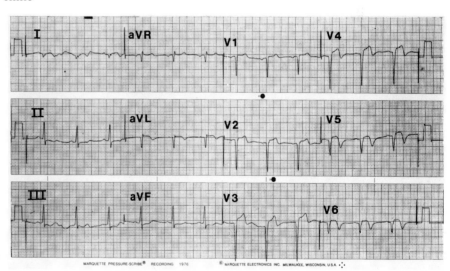

72. A 62-year-old woman after cholecystectomy

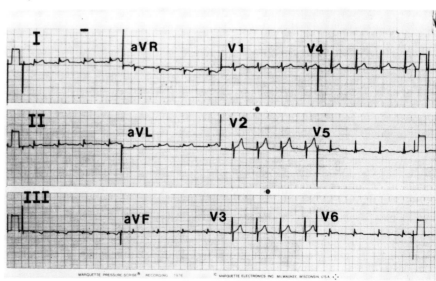

73. A 44-year-old asymptomatic woman having a routine
    evaluation

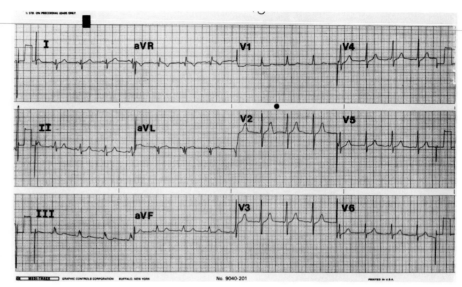

74. A 44-year-old woman with dyspnea

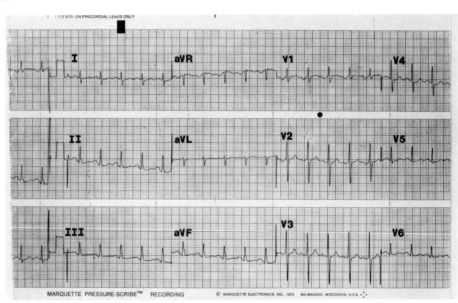

75. A 72-year-old man with dizziness

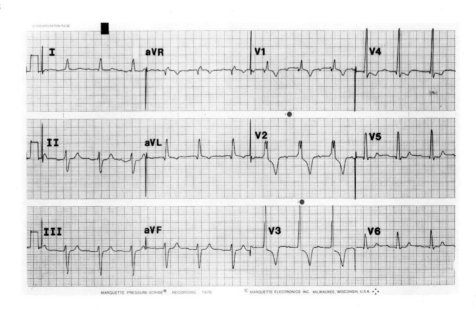

76. A middle-aged man with palpitations

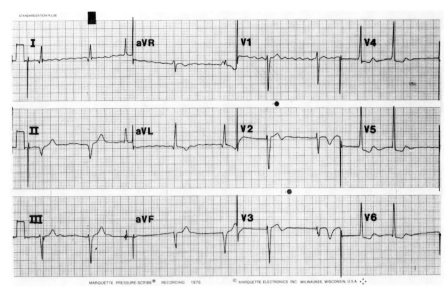

77. A 36-year-old woman in acute pulmonary edema

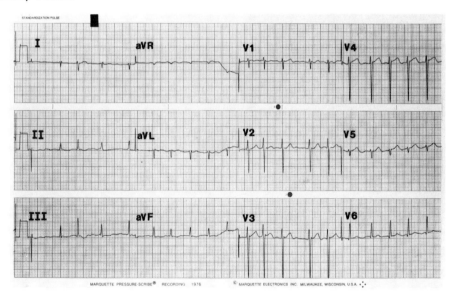

78. A young man in the cardiology clinic

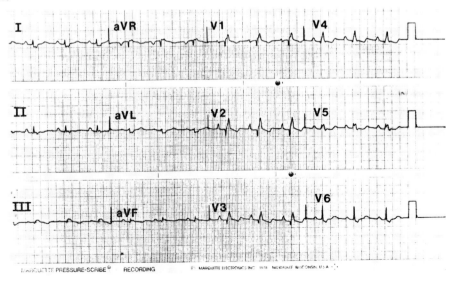

79. A 56-year-old man in the CCU

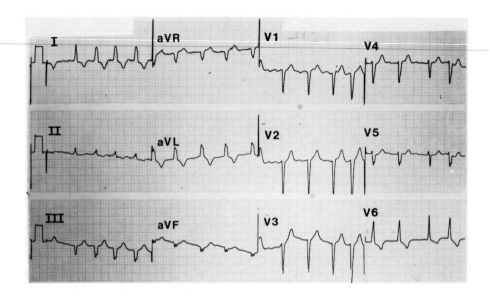

80. A 42-year-old man in the emergency room with palpitations

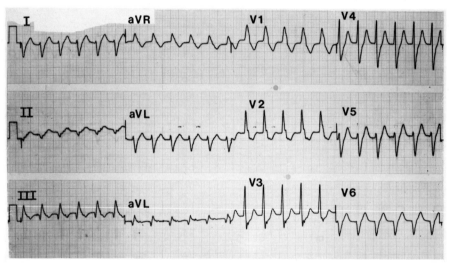

81. A 72-year-old man in the CCU

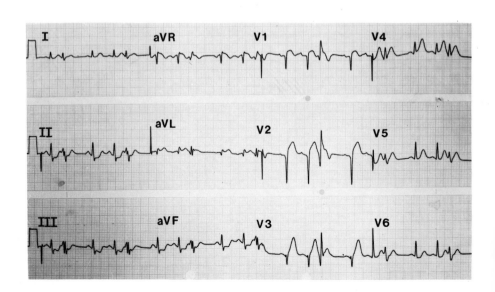

82. An asymptomatic 52-year-old man

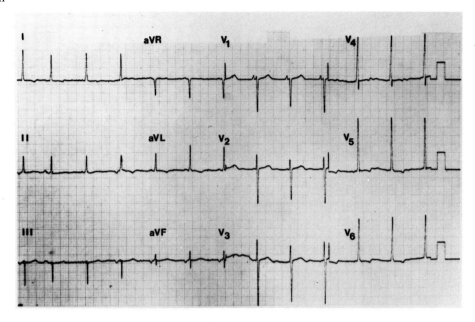

83. A 48-year-old man with a history of diabetes mellitus

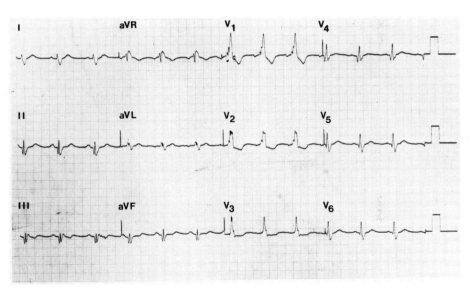

84. A 62-year-old woman in the CCU

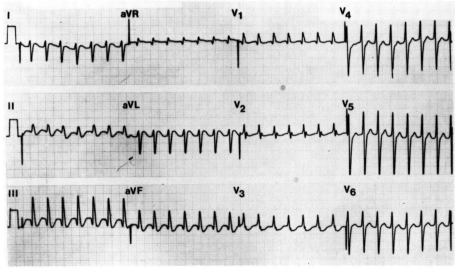

PART I: EXAMINATION OF THE PATIENT
CHAPTERS 1 THROUGH 12
ANSWERS

1-D *(Braunwald, p. 10;* Guntheroth, W.G., et al.: Physiologic studies of paroxysmal hyperpnea in cyanotic congenital heart disease. Circulation *31*:70, 1965.)

In infants or children with cardiac murmurs, knowing the age at which a murmur was first appreciated may be helpful diagnostically. Murmurs of aortic or pulmonic stenosis are usually audible within the first 2 days of life, whereas the murmur of a ventricular septal defect (VSD) usually appears a few days or weeks later. Frequent episodes of pneumonia early in infancy should suggest the presence of a sizable left-to-right shunt. Excessive diaphoresis may occur in LV failure in this age group, most often due to the presence of a VSD. Squatting, which appears to improve O_2 saturation by increasing systemic vascular resistance, is most frequently noted in tetralogy of Fallot or tricuspid atresia, especially after exertion.

Maternal illness may lead to cardiac disease in the developing fetus. Rubella in the first trimester is associated with patent ductus arteriosus, atrial and ventricular septal defect, tetralogy of Fallot, and supravalvular aortic stenosis, whereas a maternal viral illness in the last trimester may be responsible for neonatal myocarditis.

2-E *(Braunwald, p. 24)*

Pulsus paradoxus is an exaggeration of the normal tendency for arterial pulse strength to fall with inspiration, resulting from a reduced LV stroke volume and the transmission of negative intrathoracic pressure to the aorta. A fall of more than 8 to 10 mm Hg with inspiration is considered abnormal and can be observed in a variety of conditions. Pulsus paradoxus is characteristic of patients with cardiac tamponade, is seen in approximately half of patients with chronic constrictive pericarditis, and is noted as well in patients with wide intrapleural pressure swings (e.g., bronchial asthma and emphysema), pulmonary embolism, pregnancy, extreme obesity, and hypovolemic shock. Of note, AR tends to prevent the development of pulsus paradoxus even in the presence of tamponade. In HOCM an inspiratory *rise* in arterial pressure may occur, leading to *reversed* pulsus paradoxus.[1] Interestingly, pulsus paradoxus may also be present occasionally in patients with right ventricular infarction,[2] perhaps due to a combination of right ventricular

dysfunction and the restricting effects of the pericardium, in a manner analogous to that occurring in constrictive pericardial disease.

REFERENCES

1. Massumi, R. A., et al.: Reversed pulsus paradoxus. N. Engl. J. Med. 289:1272, 1973.
2. Lorell, B., et al.: Right ventricular infarction. Am. J. Cardiol. 43:465, 1979.

3-C; 4-D *(Braunwald, pp. 42–43, 57–60;* Tavel, M. E.: Clinical Phonocardiography and External Pulse Recording, 4th ed. Chicago, Year Book Medical Publishers, 1985.)

The phonocardiogram presented in *A* illustrates a widely split first sound, a relatively late peaking systolic murmur, and a soft second sound that is single. The second component of the first sound is prominent and coincides with the upstroke in the carotid tracing, consistent with an ejection sound. The murmur is long and crescendo-decrescendo in shape, and it stops just before the second sound. This second sound just precedes the dicrotic notch on the carotid pulse tracing and is best recorded at the apex, consistent with its origination from aortic closure. Of note, pulmonic closure is not seen, probably because it is "buried" in the murmur. The prolonged ejection time, as reflected in the slowly rising carotid pulse tracing, is consistent with this notion. In *B*, a prominent *fourth* heart sound is seen synchronized with an exaggerated apical *a* wave. Note also the sustained systolic wave seen in the apex cardiogram.

The data presented are most consistent with relatively severe aortic stenosis with a fixed valve orifice. The ejection sound localizes the process to the valvular level and implies that the valve is not completely immobile, but the markedly diminished second sound indicates that the valve is stiff or calcified. The presence of a prominent fourth heart sound suggests a systolic gradient of 75 mm Hg or more. A third heart sound is usually absent in uncomplicated valvular AS in adults; its presence suggests cardiac decompensation. In HOCM, A2 is usually normal, an ejection sound is rare, and the carotid pulse normally

---

Each answer in this Review and Assessment for Heart Disease *contains page references to the 3rd edition of the textbook. On occasion, a journal reference is cited initially, along with the textbook. This occurs when the reference is particularly general or historically important. All other references are given* below *the individual answers.*

shows a rapid initial upstroke. In supravalvular aortic stenosis, A2 is usually normal in intensity, an ejection sound is usually absent, and a discrepancy may often be found in the carotid upstroke between the right (normal) and left (delayed) sides. In a ventricular septal defect with a significant left-to-right shunt, the second heart sound shows wide splitting, a third sound is often present, the murmur is pansystolic, and the carotid pulse is usually normal.

The tracings in question were obtained from a patient who had three definitive findings: a prominent systolic thrill in the aortic area, a long systolic murmur heard radiating into the neck, and a fourth heart sound. Cardiac catheterization revealed a resting aortic valve gradient of 75 mm Hg which rose to 90 mm Hg with exercise, a cardiac index of 2.4 liters/min/m^2, and a left ventricular end-diastolic pressure of 24 mm Hg at rest. Pulmonary pressures were normal.

5-D (Braunwald, pp. 252–255)

The two methods routinely used to measure cardiac output at cardiac catheterization are the Fick O$_2$ method and the indicator dilution technique. The Fick principle, as applied to measurement of systemic blood flow, states that the total uptake of O$_2$ (O$_2$ consumption) divided by the difference in O$_2$ content between arterial and mixed venous blood gives a measure of pulmonary blood flow which, in the absence of intracardiac shunting, is equal to systemic blood flow. This is expressed mathematically as:

$$\text{Cardiac Index (ml/min/m}^2) = \frac{\text{O}_2 \text{ consumption (ml}^1\text{/min/m}^2)}{\text{Arterio–mixed venous O}_2 \text{ difference}}$$

The normal range for cardiac index is 2.6 to 4.2 liters/min/m^2. (The cardiac output is divided by body surface area to correct for differences in O$_2$ consumption rates caused by variations in body size.) Of the available measures of cardiac output, the Fick method is most accurate in patients with a low cardiac output and corresponding wide arteriovenous O$_2$ difference. Angiographic cardiac output can be calculated as described in Answer C; the calculation is limited by the accuracy with which the systolic and diastolic volumes can be extrapolated from the angiographic data.

6-D (Braunwald, p. 67; Lisler, G., and Talner, N.S.: Oxygen transport in congenital heart disease. In Engle, M.A. [ed.]: Pediatric Cardiovascular Disease. Philadelphia, F.A. Davis, 1981.)

Cyanosis is a bluish discoloration of the skin and mucous membranes which results from either an increased amount of reduced hemoglobin or from abnormal hemoglobin perfusing these areas. Two forms of cyanosis are recognized: (1) peripheral cyanosis, which most commonly is due to cutaneous vasoconstriction (e.g., cold air or water exposure or low cardiac output), and (2) central cyanosis, characterized by a decreased arterial oxygen saturation (in Caucasians, arterial saturation is usually

≤ 85 per cent), caused by right-to-left shunting or abnormal pulmonary function. It is the *absolute* quantity of reduced hemoglobin in the blood that produces the characteristic blue discoloration. Therefore, patients with polycythemia become cyanotic at higher levels of arterial oxygen saturation, and those with severe anemia may resist cyanosis despite marked arterial desaturation. Localized peripheral cyanosis involving one extremity may be due to arterial or venous occlusion.

7-E (Braunwald, pp. 200–201)

The Ashman phenomenon is aberrancy caused by changes in the preceding cycle length. Since the duration of the refractory period is a function of the immediately preceding cycle length, the longer the preceding cycle the longer the ensuing refractory period and the more likely that the next impulse will be conducted with delay.[1] Normally the refractory period of the conduction system is right bundle branch block > left bundle branch block = AV node >> His bundle; therefore, it would be very unusual for the bundle of His to be the site of conduction delay.[2]

REFERENCES

1. Gouaaux, J.L., and Ashman, R.: Auricular fibrillation with aberration simulating ventricular paroxysmal tachycardia. Am. Heart J. 34:366, 1947.
2. Fisch, C., Zipes, D.P., and McHenry, P.L.: Rate-dependent aberrancy. Circulation 48:714, 1973.

8-B (Braunwald, pp. 242–247)

Most cardiac catheterizations at present are performed using either direct exposure of the artery and vein (e.g., brachial vessels) or by the percutaneous approach (brachial or femoral vessels, including transseptal catheterizations). In selected patients, outpatient catheterization is now being used because it is practical, cost-effective, and safe. In this setting the brachial approach is most often used because the patient may ambulate easily shortly after the procedure. The brachial approach may be used either with direct exposure of the appropriate vessels or percutaneously, utilizing the Seldinger technique and No. 5 French catheters.[1] In patients in whom the aortic valve should not be crossed by a retrograde approach from the aorta, including those with a tilting-disc prosthetic aortic valve,[2] transseptal catheterization may be utilized. This approach may also be used when a severely stenotic aortic valve cannot be crossed, as well as in patients with suspected mitral valve stenosis in whom a confirmed wedge pressure cannot be obtained. Transseptal left heart catheterization is not necessary with bioprostheses or ball-and-cage prosthetic valves in the aortic position, which can be crossed safely in retrograde fashion.

REFERENCES

1. Fergusson, D.J.G., and Karnada, R.O.: Percutaneous entry of the brachial for left heart catheterization using an arterial sheath: Further experience. Cathet. Cardiovasc. Diagn. 12:209, 1986.

2. Karsh, D.L., et al.: Retrograde left ventricular catheterization in patients with an aortic valve prosthesis. Am. J. Cardiol. 41:893, 1978.

9-B   (Braunwald, pp. 358–360)

The major advantage of digital ventriculography is that, despite some decrease in spatial resolution, image enhancement allows small amounts of contrast medium to be utilized with a resulting decreased incidence of arrhythmias and dye-induced complications.[1] Digital intravenous ventriculography for evaluation of exercise-induced wall motion abnormalities has better spatial resolution than radionuclide angiography,[2] but is considerably more cumbersome. Digital coronary angiography has had limited application because of several problems: (1) difficulty in subtracting the large contrast pool within the left ventricle and pulmonary veins from the image; (2) low-level contrast enhancement of the coronary arteries; (3) overlapping of vessels; and (4) poor spatial resolution on standard matrix. However, with more detailed analysis on 512 × 512 matrices, digital techniques have found a role in evaluating the efficacy of PTCA.[3] Furthermore, the study of flow reserve, which is a physiological measurement of the significance of a coronary artery stenosis, is an area of great potential for digital subtraction angiography.[4, 5]

REFERENCES

1. Nichols, A.B., Martin, E.C., Fles, T.P., Stugensky, K.M., Balancio, L.A., Casarella, W.J., and Weiss, M.B.: Validation of the angiographic accuracy of digital left ventriculography. Am. J. Cardiol. 51:224, 1983.
2. Goldberg, H.L., Moses, J.W., Borer, J.S., Fisher, J., Tamari, I., Skelly, N.T., and Cohen, B.: Exercise left ventriculography utilizing intravenous digital angiography. J. Am. Coll. Cardiol. 2:1092, 1983.
3. Tobis, J., Nalcioglu, O., Johnston, W.D., Qu, L., Reese, T., Sato, D., Roeck, W., Montelli, S., and Henry, W.L.: Videodensitometric determination of minimum coronary artery luminal diameter before and after angioplasty. Am. J. Cardiol. 59:38, 1987.
4. Hodgson, J.M., LeGrand, V., Bates, E.R., Mancini, G.B.J., Aueron, F.M., O'Neill, W.W., Simon, S.B., Beauman, G.J., LeFree, M.T., and Vogel, R.A.: Validation in dogs of a rapid digital angiographic technique to measure relative coronary blood flow during routine cardiac catheterization. Am. J. Cardiol. 55:188, 1985.
5. Nissen, S.E., Elion, J.L., Booth, D.C., Evans, J., and DeMaria, A.N.: Value and limitations of computer analysis of digital subtraction angiography in the assessment of coronary flow reserve. Circulation 73:562, 1986.

10-B   (Braunwald, pp. 87–88, 96–102; Nishimura, R.A., et al.: Doppler echocardiography: Theory instrumentation, technique and application. Mayo Clin. Proc. 60:321, 1985.)

Calculation of the pressure gradient across a cardiac value is determined by the following equation. Δ Pressure = 4 × (velocity)². In this instance, the pressure gradient is 64 mm Hg (4 × 4²). With a right atrial pressure of 4 mm Hg and a pressure gradient of 64 mm Hg, the right ventricular pressure equals 68 mm Hg (64 + 4 = 68

mm Hg). Pressure gradients across other cardiac valves can be calculated in a similar manner.

11-A   (Braunwald, pp. 103–105)

The echocardiographic hallmarks of mitral stenosis are the same for M-mode and two-dimensional echocardiography and consist of decreased valve motion, increased thickness of the valve leaflets, inadequate separation of the anterior and posterior leaflets of the valve during diastole, and increase in left atrial size. However, doming of the mitral leaflets, which is indicative of restricted motion, is a characteristic sign of stenosis seen only on two-dimensional echocardiography. The presence of doming is particularly helpful because it may help distinguish a valve that is truly stenotic from one that opens poorly because of low flow.

12-A   (Braunwald, pp. 183–186)

Limb lead reversal is a relatively common cause of a bizarre QRS axis. It is useful to remember Einthoven's law, which allows one to derive the relationship that a complex in lead 2 is equal to the sum of the corresponding complexes in leads 1 and 3 (2 = 1 + 3). Thus, if the P wave is upright in all three leads, the lead with the tallest P is lead 2. The most common error is reversal of the arm leads (as shown). This is readily detected as a result of inversion of all complexes in lead 1. Thus, "1" is the mirror image of 1, "R" is L, and "L" is R.

13-A   (Braunwald, pp. 235–239)

The Lipid Research Clinics Study[1] analyzed results of exercise tolerance tests on 3640 men over a period of 8.4 years. Of 185 asymptomatic men with positive tests, 18 per cent developed coronary artery disease compared with 3.2 per cent of 2993 men with negative tests, yielding a relative risk of 5.6/1. The incidence of left main coronary artery disease in asymptomatic patients was very low (< 0.1 per cent); ST-segment elevation due to any cause occurred in only 3 to 5 per cent of those with ETT. This test method is quite safe, with an estimated mortality rate of 10 per 100,000 tests.[2]

REFERENCES

1. Gordon, D.J., Ekelund, L.G., Karon, J.M., Probstfield, J.L., Rubenstein, C., Sheffield, T., and Weissfeld, L.: Predictive value of the exercise tolerance test for mortality in North American men: The Lipid Research Clinics mortality follow-up study. Circulation 74:252, 1986.
2. Atterhog, J.H., Jonsson, B., and Samuelsson, R.: Exercise testing: A prospective study of complication rates. Am Heart J. 98:572, 1979.

14-D   (Braunwald, pp. 315–325)

A major advantage of radionuclide angiography is that it provides a noninvasive assessment of both systolic function and regional wall motion abnormalities.[1] Although spatial resolution is poor, the image data are directly proportional to ventricular volume after background subtraction and hence no assumptions are required concerning ventricular shape or position, an important consideration in patients with asynergy.[2] Thus, despite resolution problems, accurate assessment in an individual patient of changes in systolic function and regional wall motion is possible. Future improvements in imaging quality may allow characterization and localization of foci of premature ventricular activation.[3]

REFERENCES

1. Bacharach, S.L., Green, M.V., Borer, J.S., Hyde, J.E., Farkas, S.P., and Johnson, G.S.: Left-ventricular peak ejection rate, filling rate, and ejection fraction-frame rate requirements at rest and exercise. J. Nucl. Med. 20:189, 1979.
2. Maddox, D.E., Holman, B.L., Wynne, J., Idoine, J., Parker, J.A., Uren, R., Neill, J.M., and Cohn, P.F.: The ejection fraction image: A noninvasive index of regional left ventricular wall motion. Am. J. Cardiol. 41:1230, 1978.
3. Johnson, L.L., Seldin, D.W., Yeh, H.L., Spotnitz, H.M., and Reiffel, J.: Phase analysis of gated blood pool scintigraphic images to localize bypass tracts in Wolff-Parkinson-White syndrome. J. Am. Coll. Cardiol. 8:67, 1986).

15-D (Braunwald, pp. 328–334)

Thallium-201 is a potassium analog that is metabolically concentrated by the myocardium. During thallium-201 scintigraphy, approximately 3.5 per cent of the injected dose localizes to heart tissue.[1, 2] The final cardiac concentration is unaffected by inhibition of the Na^+,K^+-ATPase and increases to about 8 to 10 per cent as coronary blood flow rises after administration of dipyridamole. Unlike microspheres, thallium-201 does *not* stay trapped in myocardial tissue, and redistribution begins within 10 minutes after injection.[3] Thallium is retained in regions of hypoperfusion,[4] and its clearance rate is proportional to the heart rate at the time of injection.

REFERENCES

1. Melin, J.A., and Becker, L.C.: Quantitative relationship between global left ventricular thallium uptake and blood flow: Effects of propranolol, ouabain, dipyridamole, and coronary artery occlusion. J. Nucl. Med. 27:641, 1986.
2. Weich, H.F., Strauss, H.W., and Pitt, B.: The extraction of T1-201 by the myocardium. Circulation 56:188, 1977.
3. Schwartz, J.S., Ponto, R., Carlyle, P., Forstrom, L., and Cohn, J.N.: Early distribution of thallium-201 after temporary ischemia. Circulation 57:332, 1978.
4. Grunwald, A., Watson, D., Holzgrefe, H., Irving, J., and Beller, G.A.: Myocardial thallium-201 kinetics in normal and ischemic myocardium. Circulation 64:610, 1981.

16 A-Y, B-Y, C-Y, D-Y, E-Y (Braunwald, p. 255); Swan, H.J.C., and Wood, E.H.: Localization of cardiac defects by dye dilution curves recorded after injection of T-1824 at multiple sites in the heart and great vessels during cardiac catheterization. Proc. Staff Meet. Mayo Clin. 28:95, 1953.)

Detection and localization of intracardiac shunts is usually possible at catheterization by the traditional oximetry run in which samples are drawn at numerous sites in the right side of the heart and adjacent vessels. The technique involves measurement of O_2 saturations in order to identify a significant step-up between consecutive chambers. Using averaged samples, an O_2 saturation step-up of ≥ 7 per cent is necessary to diagnose a left-to-right shunt at the atrial level, while ≥ 5 per cent suffices at the level of the right ventricular or pulmonary artery levels. Because of normal variability in O_2 saturation, shunts with $Qp/Qs \leq 1.3$ at the pulmonary artery or right ventricular levels and those with $Qp/Qs < 1.5$ at the atrial level are not detected. The data obtained in the course of an oximetry run may be used to quantify shunt size. Pulmonary and systemic blood flows can be calculated using the standard Fick equation appropriately written for the system in question. For unidirectional shunts, the magnitude is given by $Qp-Qs$; from this it can be deduced that a negative value will occur with pure right-to-left shunts, as often is seen in tetralogy of Fallot. More sensitive techniques, including hydrogen-sensitive electrode placement used with inhaled hydrogen gas or indocyanine green dye curve methods, may be used to detect small shunts.

17 A-N, B-Y, C-Y, D-Y, E-Y (Braunwald, pp. 368–375)

The MRI shown is taken from a patient with a lymphoma[1] and demonstrates the unique capabilities of this technique. This image depicts the midlevel of both ventricles in the short axis. The RV is anterior to the LV. The open arrows delineate a large mass involving the wall of the heart both within and outside the epicardial fat line. There is also a pericardial effusion present which could contain either blood or fluid. Although in this patient the lymphoma originated from the epicardium, most commonly lymphomatous involvement of the heart is metastatic (see Braunwald, p. 374). MRI is superior to computed tomography for assessing mediastinal masses, especially those anterior to the heart. Furthermore, the intensity of spin-echo images can be used to differentiate paracardiac masses (medium to high signal intensity) from lipomas (low signal intensity), loculated pericardial effusions, pericardial cysts, and abnormalities of the myocardium.[2] In this case, the paracardiac mass appears to have a high signal intensity consistent with a tumor rather than a lipoma.

REFERENCES

1. Levine, H.J., and Southern, J.F.: A 58-year-old woman with progressive pericardial disease. N. Engl. J. Med. 316:1394, 1987.
2. Go, R.T., O'Donnell, J.K., Underwood, D.A., Feiglin, D.H., Salcedo, E.E., Pantoja, M., MacIntyre, W.J., and Meaney, T.F.: Comparison of gated cardiac MRI and two-dimensional echocardiography of intracardiac neoplasms. Am. J. Roentgenol. 145:21, 1985.

18 A-Y, B-N, C-N, D-Y, and E-N (Braunwald, pp. 121–123)

The ventricular wall normally thickens during systole. During ischemia the ability of the myocardium to thicken during systole is impaired. Myocardial infarction is manifested by a decrease in diastolic wall thickness and an increase in the echo intensity consistent with the presence of scar. Echocardiography is only moderately sensitive in the detection of ventricular aneurysms, which are localized areas of dilated ventricular wall. A pseudoaneurysm is a serious complication representing rupture of the free wall; in this condition the blood actually escapes from the myocardium and is trapped within the pericardial sac. This occurs most commonly in inferior wall infarctions. Indications for surgery are urgent with pseudoaneurysm; therefore, the diagnosis is critical.

Mural thrombi are a common complication of MI and are especially common following anterior MI. When these thrombi are elongated they have a higher incidence of embolizing; more typically they are flat and line the ventricular wall. In general, re-endothelialization of mural thrombi occurs within 2 weeks after acute MI. Although perforation of the ventricular septum is commonly observed in two-dimensional echocardiography, the best technique for making the diagnosis is Doppler echocardiography. Sampling on the RV side of the interventricular septum, one can record a high velocity systolic flow in a positive direction—that is, moving from the LV to the RV through the ruptured septum.

19-D *(Braunwald, pp. 287–289;* Levin, P.C., Harrington, D.P., Bettman, M.A., Garnick, J.D., Davidoff, A., and Lois, J.: Anatomic variations of the coronary arteries supplying the anterolateral aspect of the left ventricle. Invest. Radiol. *17:458, 1982.)*

A knowledge of the anatomy of the human coronary circulation is important in the diagnosis and management of ischemic syndromes. The left main coronary artery gives rise to the left anterior descending artery and the left circumflex artery and, in approximately 37 per cent of patients, a branch lying between these two vessels called the ramus medianus branch. The major components of the LAD are the septal and diagonal branches. The septal branches supply the interventricular septum, the most densely vascularized area of the heart, and the first septal serves as the most important potential collateral channel. Over 90 per cent of patients have one to three diagonal branches that arise from the LAD; the absence of identifiable diagonal branches on angiography should suggest the possibility of one or more diagonal occlusions. The circumflex artery runs in or near the atrioventricular groove and supplies the lateral free wall of the left ventricle via obtuse marginal branches. While the majority of patients have a right dominant system, in 10 to 23 per cent of humans the posterior diaphragmatic myocardium is supplied via branches of the left coronary system.

20 A-Y, B-Y, C-Y, D-N, E-Y *(Braunwald, pp. 203–210)*

Various studies have shown that ECGs in the emergency room are diagnostic in 50 to 70 per cent of patients with myocardial infarction and that serial ECGs increase the sensitivity significantly to > 80 per cent.[1] Within 6 to 12 months about 30 per cent of patients with Q wave infarcts will lose their Q waves. Patients with inferior infarcts and anterior ST segment depressions have been

shown to have a worse prognosis than those with inferior myocardial infarctions without such ST segment depressions. This has been shown to be due to a high probability of associated left anterior descending artery disease in the presence of ST depressions in this situation.[2–4] ST segment elevation equal to or greater than 1 mm in V_4R has a sensitivity and specificity for right ventricular infarction of approximately 90 per cent.[5]

REFERENCES

1. Behar, S., Schor, S., Kariv, I., Barell, V., and Modan, B.: Evaluation of electrocardiogram in emergency room as a decision-making tool. Chest *71*:486, 1977.
2. Tzivoni, D., Chenzbraun, A., Keren, A., Benhorin, J., Gottlieb, S., Lonn, E., and Stern, S.: Reciprocal electrocardiographic changes in acute myocardial infarction. Am. J. Cardiol. *56*:23, 1986.
3. Pierard, L.A., Sprynger, M., Gilis, F., and Carlier, J.: Significance of precordial ST segment depression in inferior acute myocardial infarction as determined by echocardiography. Am. J. Cardiol. *57*:82, 1986.
4. Quyyumi, A.A., et al.: Importance of "reciprocal" electrocardiographic changes during occlusion of left anterior descending coronary artery. Lancet *1*:347, 1986.
5. Lopez-Sendon, J., Coma-Canella, I., Alcasena, S., Seoane, J., and Gamallo, C.: Electrocardiographic findings in acute right ventricular infarction. Sensitivity and specificity of electrocardiographic alterations in right precordial leads V_4R_1, $V_3R_1V_1$, V_2 and V_3. J. Am. Coll. Cardiol. *6*:1273, 1985.

21 A-Y, B-Y, C-Y, D-Y, E-N *(Braunwald, pp. 19–20;* Swartz, M.H.: Jugular venous pressure pulse: Its value in cardiac diagnosis. Primary Cardiol. *8*:197, 1982.)

The JVP is best examined on the right side of the neck, with the patient lying in the 45-degree position. The JVP, which reflects the distention of the internal jugular vein, provides a measure of right-sided cardiac dynamics, including the level of venous pressure and the pattern of the venous waves, which may give important information about the underlying cardiac pathology. Whereas the *a* wave results from venous distention in response to atrial systole, the *v* wave is created by venous return to the right atrium when the tricuspid valve is closed (i.e., during ventricular systole). Giant (cannon) *a* waves are seen when atrial systole occurs against a closed tricuspid valve in the presence of atrioventricular dysynchrony. During inspiration, the height of the JVP normally declines while the amplitude of the pulsations increases.

In Kussmaul's sign, inspiration leads to a paradoxical *rise* in the height of the JVP with inspiration; it is seen frequently in chronic constrictive pericarditis and may also occur in congestive heart failure and tricuspid stenosis. A positive abdominojugular reflux augments already elevated right-sided pressures (as might be seen in RV failure or tricuspid regurgitation) and leads to a sustained elevation in the jugular venous column. Interestingly, an elevated JVP and Kussmaul's sign have been shown to be sensitive indicators for the bedside diagnosis of RV infarction.[1]

REFERENCES

1. Dell'italia, L.J., Sterling, M.R., and O'Rourke, R.A.: Physical examination for exclusion of hemodynamically important right ventricular infarction. Ann. Intern. Med. *99*:608, 1983.

22 **A-Y, B-Y, C-Y, D-N, E-Y** (*Braunwald, pp. 261–262;* Kennedy, J.W.: Complications associated with cardiac catheterization and angiography. Cathet. Cardiovasc. Diagn. 8:5, 1982.)

The Registry of the Society for Cardiac Angiography has reported the incidence of various complications in 53,581 patients undergoing cardiac catheterization over a 14-month period beginning October, 1979. The overall death rate was 0.14 per cent, the rate of acute MI was 0.07 per cent, and the greatest incidence of death occurred in patients under 1 year of age (1.75 per cent). Coronary angiography led to a mortality of 0.86 per cent in patients with significant left main coronary artery disease, in contrast to zero in patients with normal coronary arteries. The mortality rate was also increased in patients over 60 (0.25 per cent). Other patient characteristics that have been associated with an increased mortality from catheterization include elevated functional class and valvular heart disease (especially if coexisting with CAD, left ventricular dysfunction, or severe noncardiac disease). Of note, patients with an LV ejection fraction < 30 per cent have a risk of death > 10 times those with a normal ejection fraction. Strict attention to technique, use of low volumes of radiographic contrast medium, and careful therapeutic intervention when arrhythmias or abnormal hemodynamics occur all may help minimize morbidity and mortality from the procedure.

23 **A-Y, B-N, C-Y, D-Y, E-Y** (*Braunwald, pp. 232–235*)

The conventional criterion for ECG diagnosis of ischemia (0.1 mV ST-segment depression) was standardized postexercise and does not necessarily apply to tracings recorded during exercise. However, some authors have proposed that during exercise greater degrees of ST-segment depression (≥ 0.2 mV), perhaps proportional to heart rate, are more specific for ischemia.[1] During normal exercise there is frequently J-point depression, but this is associated with an upsloping ST-segment. Because of the large coronary vasodilator reserve which normally exists, patients with a 50 per cent stenosis are unlikely to develop characteristic symptoms or ECG changes.[2] The normal peak-pressure product (HR × systolic BP) is 20,000 to 35,000 mm Hg × beats/min. Heart rate is linearly related to cardiac output and hence to exercise capacity. As maximal aerobic capacity is approached, heart rate approaches a plateau just as oxygen consumption does. Maximal heart rate decreases linearly with age over 20.[3]

REFERENCES

1. Lozner, E.C., and Morganroth, J.: New criteria for evaluation of "positive" exercise tests in asymptomatic patients. Am. J. Cardiol. 39:288, 1977.
2. Gould, L.K., Hamilton, G.W., Lipscomb, K., Ritchie, J.L., and Kennedy, J.W.: Method for assessing stress-induced regional malperfusion during coronary arteriography. Experimental validation and clinical application. Am. J. Cardiol. 34:557, 1974.
3. Gould, F.L., Nordstrom, L.A., Nelson, R.R., Jorgensen, C.R., and Wang, Y.: The rate-pressure product as an index of myocardial oxygen consumption during exercise in patients with angina pectoris. Circulation 57:549, 1978.

24 **A-Y, B-N, C-Y, D-Y, E-N** (*Braunwald, pp. 315–322*)

Both first-pass and equilibrium angiography provide reliable measures of global function. However, equilibrium techniques, which yield high counts by virtue of "gating" strategies, provide greater spatial resolution and accuracy for regional wall motion abnormalities. Thus, alterations in systolic function in response to inotropes or vasodilators maintained over several minutes can be assessed using an equilibrium study. On the other hand, rapid changes in left ventricular function are better assessed by first-pass techniques, which require only five or six cardiac cycles, in contrast to at least 2 minutes for gated studies. Furthermore, because a radiopharmaceutical must be administered each time for a first-pass study, background counts and radiation dosage limits preclude serial studies.

25 **A-N, B-Y, C-Y, D-Y, E-N** (*Braunwald, pp. 341–345*)

^{99m}Tc-PYP is "infarct-avid" and its uptake is related to the degree of tissue damage; however, the pharmaceutical must first reach the damaged tissue before it can be extracted. Normally, uptake increases after 4 hours, peaks at 48 hours, and persists for up to 7 days.[1] Concentration ratios may be as great as 18:1 in areas of fresh infarction but are frequently lower in zones of necrosis where blood flow is lowest, giving a "bull's eye" appearance.[2] Since metabolically active bone receives substantial blood flow and is also capable of utilizing pyrophosphate, a significant percentage of early uptake is in bone.

REFERENCES

1. Holman, B.L., Lesch, M., and Alpert, J.S.: Myocardial scintigraphy with technetium-99m pyrophosphate during the early phase of acute infarction. Am. J. Cardiol. 41:39, 1978.
2. Zaret, B.L., DiCola, V.C., Donabedian, R.K., Puri, S., Wolfson, S., Freedman, G.S., and Cohen, L.S.: Dual radionuclide study of myocardial infarction. Relationships between myocardial uptake of potassium-43, technetium-99m stannous pyrophosphate, regional myocardial blood flow and creatine phosphokinase depletion. Circulation 53:422, 1976.

26-A (1, 2, and 3 are correct) (*Braunwald, p. 336*)

Transient perfusion defects occur whenever the blood flow is inadequate for myocardial demand. The most common cause for "false-positive" defects is probably subcritical (< 50 per cent) coronary artery disease. Other causes for transient defects include diffuse myocardial disease, aortic valve stenosis,[1] and myocardial bridges.[2] Most studies have shown no transient defects in patients with mitral valve prolapse.[3, 4]

REFERENCES

1. Bailey, I.K., Come, P.C., Kelly, D.T., Burow, R.D., Griffith, L.S.C., Strauss, H.W., and Pitt, B.: Thallium-201 myocardial perfusion imaging in aortic valve stenosis. Am. J. Cardiol. 40:889, 1977.
2. Ahmad, M., Merry, S.L., and Harbach, H.: Thallium-201 scinti-

graphic evidence of ischemia in patients with myocardial bridges. Am. J. Cardiol. 45:482, 1980.

3. Gaffney, F.A., Wohl, A.J., Glomqvist, C.G., Parkey, R.W., and Willerson, J.T.: Thallium-201 myocardial perfusion studies in patients with mitral valve prolapse syndrome. Am. J. Med. 64:21, 1978.
4. Massie, B., Botvinick, E.H., Shames, D., Taradash, M., Werner, J., and Schiller, B.N.: Myocardial perfusion scintigraphy in patients with mitral valve prolapse. Circulation 57:19, 1978.

27-E   (All are correct) *(Braunwald, pp. 3–6;* Walsh, R.A., and O'Rourke, R.A.: Clues to the evaluation of chest pain in the patient's history. Pract. Cardiol. 4:41, 1978.)

Chest pain or discomfort may arise from a variety of cardiac and noncardiac structures, either intrathoracic or subdiaphragmatic in location. The history is the single most important mode of examination providing data for the differential diagnosis of chest pain. The chest discomfort of pulmonary hypertension may be caused by dilatation of the pulmonary arteries, acute pulmonary embolism, or right ventricular ischemia and may be identical to that of typical angina.[1] A lower esophageal tear due to protracted vomiting (the Mallory-Weiss syndrome) may elicit a chest pain syndrome that is difficult to distinguish from acute MI without a careful history. The thoracic outlet, or scalenus anticus syndrome, is an uncommon cause of chest or arm discomfort due to compression of the neurovascular bundle by a cervical rib or the anterior scalenus muscle. Paresthesias may occur along the ulnar distribution of the forearm in this syndrome and may be confused with angina despite the nonexertional nature of the pain. Congenital absence of the pericardium is a rare anomaly that may produce fleeting chest pain precipitated by lying on the left side and relieved by changing position. While difficult, the diagnosis may be made by standard chest roentgenography.[2]

REFERENCES

1. Viar, W.N., and Harrison, T.R.: Chest pain in association with pulmonary hypertension; its similarity to the pain of coronary disease. Circulation 5:1, 1952.
2. Glover, L.B., Barcia, A., and Reeves, T.J.: Congenital absence of the pericardium. Am. J. Roentgenol. 82:125, 1959.

28-A   (1, 2, and 3 are correct) *(Braunwald, pp. 48–50;* Mills, P.G., Brodie, B., McLaurin, L.P., Schall, S., and Craige, E.: Echocardiographic and hemodynamic relationships of ejection sounds. Circulation 56:430, 1977.)

Ejection sounds are high-frequency "clicks" that occur in early systole. They may be either aortic or pulmonic in origin, require a mobile valve for their generation, and begin at the exact time of maximal opening of the semilunar valve in question. If the valve is abnormal, as is frequently the case, the ejection sound is "valvular," and it is generally accepted that halting of the "doming" valve generates the sound. If the valve associated with the ejection sound is normal, it is called a "vascular" ejection sound; the origin of the sound is not clearly defined. In either case, the ejection sound starts at the moment of full opening of the aortic (0.12 to 0.14 sec after the Q wave on the ECG) or pulmonic (0.09 to 0.11 sec after the Q wave) valve. In valvular pulmonic stenosis, the ejection sound is loudest during expiration. With inspiration, increased venous return augments atrial systole and results in partial opening of the pulmonic valve before ventricular systole commences. In contrast, with expiration, the pulmonic valve opens quickly from a fully closed position, generating a louder ejection sound from the sudden halt to the valve's opening movement.[1]

REFERENCES

1. Hultgren, H.N., et al: The ejection click of valvular pulmonic stenosis. Circulation 40:631, 1969.

29-A   (1, 2, and 3 are correct) *(Braunwald, pp. 249–252;* Grossman, W., et al.: Left ventricular stiffness associated with chronic pressure and volume overload in man. Circ. Res. 35:793, 1974)

Pressure tracing recordings at cardiac catheterization remain the "gold standard" for diagnosis of hypertrophic obstructive cardiomyopathy (HOCM). In the tracing provided, a large gradient between the body of the left ventricle (LVB) and the root of the aorta (Ao) is seen on the left of the tracing. As the catheter is withdrawn into the LV outflow tract (LVOT), the gradient is no longer present and the diagnosis is confirmed, while that of *valvular* aortic stenosis is excluded. The bifid aortic pulse contour with a characteristic notch on the upstroke and a rapid initial upstroke of the LVB tracing is also demonstrated. This is in marked contrast to the slow and delayed rise in the aortic pressure pulse in valvular aortic stenosis. In HOCM, left ventricular diastolic dysfunction is often present; this may lead to a prominent *a* wave and an elevation of left ventricular end-diastolic pressure. Interestingly, recent studies of LV diastolic function in this condition have identified abnormalities in both LV distensibility and relaxation leading to impaired diastolic filling.[1] Many investigators believe that the outflow tract gradient in HOCM results from true mechanical impedance to ejection by anterior movement of the mitral valve across the outflow tract and subsequent contact of the valve with the ventricular septum in early systole.[2]

REFERENCES

1. Maron, B.J., et al: Hypertrophic cardiomyopathy. N. Engl. J. Med. 316:780, 1987.
2. Yock, P.G., et al.: Patterns and timing of Doppler-detected intracavitary and aortic flow in hypertrophic cardiomyopathy. J. Am. Coll. Cardiol. 8:1047, 1986.

30-E   (All are correct) *(Braunwald, pp. 185–186)*

The heart may be considered to maintain two axes— an anteroposterior axis, which defines whether the apex of the heart faces the left arm (horizontal) or the left foot (vertical), and a longitudinal, apex-to-base axis, which defines whether the left ventricle is anterior or posterior. The direction of rotation for the latter axis is described by viewing the heart from a position below the diaphragm. Clockwise rotation results in a more posterior position of the left ventricle and the right ventricular QRS complex (rS) is displaced to the left. Counterclockwise rotation results in a more anterior shift of the left ventricle, and the left ventricular QRS (qR) pattern is observed in the right precordial leads.

31-E (All are correct) (*Braunwald, pp. 341–344*)

Focal uptake of ^{99m}Tc-pyrophosphate may be seen after myocardial contusion[1] and repeated DC cardioversion.[2] Although uptake in regions of MI is usually absent by 2 weeks, about 40 per cent of patients will have a much slower disappearance of the radiotracer lasting for several months. Right ventricular infarction is well demonstrated with pyrophosphate scanning, with high sensitivity.[3]

REFERENCES

1. Go, R.T., et al: Radionuclide imaging of experimental myocardial contusion. J. Nucl. Med. *15*:1174, 1974.
2. Pugh, B.R., Buja, L.M., Parkey, R.W., Poliner, L.R., Stokely, E.M., Bonte, F.J., and Willerson, J.T.: Cardioversion and "false-positive" technetium-99m stannous pyrophosphate myocardial scintigrams. Circulation *54*:399, 1976.
3. Sharpe, D.N., Botvinick, E.H., Shames, D.M., Schiller, N.B., Massie, B.M., Chatterjee, K., and Parmley, W.W.: The noninvasive diagnosis of right ventricular infarction. Circulation *57*:483, 1978.

32-A (1, 2, and 3 are correct) (*Braunwald, pp. 252–258; Gorlin, R., and Gorlin G.: Hydraulic formula for calculation of area of stenotic mitral valves, other valves, and central circulatory shunts. Am. Heart J. 41:1, 1951.*)

The pioneering work of Gorlin (see reference) has provided equations using measured pressure gradient and flow across the stenotic valve that allow for calculation of valve orifice area:

$$\text{valve area} = \frac{F}{K \cdot (P)^{1/2}}$$ where F is flow in ml/sec, P is the

mean pressure gradient in mm Hg across the orifice, and K is an empirical constant for the valve in question.

There are a number of assumptions and potential pitfalls in the determination of valve area by catheterization techniques. Since flow in the Gorlin equation is assumed to be systemic cardiac output, the presence of valvular regurgitation results in a falsely low flow substituted in the Gorlin equation. Therefore, the valve area calculated is falsely low. In measuring the valve area of a stenotic orifice, the calculated valve area represents the *lower* limit of the true valve area, since any coexisting regurgitation would provide for a larger flow than the calculated cardiac output used as F in the equation above.

In calculations of mitral valve area, a confirmed pulmonary capillary wedge pressure may be substituted for left atrial pressure. This confirmation requires (1) that the measured mean wedge pressure is lower than the mean pulmonary artery pressure and (2) that the blood drawn from a wedged catheter has an O_2 saturation ≥ 95 per cent (or at least equal in saturation to arterial blood).

33-A (*Braunwald, pp. 341–344*)

In the normal scintigram (*A*) there is homogeneous distribution of tracer in the apical and apical-inferior segments, in which activity can normally be slightly lower. In the abnormal scintigram (*B*), inferior and apical defects are seen on the initial anterior (ANT) view and septal and apical-inferior defects on the initial left anterior oblique (LAO) view. There is complete redistribution into the septal and apical-inferior segments (transient defect), partial redistribution into the inferior segment, and no redistribution into the apical defect (persistent defect). When an increase in lung activity is observed, it correlates both with increased pulmonary capillary wedge pressure and multivessel disease.

The images can be evaluated as follows: (1) a reversible or transient defect corresponds to transient ischemia; (2) an irreversible defect, interpreted as scar, corresponds to prior infarct (segments involving the apex can normally have reduced activity because of myocardial thinning and must be interpreted with caution); and (3) normal anatomic variations such as apical thinning and decreased perfusion at the base due to the aortic and mitral valves.

34-A (*Braunwald, pp. 360–367*)

Computed tomography (CT) provides distinct visualization of the pericardium based on the presence of the pericardial line, which is probably due to epicardial fat and is always less than 4 mm in width.[1] Thus, the presence or absence of pericardium, its thickness and density, and fluid collections outside the pericardium can readily be discerned. CT is particularly useful for differentiating benign from malignant tumors on the basis of density, but mucoid-secreting pericardial cysts have the same density as solid tumors and usually cannot be distinguished.[2] CT can aid in the diagnosis of constrictive pericarditis by documentation of increased pericardial thickness (> 4 mm) and coexisting effusions and calcification.

REFERENCES

1. Silverman, P.M., and Harell, G.S.: Computed tomography of the normal pericardium. Invest. Radiol. *18L141*, 1983.
2. Isner, J.M., Carter, B.L., Bankoff, M.S., Konstum, M.A., and Salem, D.N.: Computed tomography in the diagnosis of pericardial heart disease. Ann. Intern. Med. 97:473, 1982.

35-A, 36-C, 37-D, 38-B (*Braunwald, pp. 154–158, 166*)

The chest roentgenogram in patients with abnormalities of the mitral valve commonly displays evidence of dilatation of the left atrium, whether the lesion in question is mitral stenosis or mitral regurgitation. The characteristic chest film in mitral stenosis displays a heart that is often normal in size, except for the enlargement of the left atrium, which is more prominent in patients with atrial fibrillation. Extensive calcification of the mitral valve may also be visible on chest films and must be distinguished from calcification of the mitral valve annulus. Severe mitral stenosis commonly occurs with pulmonary hypertension, which may be associated with right ventricular dilatation that is often reflected on the chest roentgenogram. In many patients with progressive mitral stenosis, a sequence of alterations in the pulmonary vascular pattern up to and including frank interstitial edema is seen.

More unusual findings on the chest roentgenogram that are relatively specific for mitral stenosis include calcification of the left atrium, pulmonary hemosiderosis from chronic intraalveolar hemorrhages, and pulmonary ossification, probably also from intraalveolar hemorrhage.

A number of findings may be present on the chest roentgenogram in patients with aortic regurgitation. Enlargement of the left ventricle causing elongation and dilatation on the chest film may be present. This results in displacement of the cardiac apex downward, to the left, and posteriorly. In addition, the ascending aorta may be dilated, and fluoroscopic examination in such cases may reveal an increase in the amplitude of the aortic pulsations. In contrast, aortic stenosis tends to be more difficult to recognize on plain chest films. Abnormalities in the shape of the heart, while sometimes present, tend to be subtle. Significant left ventricular dilatation occurs only with myocardial failure in end-stage aortic stenosis. While calcification of the aortic valve is common in aortic stenosis, it may not be appreciated on routine chest films. Similarly, such routine views may obscure the poststenotic dilatation of the ascending aorta that occurs in this disease.

The ostium secundum type of atrial septal defect is an extremely common congenital cardiac lesion of adult life. This lesion may be difficult to diagnose from chest roentgenograms in younger patients, but as time passes the characteristic findings of the ASD appear. These include dilatation of the main pulmonary artery, enlargement of the right ventricle, and a generalized increase in the pulmonary vascularity. Right atrial enlargement may be present as well. It is usually not possible to distinguish between an ostium primum ASD and an ostium secundum ASD on the plain chest film. Although the chest film in patients with a secundum ASD may be similar to that of the patient with mitral stenosis, in the latter condition there is usually left atrial enlargement and redistribution of pulmonary blood flow with dilatation of upper lobe vessels and constriction of the vessels at the lung bases. In contrast, when significant left-to-right shunting is present in an atrial septal defect, all the pulmonary vessels—including those at the bases—are dilated.

The presence of pericardial fluid leads to a characteristic set of changes in the chest roentgenogram. With increasing volumes of pericardial fluid, enlargement of the cardiac silhouette with smoothing out and loss of the normal cardiac contours occurs, leading to a smoothly distended flask-shaped cardiac shadow. While such a pattern may be seen with the generalized dilatation that occurs in heart failure, the appearance of the pulmonary hila distinguishes between these two conditions. In pericardial effusion, the pericardial sac tends to cover the shadows of the hilar vessels as it is further distended. In contrast, the failing heart is usually associated with abnormally prominent hilar vessels in the setting of pulmonary vascular congestion. In some instances displacement of the epicardial fat line may be visible, a sign that is pathognomonic of pericardial effusion.

39-E, 40-A, 41-B, 42-C *(Braunwald, p. 22; Sapira, J.D.: Quincke, de Musset, Duroziez, and Hill: Some aortic regurgitations. South Med. J. 74:459, 1981.)*

Chronic, severe AR may lead to a variety of characteristic physical signs, most of which have eponyms. In each instance these physical findings arise as a direct consequence of the widened pulse pressure that characterizes AR. The most predictive such sign is *Duroziez's sign,*[1] demonstrated by placing a stethoscope over the femoral artery in the groin and applying first proximal and then distal pressure to hear, respectively, a systolic murmur and then a diastolic one. Placing a stethoscope over the femoral artery may also reveal the "pistol shot" sounds described by *Traube.* The exaggerated pulse pressure of AR may lead to transmission of a visible bobbing pulsation to the entire head with each heartbeat, known as *de Musset's sign. Hill's sign,* a systolic pressure in the legs that is greater than 20 mm Hg of that in the arms, usually indicates the presence of AR. *Quincke's pulse* or *sign,* which was not described above, is the alternating blanching and flushing of the skin as observed, for instance, in the nail beds, in response to wide swings in arterial pulse pressure. While it is most commonly seen in patients with AR, it is rarely observed in normal subjects with vasodilation as well.

REFERENCE

1. Rowe, G.G., et al.: The mechanism of the production of Duroziez's murmur. N. Engl. J. Med. 272:1207, 1965.

43-A, 44-C, 45-B, 46-E, 47-D *(Braunwald, 272–276, 284–285, 287–295)*

Corony arteriography remains the benchmark by which the coronary anatomy and circulation may be assessed. Coronary artery spasm may be due to organic disease or may be induced by the mechanical stimulation of the coronary artery by the catheter tip. In 1 to 3 per cent of patients who do not receive vasodilators (e.g., nitroglycerin) prior to arteriography, spasm may be seen.[1] While the major coronary arteries usually pass along the epicardial surface of the heart, occasional short segments pass down into the myocardium, leading to myocardial bridging, as demonstrated in example A above. Edwards et al. identified such bridging in 5.4 per cent of human hearts at autopsy.[2] Angiographic identification of a myocardial bridge usually occurs in the LAD artery.

Intercoronary collaterals in the interventricular septum are normally less than 1 mm in diameter, are characterized by moderate tortuosity, and tend to serve as connections between numerous septal branches of the LAD and smaller posterior septal branches that arise from the posterior descending artery. Recruitment and development of such collaterals due to occlusion of the LAD artery are demonstrated in *B* above.

The most prevalent hemodynamically significant congenital coronary artery anomaly is the coronary arteriovenous fistula. When the fistula drains into any of several areas—the coronary sinus, SVC, pulmonary artery, or a right-sided cardiac chamber—a left-to-right shunt is created. Seen in infancy and childhood, approximately half of such patients develop symptoms of CHF, but the majority come to catheterization at some point due to the presence of a loud continuous murmur.[3]

The most common *anomalous* aortic origin of a coronary artery is anomalous origin of the circumflex artery from the right sinus of Valsalva. The artery passes around the posterior aspect of the aortic root toward the left atrioventricular groove and resumes a normal circumflex course. This anomaly accounts for between one-half and two-thirds of all anomalous coronary artery origins from the aorta.

REFERENCES

1. Cheng, T.O., et al.: Variant angina of Prinzmetal and normal coronary arteriograms: A variant of the variant. Circulation *47*:476, 1973.
2. Edwards, J., et al.: Arteriosclerosis in intramural and extramural portions of coronary arteries in the human heart. Circulation *13*:235, 1956.
3. Levin, D.C., Fellows, K.E., and Abrams, H.L.: Hemodynamically significant primary anomalies of the coronary arteries. Angiographic aspects. Circulation *58*:25, 1978.

48-A, 49-D, 50-C   *(Braunwald, pp. 87–88, 99–101)*

Calculation of transvalvular gradients can be performed with continuous-wave Doppler by using a modification of the Bernoulli principle, which states that the pressure difference across a stenotic site is equal to the convective acceleration + the flow acceleration + the viscous friction. At pressures and flows observed clinically, the contributions from flow acceleration and viscous friction are negligible so that the equation can be simplified to: $P_1 - P_2 = \frac{1}{2} \times p \times (V_2^2 - V_1^2)$ where p equals the mass density of blood, which is approximately 8. Since the square of the velocity of blood upstream to the stenosis (V_1^2) is usually negligible in comparison with the square of the downstream velocity (V_2^2), one can eliminate the former term. Therefore, the simplified equation used to estimate the pressure gradient across the stenotic lesion and across the cardiac chambers is: $P_1 - P_2 = 4 \times V_2^2$.

In the figure on p. 9, with a peak velocity of 3.3 meters/second, the pressure gradient would be 40 mm Hg (3.3 × 3.3 × 4).

It is critically important that a true maximal Doppler flow signal be obtained. This requires frequent interrogation and appropriate alignment between the Doppler beam and the blood jet; any angle less than 30° will give an accurate measurement. If the Doppler flow signal has an angle greater than 30°, the equation for Doppler velocity becomes inaccurate and a decrease in the maximal signal will be obtained.

It should be noted that the Doppler-derived aortic valve gradient is the *maximal instantaneous* pressure gradient between the left ventricle and aorta. This value is higher than the catheterization derived gradient, in which the difference between the peak aortic and peak left ventricular pressures is reported, because these occur at different points in time during systole. This difference is greater with mild to moderate degrees of stenosis, in which the Doppler derived gradient may exceed the peak-to-peak gradient measured at catheterization by 20 to 30 mm Hg.

REFERENCE

1. Nishimura R.A., Miller, F.A., Callahan, M.J., Benassi, R.C., Seward, J.B., and Tajik, A.J.: Doppler echocardiography: Theory, instrumentation, technique, and application. Mayo Clin. Proc. *60*:321, 1985.

51-B, 52-A, 53-C, 54-D   *(Braunwald, pp. 14–19, 1624, 1627, 1628, 1792)*

In trisomy 21 or the *Down syndrome*, a characteristic facies includes hypoplastic mandible, poorly formed nasal bridge, large protruding tongue, prominent medial epicanthus, and low-set ears. This is accompanied by mental deficiency and a variety of congenital cardiac disorders in up to 50 per cent of cases. The two most common cardiac lesions are ventricular septal defect (VSD) and endocardial cushion defect. Most patients have a single lesion, but up to 30 per cent of those with heart disease have multiple defects.[1]

Ellis–van Creveld syndrome is a rare autosomal recessive illness characterized by small stature, with striking shortening in the distal extremities, bilateral polydactyly and ectodermal dysplasia, with, for example, hypoplastic nails. Fifty to sixty per cent of patients have congenital heart disease, a frequent cause of death. Congenital malformations include large atrial septal defects (ASD) or a single atrium, with or without associated defects, including aortic atresia, hypoplastic ascending aorta, and hypoplastic left ventricle.[2] Of note, most cases of the disorder in the U.S. occur in the Old Order Amish, an inbred religious isolate in Lancaster County, PA, where 13 per cent of the population carries the mutant gene.[3]

Werner syndrome is a rare recessively inherited autosomal disorder characterized by cataract formation, proptosis, frontal balding, beaking of the nose, premature graying of the hair, and early coronary and peripheral atherosclerosis. Patients may also develop primary hypogonadism. The incidence of Werner syndrome is approximately 1 in 500,000, in contrast with more common single-gene disorders predisposing to atherosclerosis, such as heterozygous familial hypercholesterolemia, with an estimated population frequency of 1 in 500.[4]

Kearns-Sayre syndrome is characterized by the triad of external ophthalmoplegia, atypical pigmentary retinopathy, and heart block, first described in 1958 by Kearns and Sayre. In many instances, there is evidence of a widespread neurological disorder in affected patients. There appear to be two distinct alterations in conduction in this abnormality: (1) a gradual impairment of infranodal conduction and (2) a concomitant enhancement of AV nodal conduction. Current evidence suggests that the disorder is "neurogenic" rather than myopathic.[5]

Holt-Oram syndrome, which is *not* described in the questions above, is characterized by an upper limb deformity in association with congenital heart disease, usually a secundum ASD or a VSD. The upper limb deformities vary, but the most characteristic (but not pathognomonic) anomaly involves the thumbs, which may be "digitalized" or finger-like, with the presence of an extra phalynx. The most specific upper limb abnormalities are an abnormal scaphoid bone and/or accessory carpal bones seen on radiography of the wrist.[6]

REFERENCES

1. Tandon, R., and Edwards, J.E.: Cardiac malformations associated with Down's syndrome. Circulation 47:1349, 1973.
2. da Silva, E.O., Janovitz, D., and deAlbuquerque, S.C.: Ellis–van Creveld syndrome. J. Med. Genet. 17:349, 1980.
3. McKusick, V.A., Egeland, J.A., Eldridge, R., and Krusen, D.E.: Dwarfism in the Amish. I. The Ellis–van Creveld syndrome. Bull. Johns Hopkins Hosp. 115:306, 1964.
4. Zackai, A.H., Weber, D., and Noth, R.: Cardiac findings in Werner's syndrome. Geriatrics 29:141, 1974.
5. Roberts, N.K., Perloff, J.K., and Kark, P.: Cardiac conduction in Kearns-Sayre syndrome. Am. J. Cardiol. 44:1396, 1979.
6. Poznanski, A.K., Stern, A.M., and Gall, J.C., Jr.: Skeletal anomalies in genetically determined congenital heart disease. Radiol. Clin. North Am. 9:435, 1971.

55-D, 56-C, 57-B, 58-A   *(Braunwald, pp. 191–202)*

In contrast to left ventricular (LV) hypertrophy, right ventricular (RV) hypertrophy is not simply an exaggeration of normal; rather, the RV mass must become so large as to overcome the LV forces. Thus, the specificity of the ECG pattern of RV hypertrophy is high but the sensitivity is low, varying from 25 to 40 per cent. In RV hypertrophy there is right axis deviation ($\geq 110°$), a vertical position with rS pattern in leads I, II, and III and rS pattern in V_5 and V_6, and counterclockwise rotation (R/S ratio in V_1 ≥ 1, R/S V_5: R/S $V_1 \leq 0.4$, qR in V_1, R in V_5 or $V_6 \leq 5$ mm). Based on the QRS pattern in lead V_1, RVH can be generally separated into three groups: a dominant R wave (R, qR, rR, rsR), Rs (Rs, Rsr), and rS. In general, the following hemodynamics for RV and LV systolic pressures are correlated with three patterns in V_1: qRS implies RV $>$ LV; prominent R implies RV $=$ LV, and rSr or RVH with incomplete RBBB implies RV $<$ LV.

The left bundle branches into two fascicles, one lying anterior and superior with the other posterior and inferior. Thus, conduction delay in the anterior fascicle, left anterior hemiblock (LAHB), results in initial septal activation that proceeds inferiorly, anteriorly, and usually to the right; followed by activation of the inferior and apical areas with the vector oriented inferiorly, to the left, and anteriorly. The remainder of the QRS vector is then oriented posteriorly, superiorly, and to the left. The ECG pattern includes axis $\geq -45°$, qR in I, rS in III, small s

in $V_5 + V_6$ reflecting the initial inferior activation and later, unopposed, LV anterolateral activation.

Left posterior fascicular block (left posterior hemiblock) (LPHB) is rare and usually associated with myocardial damage, and its pattern is nonspecific. Activation begins in midseptum, generating an initial vector directed to the left, anteriorly and superiorly. This is followed by activation of the anterior and anterolateral walls of the LV, with the QRS vector directed left and anteriorly. Finally, inferior and posterior walls are activated. The characteristic pattern includes axis $+90°$ to $140°$; small R in I followed by deep S reflecting inferior, posterior, and rightward orientation of activation; QR in leads II, III, and aVF.

Wolff-Parkinson-White syndrome is characterized by a short P-R (≤ 0.12 sec) interval, prolonged QRS (≥ 0.12 sec) complex, and a slur on the upstroke of the QRS (delta wave), with secondary ST-segment and T-wave changes frequently present.

RBBB with LAHB is the most common combination of the left divisional and bundle branch blocks. The activation during the first 0.08 sec determines the axis and identifies LAHB. The delay of depolarization due to RBBB results in a final activation of the RV to the right and anteriorly.

ELECTROCARDIOGRAPHIC INTERPRETATIONS

59.   Artifact due to tremor
Sinus bradycardia with atrial premature complexes
Nonspecific ST and T wave abnormalities (Parkinson's disease)

60.   Atrial fibrillation with a controlled ventricular response
Right bundle branch block
Right axis deviation
Right ventricular hypertrophy
(Patient with longstanding mitral stenosis and elevated pulmonary pressures)

61.   Sinus tachycardia
Marked QT interval shortening
Nonspecific ST and T wave abnormalities
(Patient with hypercalcemia)

62.   Sinus rhythm with abnormal intraventricular conduction
Preexcitation syndrome pattern
(False-positive ETT due to WPW syndrome)

63.   Normal sinus rhythm
Left atrial abnormality
Right axis deviation ($> +100°$)
Left posterior fascicular block
Extensive anterior and lateral Q wave myocardial infarction (age indeterminate or probably old)
Nonspecific ST and/or T wave abnormalities
(Coronary artery disease suggested)

64. Normal sinus rhythm
    Left atrial abnormality
    Right axis deviation (> +100°)
    Complete right bundle branch block
    Left posterior fascicular block

65. Normal variant
    Juvenile T wave pattern

66. Normal sinus rhythm (without other abnormalities
        of rhythm or AV conduction)
    Right bundle branch block (complete)
    ST-T segment abnormalities secondary to the intra-
        ventricular conduction disturbance
    (Congenital right bundle branch block or atrial septal
        defect suggested)

67. Sinus rhythm with aberrant intraventricular con-
        duction due to the presence of a bypass tract
    Preexcitation pattern

68. Sinus rhythm with first-degree AV block
    Left axis deviation
    Complete left bundle branch block, with ST-T
        waves suggestive of acute myocardial injury or
        infarction
    Intraventricular conduction disturbance, nonspe-
        cific type (note "notched QRS" in II, III, and F)
    Q wave myocardial infarction, of recent age (note
        Q wave in lead aVL)
    ST-T segment abnormalities secondary to the intra-
        ventricular conduction disturbance
    (Coronary artery disease suggested)

69. Atrial fibrillation
    Fusion complexes
    Left ventricular hypertrophy by voltage
    Acute inferolateral Q wave myocardial infarction
    ST and/or T wave abnormalities suggesting myocar-
        dial injury
    (Coronary artery disease suggested)

70. Nonspecific atrial abnormality
    Normal sinus rhythm
    Right axis deviation
    Left posterior fascicular block
    Old inferior Q wave myocardial infarction
    Posterior Q wave myocardial infarction, age inde-
        terminate
    Nonspecific ST and T wave abnormalities
    (Coronary artery disease suggested)

71. Normal sinus rhythm
    Left atrial abnormality
    Right axis deviation
    Left posterior fascicular block
    Old anterior MI
    Lateral ST and T wave abnormalities consistent
        with acute ischemia
    Anterior ST segment elevation consistent with ven-
        tricular aneurysm
    (Coronary artery disease suggested)

72. Left atrial abnormality
    Normal sinus rhythm
    Low voltage (limb leads only)
    Acute lateral Q wave myocardial infarction
    Old inferoposterior Q wave myocardial infarction
    ST and T wave abnormalities suggesting myocardial
        injury
    (Coronary artery disease suggested)

73. Sinus rhythm with aberrant intraventricular con-
        duction due to the presence of a bypass tract
    Preexcitation pattern
    Right axis deviation

74. Left atrial abnormality
    Sinus tachycardia
    Right axis deviation
    Right ventricular hypertrophy
    Nonspecific ST and T wave abnormalities
    (Mitral valve disease suggested)

75. Left atrial abnormality
    Sinus rhythm with marked first-degree AV block
    Left axis deviation
    Left ventricular hypertrophy by both voltage and
        ST-T segment abnormalities
    Right bundle branch block, complete
    Left anterior fascicular block
    ST-T segment abnormalities secondary to intraven-
        tricular conduction disturbance or hypertrophy

76. Atrial fibrillation with variable, slow ventricular
        response and ventricular escape complexes
    Fusion complexes
    Nonspecific ST and T wave abnormalities

77. Atrial fibrillation with intermittent aberrant intra-
        ventricular conduction
    Right axis deviation
    Right bundle branch block (incomplete)
    Nonspecific ST and T wave abnormalities
    (Mitral valve disease suggested)

78. Right atrial abnormality
    Normal sinus rhythm with first-degree AV block
    Low voltage (limb leads only)
    Right axis deviation
    Right bundle branch block (complete)
    ST-T segment abnormalities secondary to the intra-
        ventricular conduction disturbance
    (The patient had Ebstein's anomaly of the tricuspid
        valve; note in particular the abnormal P-wave
        morphology.)

79. Atrial fibrillation with intermittent aberrant conduc-
        tion of a left bundle branch type
    Left axis deviation
    Poor precordial R wave progression consistent with
        old anteroseptal/anterior myocardial infarction
        and/or intraventricular conduction defect
    Possible old inferior myocardial infarction
    Nonspecific ST and wave abnormalities

80. Ventricular tachycardia

81. Sinus tachycardia
    Ventricular premature complexes with fixed coupling
    Fusion complexes
    Anteroseptal Q wave infarction of recent age
    ST and T wave abnormalities suggesting myocardial ischemia, inferior leads
    ST and T wave abnormalities suggesting myocardial injury, anteroseptal leads
    (Coronary artery disease suggested)

82. Wandering atrial pacemaker
    Left ventricular hypertrophy with accompanying ST and T wave abnormalities

83. Normal sinus rhythm
    Right bundle branch block with associated ST and T wave abnormalities
    Inferoposterolateral Q wave myocardial infarction
    (Coronary artery disease suggested)

84. Left anterior fascicular tachycardia at a rate of 150
    Right axis deviation
    Right bundle branch block
    Left posterior fascicular block
    ST and T wave abnormalities secondary to the intraventricular conduction disturbances

PART II: NORMAL AND ABNORMAL CIRCULATORY FUNCTION
CHAPTERS 13 THROUGH 29

DIRECTIONS: Each question below contains five suggested responses. Select the ONE BEST response to each question.

85. True statements about paroxysmal supraventricular tachycardia (PSVT) due to reentry over a concealed accessory pathway include all of the following EXCEPT:

    A. In patients referred for electrophysiological evaluation of apparent PSVT, the prevalence of concealed accessory pathway is approximately 30 per cent
    B. Most accessory pathways that participate in concealed conduction are located between the RV and RA
    C. The PSVTs caused by retrograde conduction over an accessory pathway tend to be somewhat faster than those occurring in AV nodal reentry tachycardias
    D. Atrial fibrillation (AF) in patients with a concealed accessory pathway may be approached therapeutically as patients with AF without such a pathway
    E. Under some circumstances, anterograde conduction down a concealed accessory pathway may occur

86. True statements with respect to diastolic left ventricular function in patients with hypertrophic cardiomyopathy include all of the following EXCEPT:

    A. Increasing heart rate worsens function
    B. Myocardial ischemia worsens function
    C. Atrial fibrillation worsens function
    D. Administration of dopamine may worsen function
    E. Administration of an acute volume load (e.g., 500 ml normal saline) will result in only a small fall in left ventricular diastolic pressure

87. An increased resistance to pulmonary venous drainage may lead to secondary pulmonary hypertension. True statements about secondary pulmonary hypertension due to such a cause include all of the following EXCEPT:

    A. Generation of RV systolic pressures ≥80 to 100 mm Hg requires RV hypertrophy
    B. Vasodilatation and plexiform lesions are characteristic of the pulmonary response to acquired pulmonary venous hypertension
    C. Pulmonary blood volume is one determinant of pulmonary artery pressure in patients with increased resistance to pulmonary venous drainage

    D. Congenital pulmonary venous hypertension is pathologically different from acquired pulmonary venous hypertension
    E. Considerable variability in pulmonary arterial vasoconstriction occurs in response to pulmonary venous hypertension

88. True statements about the use of Holter monitoring in the detection of cardiac arrhythmias include all of the following EXCEPT:

    A. Wenckebach second-degree AV block may be seen in normal subjects
    B. The frequency of PVCs after MI increases over the first several weeks
    C. Holter monitoring has proven useful in the detection of potentially serious arrhythmias in patients with mitral valve prolapse
    D. The sensitivity of long-term ECG recordings for the detection of ventricular arrhythmias is somewhat less than that of programmed stimulation studies
    E. In normal subjects the cardiac rhythm detected by ambulatory monitoring shows little variation from one recording period to the next

89. True statements about the use of rest as a therapeutic strategy in the treatment of heart failure include all of the following EXCEPT:

    A. Reduction in physical activity is critical in the care of patients with heart failure throughout the entire course of their illness
    B. In chronic heart failure, the patient is urged to remain active short of becoming symptomatic, whereas acute cardiac decompensation requires rigid restriction of physical activity
    C. A program of complete physical rest should be based upon complete bed rest
    D. Patients with marked impairment of ventricular function are at particularly high risk for systemic and pulmonary embolization when their activity is restricted
    E. As a general rule the presence of edema or moist pulmonary rales is an indication to maintain the patient at rest

90. A 9-year-old girl is brought in for evaluation because of several episodes of fainting. During one episode, which occurred while she was reading a book with her mother, she turned blue and was resuscitated. Her past medical history is unremarkable except for congenital deafness. The family history is remarkable for a sister who died suddenly at the age of 3 years. The most likely diagnosis is:

    A. sudden infant death syndrome
    B. Jervell and Lange-Nielsen syndrome
    C. Romano-Ward syndrome
    D. Lown-Ganong-Levine syndrome
    E. Barlow's syndrome

91. True statements about the Eisenmenger syndrome as a cause of secondary pulmonary hypertension include all of the following EXCEPT:

    A. The term Eisenmenger *syndrome* was first used to refer to patients with congenital cardiac lesions with severe pulmonary hypertension in whom reversal of a left-to-right shunt has occurred
    B. Eisenmenger *complex* refers specifically to patients with ventricular septal defect, severe pulmonary hypertension, and a right-to-left shunt through the defect
    C. Plexiform lesions of the muscular pulmonary arteries are a pathological indication of end-stage alterations in the pulmonary vasculature
    D. The emergence of plexiform lesions, or angiomatous or cavernous lesions, is a strong indication for surgical closure of the intracardiac communication
    E. The classification of Heath and Edwards of six grades of obstructive change in the pulmonary vasculature is widely employed to assess the potential reversibility of pulmonary vascular disease

92. Each of the following statements about the pathophysiology of cardiac and pulmonary dyspnea is true EXCEPT:

    A. Since most bronchial capillaries drain by way of the pulmonary veins, congestion tends to develop in alveolar and bronchial vasculature simultaneously
    B. Paroxysmal nocturnal dyspnea (PND) reflects the presence of interstitial edema, while pulmonary edema reflects the presence of alveolar edema
    C. The difficulty in distinguishing between cardiac and pulmonary dyspnea may be compounded by their simultaneous presence in some patients
    D. Sudden awakening at night occurs in patients with chronic obstructive pulmonary disease (COPD) and is commonly accompanied by sputum production
    E. Acute cardiac asthma often occurs in patients with subclinical heart disease and less commonly leads to cyanosis than does acute bronchial asthma

93. True statements about the pulmonary vasculature include all of the following EXCEPT:

    A. Acute hypoxemia leads to pulmonary vasoconstriction
    B. Acidemia causes vasoconstriction of pulmonary arteries and arterioles
    C. Beta-adrenoceptor stimulation elicits pulmonary vasoconstriction
    D. Acetylcholine is a potent relaxant of pulmonary arteries and arterioles
    E. While serotonin is a potent pulmonary vasoconstrictor in animals, it has little or no effect in humans

94. All the following characteristics are typical of hypertensive crisis EXCEPT:

    A. diastolic BP >140 mm Hg
    B. retinal hemorrhages
    C. normal mental status
    D. proteinuria and azotemia
    E. microangiopathic hemolytic anemia

95. A 63-year-old man who has been an insulin-requiring diabetic for 10 years presents to the office for initial management of hypertension (180/100). Urine and serum chemistries at this time are normal except for serum creatinine, 1.8 mg/dl, and blood urea nitrogen (BUN), 30 mg/dl. Because of gastroparesis you elect to initiate therapy with a potassium-sparing diuretic. When he returns in 2 weeks his serum potassium is 6.8 mEg/liter with no significant change in BUN or creatinine. The most likely explanation is:

    A. consumption of tomatoes and bananas
    B. a recent urinary tract infection
    C. primary hypoaldosteronism
    D. hyporeninemic hypoaldosteronism
    E. tuberculous adrenal hypoplasia

96. Each of the following statements about cardiac transplantation is true EXCEPT:

    A. Younger patients have better survival rates following cardiac transplantation
    B. Use of the immunosuppressant agent cyclosporine has led to improvement in results of cardiac transplantation
    C. The majority of patients who have received cardiac transplants have had end-stage heart disease due to coronary artery disease or cardiomyopathy
    D. Patients with heart transplants have limited exercise capacity because of absence of autonomic neural control
    E. Clinical signs of rejection include a fall in ECG voltage and the development of atrial arrhythmias

97. Each of the following statements about direct-current cardioversion of cardiac arrhythmias is true EXCEPT:

    A. In patients without clinical evidence of digitalis toxicity it is not necessary to withhold digitalis for 1 to 2 days before elective cardioversion
    B. In general, direct-current cardioversion of stable ventricular tachycardia requires greater energy levels than those required for atrial fibrillation
    C. Electrical cardioversion may be the therapy of choice for the treatment of rapid ventricular rates in patients with atrial fibrillation and the Wolff-Parkinson-White syndrome
    D. The occurrence of transient ventricular arrhythmias during attempted electrical cardioversion may be attenuated by administering a bolus of lidocaine before subsequent shocks
    E. Cardioversion of ventricular tachycardia by a chest "thump" may occasionally induce ventricular flutter or fibrillation

98. All of the following statements about cardiac hypertrophy in athletes are true EXCEPT:

    A. Isotonic exercise such as running and swimming increases left ventricular end-diastolic diameter
    B. Isometric exercise such as weight-lifting may cause an increase in left ventricular end-diastolic diameter
    C. Both isotonic and isometric exercise cause an increase in left ventricular mass
    D. Both isometric and isotonic exercise cause no change in left ventricular wall thickness
    E. Cardiac hypertrophy secondary to exercise usually disappears rapidly when training is discontinued

99. This hypothetical patient, a 78-year-old man who lives in a nursing home, is admitted via the emergency room because of fever and disorientation. His physical examination and ECG are normal except for sinus tachycardia and tachypnea. Laboratory results include an elevated white blood cell count, low platelet count, and prolonged prothrombin time. Urine sediment contains numerous polymorphonuclear leukocytes. A cardiology consult is obtained for evaluation of the chest x-ray shown. The most likely explanation for the *accompanying chest x-ray* findings is:

    A. left ventricular failure
    B. pneumococcal pneumonia
    C. adult respiratory distress syndrome
    D. gram-negative pneumonia
    E. posterior wall MI

100. A pacemaker's pulse generator is connected electrically to the heart via an electrode system referred to as a lead. True statements with regard to unipolar and bipolar electrodes include all of the following EXCEPT:

    A. In bipolar systems both electrodes are located in the cardiac chamber

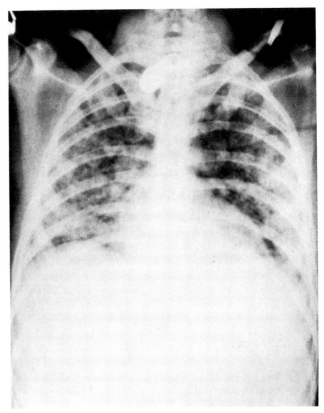

From Snider, G.L. (ed.): Acute respiratory failure. *In* Clinical Pulmonary Medicine. Boston, Little, Brown & Company, 1981, p. 378.

    B. Pacing thresholds for generation of stimuli are similar for unipolar and bipolar electrodes
    C. Unipolar electrodes are more susceptible to extracardiac interference from skeletal muscle potentials (myopotentials)
    D. The signal amplitudes of the electrograms generated by both types of electrodes are similar
    E. Electromagnetic interference causes oversensing and pacemaker malfunction more frequently with bipolar than with unipolar electrodes

101. The following statements about laboratory findings in heart failure are true EXCEPT:

    A. Serum electrolyte values are usually normal in patients with untreated heart failure
    B. Hyponatremia in heart failure may be due to a combination of dietary sodium restriction, diuretic therapy, and an elevated circulating vasopressin concentration
    C. Elevated serum glutamic oxaloacetic transaminase (SGOT) levels may accompany congestive hepatomegaly due to heart failure
    D. Acute hepatic venous congestion due to heart failure may produce a syndrome that closely resembles viral hepatitis
    E. Elevations of pulmonary capillary pressure to 17 mm Hg are commonly responsible for pulmonary vascular redistribution and interstitial edema on the chest roentgenogram

102. All of the following interventions are likely to lower BP EXCEPT:

A. a diet that reduces intake by 1000 calories per day
B. reduction of dietary sodium to 2 gm per day
C. a scheduled daily regimen of isometric exercise
D. reduction of dietary calcium by avoiding dairy products
E. reduction of ethanol consumption to less than 1.0 oz per day

103. Each of the following statements about procainamide is true EXCEPT:

A. The plasma concentration of procainamide required to suppress PVCs in patients after acute myocardial infarction may be less than that required to prevent sustained ventricular tachycardia
B. Procainamide, like quinidine, may accelerate the ventricular response in patients with atrial fibrillation or flutter
C. Procainamide may block conduction in the accessory pathway of patients with the Wolff-Parkinson-White syndrome
D. Toxic concentrations of procainamide may diminish myocardial performance
E. Procainamide is the drug of choice for the control of the tachyarrhythmias in patients with bradycardia-tachycardia syndrome

104. All of the following are primary determinants of cardiac output EXCEPT:

A. heart rate
B. left ventricular preload
C. left ventricular afterload
D. myocardial contractile or inotropic state
E. oxygen-carrying capacity of blood

105. Each of the following statements about exercise testing in the diagnosis of cardiac arrhythmias is true EXCEPT:

A. Approximately one-third of normal subjects develop ventricular ectopy during exercise testing
B. Nonsustained ventricular tachycardia of six beats or less can occur in normal patients and does not predict cardiovascular morbidity
C. Patients with ischemic heart disease develop PVCs at lower heart rates than normal subjects
D. Exercise testing should be avoided in patients with a history of serious ventricular arrhythmia
E. Exercise testing is less sensitive than prolonged ambulatory monitoring in detecting ventricular ectopy

106. With respect to renovascular disease all of the following statements are true EXCEPT:

A. Less than 2 per cent of adults with hypertension in a general practice have renovascular hypertension
B. Atherosclerotic disease most commonly involves the proximal third of the main renal artery
C. The most common form of fibroplastic renovascular disease in adults involves the media
D. The incidence of renovascular hypertension is higher in blacks than whites
E. Patients with severe, accelerated hypertension have the highest prevalence of renovascular disease

107. Each of the following statements about invasive electrophysiological study of the cardiac conduction system is true EXCEPT:

A. Ventricular tachyarrhythmia is a common explanation for syncope or presyncope in patients with an intraventricular conduction disturbance
B. The presence of an H-V interval equal to or greater than that recorded during normal sinus rhythm is consistent with the diagnosis of a ventricular tachycardia
C. In patients with sinus node dysfunction, associated impaired AV conduction is commonly found
D. Sinus node recovery time (SNRT) is defined as the difference between the spontaneous sinus node cycle length prior to pacing and the duration of the first spontaneous sinus response after termination of pacing
E. Localization of accessory pathways by endocardial mapping in patients with the Wolff-Parkinson-White syndrome is an important prerequisite for ablative surgery

108. All of the following statements with respect to primary aldosteronism are true EXCEPT:

A. The most common cause for primary aldosteronism is a solitary benign tumor
B. Hypokalemia (<3.2 mEq/liter) is present in the majority of patients
C. In patients with primary aldosteronism not receiving diuretics or supplemental potassium, urinary potassium will be >30 mEq/day
D. Patients with primary aldosteronism usually have high plasma renin activity
E. If a patient has high urinary potassium and low serum potassium but low serum aldosterone levels, licorice ingestion should be considered as a possible cause of the laboratory abnormalities

109. Comparison of left ventricular (LV) parameters in pressure- and volume-overloaded hearts reveals all of the following changes EXCEPT:

A. LV systolic stress initially is greater in pressure overload
B. Eccentric hypertrophy is characteristic of volume overload

C. Concentric hypertrophy is characteristic of pressure overload

D. LV wall thickness is greater in pressure overload

E. LV peak systolic pressure is greater in volume overload

---

110. True statements about drug interactions with digitalis include all of the following EXCEPT:

A. Amiodarone leads to decreased renal and non-renal clearance of digoxin

B. Verapamil decreases the volume of distribution of digoxin

C. Nifedipine decreases the clearance of digoxin and causes a resultant increase in serum digoxin levels

D. Erythromycin leads to an increase in bioavailability of digoxin and a resultant increase in serum levels

E. Diuretic agents may enhance the occurrence of digitalis toxicity

---

111. All of the following are correct statements with respect to management of hypertension in pregnancy EXCEPT:

A. Sodium restriction is an important component of therapy

B. Restriction of physical activity is advisable

C. Diuretics are usually contraindicated

D. Beta blockers may be useful

E. Methyldopa is frequently prescribed

---

112. A 50-year-old man who is an active tennis player presents because of symptomatic bradycardia in association with frequent episodes of paroxysmal supraventricular tachycardia (PSVT). On ambulatory (Holter) ECG, he is observed to have 9-second pauses on conversion from PSVT to sinus rhythm. His PSVT is poorly controlled despite trials of several drugs. Because of these difficulties with his management, a prophylactic pacemaker is implanted. The BEST choice would be:

A. AAI

B. VDD

C. DDD

D. rate-responsive VVI

E. DVI

---

113. Each of the following statements about the clinical manifestations of digitalis toxicity is correct EXCEPT:

A. Digitalis overdose may lead to nausea and vomiting due to central nervous system mechanisms

B. Digitalis intoxication may result in malaise, disorientation, seizures, or other neurological symptoms

C. Digitalis may occasionally induce gynecomastia in men

D. Paroxysmal atrial tachycardia with AV block (PAT with block) is virtually pathognomonic of digitalis excess

E. Common arrhythmias due to digitalis toxicity include atrioventricular junctional escape rhythms and ventricular bigeminy or trigeminy

---

114. Pulmonary parenchymal disease may lead to an increased resistance to flow through the pulmonary vascular bed and therefore to secondary pulmonary hypertension. True statements about pulmonary parenchymal disease in this regard include all of the following EXCEPT:

A. Hypoxia-induced vasoconstriction occurs in patients with chronic bronchitis and emphysema and may play a role in producing pulmonary hypertension

B. In patients with chronic obstructive lung disease, pulmonary hypertension is directly correlated with the extent of alveolar destruction

C. Progressive systemic sclerosis may lead to interstitial pulmonary fibrosis and subsequent pulmonary hypertension

D. CREST syndrome may lead to RV systolic overload secondary to pulmonary vascular disease and hypertension

E. Obstruction of the major pulmonary arteries by tumor may be a cause of pulmonary artery hypertension

---

115. Each of the following statements about vasodilator agents used in heart failure is true EXCEPT:

A. The most important adverse effect of sodium nitroprusside is hypotension

B. Sublingual nitroglycerin may be used to effect a rapid reduction in left ventricular filling pressures

C. Chronic administration of a combination of hydralazine and isosorbide dinitrate has been shown to prolong survival in patients with heart failure

D. Hydralazine appears to be most effective in patients with normal heart size

E. Angiotensin-converting enzyme inhibitors lead to a decline in left and right ventricular filling pressures with little or no change in heart rate in patients with heart failure

---

116. All of the following statements about protodiastolic gallop sounds are true EXCEPT:

A. Left ventricular gallop sounds are best heard along the left sternal border

B. Protodiastolic gallop sounds result from the sharp deceleration of ventricular inflow that occurs immediately after the early diastolic filling phase

C. The protodiastolic gallop occurring in mitral

regurgitation results from the torrential flow of blood into the left ventricle in early diastole and is not a result of underlying heart failure

D. The protodiastolic or S_3 gallop may be a normal finding in children and young adults

E. Protodiastolic gallop sounds originating from the left ventricle tend to be louder with rapid heart rates and may be elicited on occasion by a brief course of exercise

---

117. Sudden cardiac death, defined as natural death due to a cardiac event within one hour of symptoms heralded by loss of consciousness, causes what percentage of all coronary heart disease deaths?

A. 10 per cent
B. 25 per cent
C. 50 per cent
D. 75 per cent
E. Unknown

---

118. All of the statements below concerning the effects of digitalis on myocardial contractility are true EXCEPT:

A. The inotropic action of digitalis occurs in both normal and failing heart muscle

B. The relative augmentation of the velocity of myocardial contraction by digitalis may be greater in failing than in normal myocardium

C. Administration of cardiac glycosides in normal subjects leads to a rise in cardiac output

D. Recent studies have documented sustained improvement in cardiac performance in patients with chronic congestive heart failure treated with digitalis

E. Patient selection and the nature and extent of ventricular dysfunction are critical factors in the clinical response to digitalis therapy

---

119. True statements about the clinical use of lidocaine include all of the following EXCEPT:

A. Lidocaine is generally ineffective against supraventricular tachyarrhythmias

B. In patients with the Wolff-Parkinson-White syndrome, lidocaine may accelerate the ventricular response to atrial fibrillation

C. The most common side effects of lidocaine are dose-related exacerbations of cardiac rhythm disturbances

D. The use of lidocaine prophylactically in hospitalized patients with acute myocardial infarction remains a controversial subject

E. In patients resuscitated from out-of-hospital ventricular fibrillatory arrests, lidocaine is comparable to bretylium in preventing recurrent episodes of ventricular tachyarrhythmia

---

120. Each of the statements below concerning atrial fibrillation (AF) is true EXCEPT:

A. AF is commonly seen in patients following cardiac surgery

B. In patients with underlying cardiovascular disease, the development of chronic AF increases overall mortality

C. Physical findings in patients with AF include variations in the intensity of S_1 and in the amplitude of a waves in the jugular venous pulse

D. A greater frequency of right bundle branch block is noted in patients who develop AF in the year following acute myocardial infarction

E. In the absence of underlying heart disease, subjects with AF have no increase in cardiovascular risk but do display a higher incidence of stroke

---

121. The frequency of various diagnoses in hypertensive (HTN) subjects in large series is best described as:

A. essential HTN 95 per cent; chronic renal disease 4 per cent; renovascular disease 1 per cent

B. essential HTN 90 per cent; chronic renal disease 1 per cent; renovascular disease 9 per cent

C. essential HTN 80 per cent; chronic renal disease 10 per cent; renovascular disease 10 per cent

D. essential HTN 80 per cent; chronic renal disease 15 per cent; renovascular disease 5 per cent

E. essential HTN 95 per cent; chronic renal disease 1 per cent; renovascular disease 1 per cent; Cushing's disease 1 per cent; coarctation of aorta 1 per cent; primary aldosteronism 1 per cent

---

122. True statements about the syndrome of circulatory shock include all of the following EXCEPT:

A. The clinical signs of shock reflect a decrease in blood flow to a variety of organs

B. ECG signs of myocardial ischemia may appear in patients with apparently normal hearts due to a reduction in regional coronary blood flow

C. Circulatory shock in the first 3 months of life is often due to gram-negative bacteremia

D. Increases in capillary hydrostatic pressure during circulatory shock lead to a depletion of plasma water and hemoconcentration

E. During circulatory shock, pulmonary blood flow is often protected at the expense of cerebral and renal perfusion

---

123. All of the following statements regarding quinidine are true EXCEPT:

A. Quinidine may be used to treat fetal arrhythmias because it can cross the placenta

B. Quinidine may cause significant hypotension because of its alpha-adrenoreceptor blocking effects

C. Quinidine is cleared from the circulation primarily by the kidneys

D. In patients with the Wolff-Parkinson-White syndrome quinidine may prevent reciprocating tachycardias and slow the ventricular response to atrial fibrillation

E. Quinidine therapy may cause a paradoxical increase in the ventricular response to atrial flutter or fibrillation

124. Each of the following statements about edema in heart failure is correct EXCEPT:

A. Edema in heart failure does not correlate well with the level of systemic venous pressure

B. Peripheral edema may be detected when extracellular fluid volume has increased by as little as 1 to 2 liters

C. Severe edema may cause rupture of the skin and extravasation of fluid

D. In patients with acute heart failure, edema may not be present initially

E. In patients with hemiplegia due to a cerebral vascular accident, edema is usually more apparent on the paralyzed side

125. True statements about the increased cardiac output that occurs during anemia include all of the following EXCEPT:

A. A decrease in blood viscosity contributes to the high cardiac output noted in anemia

B. Clinical evidence of impaired cardiac function may occur in patients without apparent underlying heart disease when the hematocrit falls below 25 per cent

C. Patients with sickle cell anemia may manifest heart failure with less severe degrees of anemia than those seen in patients with iron deficiency anemia

D. In patients with anemia, exercise may lead to an exaggerated increase in cardiac output

E. The rate of development of anemia plays an important role in the degree to which anemia affects cardiac output

126. Loop diuretics are used extensively in the treatment of heart failure. All of the following statements about loop diuretics are correct EXCEPT:

A. Loop diuretics are among the most potent diuretic agents known and may induce natriuresis amounting to 20 per cent of the filtered sodium load

B. Loop diuretics are secreted into the tubular lumen by the organic acid secretory pathway and may therefore be competitively inhibited by agents such as probenecid and indomethacin

C. Bioavailability of orally administered loop diuretics such as furosemide is usually 80 to 90 per cent

D. Nonsteroidal antiinflammatory drugs may limit the response to loop diuretics by preventing the

rise in renal blood flow that accompanies and sustains the natriuretic response to these diuretic agents

E. Loop diuretics such as furosemide may cause changes in systemic hemodynamics before the initiation of diuresis

127. Each of the following statements about high-output heart failure is true EXCEPT:

A. Thyrotoxicosis, anemia, and pregnancy are all examples of high-output states that may lead to heart failure

B. The extremities of the patient with high-output failure are usually warm and flushed

C. The arterial–mixed venous O_2 difference may be normal in high-output failure

D. The pulse pressure in high-output failure is normal or widened

E. The arterial–mixed venous O_2 difference may be less than it was prior to the development of high-output heart failure

128. Each of the following statements about verapamil is true EXCEPT:

A. Verapamil exerts a direct myocardial depressant effect

B. Cardiac index may remain unchanged in patients on verapamil because afterload reduction produced by the drug counteracts its negative inotropic action

C. Verapamil is the drug of choice in the treatment of atrial fibrillation in patients with the Wolff-Parkinson-White syndrome

D. Verapamil is the drug of choice for terminating sustained AV nodal reentrant tachycardias

E. Verapamil is not as effective as quinidine in establishing and maintaining sinus rhythm in patients with chronic atrial fibrillation

129. Each of the following statements about physical findings in heart failure is true EXCEPT:

A. Chronic marked elevation of systemic venous pressure may produce exophthalmos or even visible systolic pulsation of the eyes

B. Pallor and coldness of the extremities are primarily due to elevation of adrenergic nervous system activity

C. A positive abdominojugular reflux test reflects the combination of hepatic congestion and the inability of the right side of the heart to accept or reject an increased venous return

D. The presence of hepatic tenderness reflects longstanding right-sided heart failure with chronic stretching of the liver capsule

E. Protein-losing enteropathy may occur in patients with visceral congestion and may result in a reduced plasma oncotic pressure

130. Each of the following statements about the antiarrhythmic agent disopyramide is true EXCEPT:

   A. Disopyramide, unlike quinidine and procainamide, is not capable of creating 1:1 conduction during atrial flutter by a direct vagolytic effect
   B. The mean elimination half-life of disopyramide is 8 to 9 hours, and peak blood levels of the agent after oral administration occur in 1 to 2 hours
   C. Disopyramide may be useful in reducing the frequency of PVCs as well as in preventing recurrence of ventricular tachycardia
   D. Disopyramide may have negative inotropic effects, especially in patients with preexisting abnormal ventricular function
   E. Important side effects of disopyramide include antiparasympathetic autonomic effects and torsades de pointes

DIRECTIONS: Each question below contains five suggested answers. For EACH of the FIVE alternatives listed you are to respond either YES (Y) or NO (N). In a given item ALL, SOME, OR NONE OF THE ALTERNATIVES MAY BE CORRECT.

131. Correct statements regarding common features in the clinical presentation of renovascular hypertension secondary to fibromuscular hyperplasia, as opposed to atherosclerosis, include which of the following?

   A. Age less than 50
   B. Female gender
   C. Coexisting cardiomegaly
   D. No family history of hypertension
   E. Presence of carotid bruits

132. Correct statements regarding arrhythmias as a precipitant of heart failure include:

   A. Tachyarrhythmias may precipitate heart failure by increasing myocardial oxygen demand and inducing ischemia
   B. Tachyarrhythmias may precipitate heart failure by increasing ventricular filling time
   C. Bradycardia may precipitate heart failure by depressing cardiac output
   D. Dissociation between atrial and ventricular contraction may precipitate heart failure, especially in patients with concentric ventricular hypertrophy
   E. Abnormal intraventricular conduction may precipitate heart failure by impairing myocardial performance

133. True statements concerning treatment of digitalis intoxication include which of the following?

   A. Lidocaine and phenytoin are both useful agents in treating arrhythmias due to digitalis excess
   B. Quinidine is useful in suppressing ventricular irritability due to digitalis excess
   C. Direct-current countershock is generally inadvisable in digitalis intoxication because severe arrhythmias may result from this procedure
   D. Elective DC cardioversion for atrial fibrillation appears to be safer in patients without digitalis-induced rhythm disturbances than in those with these disturbances
   E. No effective treatment is available for patients with potentially life-threatening digoxin or digitalis toxicity

134. With reference to myocardial function in shock (acute circulatory failure), true statements include which of the following?

   A. Peripheral vasoconstriction in circulatory shock initially helps to maintain coronary perfusion by increasing diastolic aortic pressure
   B. In shock, reductions in LV ejection fraction and ventricular dilation occur despite the maintenance of coronary perfusion pressure and flow
   C. As circulatory shock progresses, coronary perfusion pressure and flow are reduced and a decrease in the blood flow to the endocardium occurs
   D. During shock, the oxygen requirements of the myocardium are decreased secondary to the low-flow state
   E. During shock, the presence of digitalis glycosides may help reduce cardiac arrhythmias

135. With reference to the risks of hypertension, true statements include which of the following?

   A. Hypercholesterolemia in hypertensive men poses an increased risk of coronary disease
   B. Hypertensive patients with low plasma renin activity (PRA) have a lower incidence of heart attacks and strokes
   C. Adult hypertensive blacks as compared with whites develop more severe renal damage
   D. Women suffer less cardiovascular morbidity as a consequence of hypertension than men do
   E. The higher the systolic pressure the greater the incidence of target organ damage

136. Correct statements about the use of diphenylhydantoin (phenytoin) in the treatment of cardiac arrhythmias include which of the following?

   A. Phenytoin, like disopyramide, may lead to left
      ventricular dysfunction
   B. Oral administration of phenytoin leads to peak
      plasma concentrations of the drug in 1 to 2 hours
      with an elimination half-life of approximately 8
      hours
   C. Metabolism of phenytoin occurs primarily in the
      liver and may be altered by a variety of drugs
      that compete for hepatic enzymes
   D. Therapeutic plasma concentrations of phenytoin
      may be achieved rapidly by intravenous admin-
      istration of the drug
   E. Phenytoin is an effective antiarrhythmic agent
      in the treatment of atrial and ventricular ar-
      rhythmias in patients with ischemic heart dis-
      ease or with digitalis toxicity

137. Correct statements about procainamide include
which of the following?

   A. Absorption of oral procainamide may be reduced
      in the first week after MI
   B. Procainamide is primarily effective against su-
      praventricular arrhythmias
   C. Procainamide is well absorbed after intramus-
      cular injection
   D. Elimination of procainamide is primarily
      through a renal mechanism
   E. Constant-rate intravenous infusion of procain-
      amide is given in a dose of 2 to 6 mg/min

138. With reference to clinical settings in which ventricular arrhythmias are noted, true statements include
which of the following?

   A. Patients with arrhythmogenic RV dysplasia most
      often have ventricular tachycardia (VT) with a
      contour of left bundle branch block and right-
      axis deviation
   B. The presence of ventricular arrhythmias in pa-
      tients with mitral valve prolapse may be a
      warning sign for sudden cardiac death
   C. Patients with dilated cardiomyopathy and a re-
      duced ejection fraction are at increased risk of
      sudden death if ventricular couplets are noted
      on a 24-hour ECG recording
   D. Patients with hypertrophic cardiomyopathy are
      at increased risk for sudden death
   E. Patients with a history of repair of tetralogy of
      Fallot are at particular risk for the development
      of ventricular arrhythmias

139. Which of the following statements concerning minoxidil are correct?

   A. Its relative actions on veins are greater than on
      arteries

   B. Facial hirsutism is a complication of its use,
      particularly in women
   C. Pericardial effusions occur in 20 per cent of
      patients receiving this drug
   D. A lupus-like syndrome occurs in 10 per cent of
      patients
   E. Fluid retention in the absence of diuretic use is
      common

140. With reference to the use of amiodarone in the
treatment of cardiac arrhythmias, true statements
include which of the following?

   A. Intravenous amiodarone may exert a negative
      inotropic action and must be given with great
      caution to patients with depressed ejection frac-
      tions
   B. Amiodarone's efficacy in general equals or ex-
      ceeds that of other antiarrhythmic agents
   C. Adverse effects of amiodarone occur in approx-
      imately 30 per cent of patients treated with
      maintenance doses of the drug
   D. Pulmonary toxicity, while not uncommon, is
      rarely serious
   E. Amiodarone leads to hyperthyroidism in ap-
      proximately 15 per cent of patients receiving
      maintenance therapy

141. With regard to cor triatriatum, true statements
include which of the following?

   A. Pulmonary hypertension secondary to pulmo-
      nary venous obstruction may occur
   B. Partitioning of the left atrium creates two left
      atrial subchambers in this disorder
   C. The posterior subchamber receives pulmonary
      venous inflow
   D. When this disorder leads to pulmonary hyper-
      tension, pressure in the anterior subchamber is
      usually markedly elevated
   E. No specific therapy for this disorder exists

142. Atrioventricular block exists when the atrial impulse
is conducted with delay or is not conducted at all
to the ventricle. True statements about second-
degree AV block include which of the following?

   A. Type I AV block is associated with a benign
      clinical course in all age groups
   B. Type II AV block in inferior MI is not associated
      with an increase in mortality
   C. Type I AV block with a normal QRS complex
      occurs at the level of the AV node or in the His
      bundle
   D. Type II AV block in association with bundle
      branch block occurs at the level of the AV node
      or the His bundle
   E. 2:1 AV block may be either Type I or Type II
      second-degree AV block and is more likely to
      be type I if the QRS complex is normal

143. Correct statements with regard to the contractile proteins of cardiac cells include which of the following?

   A. The thick filaments are composed of aggregates of myosin filaments
   B. The thin filaments are composed largely of actin molecules
   C. Troponin C is a regulatory protein which binds Ca^{++}
   D. Troponin C normally interacts with actomyosin to inhibit the Mg^{++}-stimulated ATPase
   E. When a cardiac cell is depolarized, intracellular Ca^{++} concentration falls from $10^{-5}M$ to $10^{-7}M$ with release of Ca^{++} from troponin C

144. Which of the following are compensatory physiological responses to heart failure?

   A. Decreased blood flow to cutaneous, splanchnic, and renal vascular beds
   B. Increased sodium retention
   C. Increased water retention
   D. An increase in the affinity of hemoglobin for O_2
   E. Constriction of veins in the extremities

145. A 74-year-old man with a long history of left ventricular failure secondary to several myocardial infarctions comes to the emergency room acutely short of breath 2 hours after eating a large holiday meal. Physical examination and chest x-ray are consistent with acute pulmonary edema. ECG shows a narrow complex junctional tachycardia at a rate of 130/min with 1 mm ST-segment depression in V_4–V_6. BP is 170/100; respiration, 32. His current medical treatment includes nitrates, calcium channel antagonists, digoxin, and chlorothiazide. Appropriate initial therapy in the emergency room would include:

   A. nasal O_2
   B. morphine sulfate
   C. intravenous furosemide
   D. intravenous digoxin
   E. sublingual nitroglycerin

146. A 60-year-old man had a pacemaker inserted 5 years ago because of sinus bradycardia with poor LV function following an anterior MI. As part of his exercise program he has been using a rowing machine. Recently, he has had several episodes of near-syncope which occurred only while rowing. An ambulatory ECG (Holter monitor) revealed an abnormal rhythm during a near-syncopal event while rowing. True statements with respect to the ECG *shown below* include:

   A. There is evidence for a dual chamber pacing system
   B. There is inappropriate inhibition of ventricular pacing
   C. There is undersensing of atrial activity
   D. There is lack of capture of the ventricles
   E. There is lack of capture of the atria

147. True statements about digoxin include:

   A. The half-life of digoxin in subjects with normal renal function is about 36 to 48 hours
   B. In patients with normal renal function who have not previously taken digitalis, institution of daily maintenance therapy without a loading dose leads to a steady-state plateau concentration of the drug in about 7 days
   C. Dialysis is a relatively effective way of removing digoxin from the body
   D. Obese patients taking digoxin who undergo dramatic weight loss must have their digoxin dosage decreased to avoid toxicity
   E. Patients taking digoxin who subsequently begin quinidine therapy often require a decrease in digoxin dosage to avoid toxicity

148. Which of the following are true statements regarding measurement of myocardial contractility?

   A. Acute changes in afterload at any level of contractility cause an inverse change in ejection fraction
   B. In mitral regurgitation the ejection fraction is inappropriately elevated
   C. In aortic regurgitation the ejection fraction is inappropriately elevated
   D. At any level of contractility, end-systolic fiber length (or end-systolic volume) varies inversely with afterload
   E. At any level of contractility, end-systolic pressure varies directly with afterload

DDD 70/min

25 mm/s

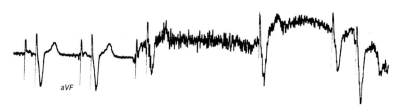

aVF

From Schuller, H. and Fahraeus, T.: Pacemaker Electrocardiograms: An Introduction to Practical Analysis. Sweden, Siemens-Elema, 1983, p. 141.

149. Insertion of a temporary pacing wire during acute myocardial infarction in patients who develop AV conduction disturbances is indicated in which of the following circumstances?

    A. New first-degree AV block
    B. New Mobitz type I second-degree AV block
    C. New Mobitz type II second-degree AB block
    D. New alternating RBBB and LBBB
    E. Preexisting RBBB

150. True statements about digitoxin include:

    A. Gastrointestinal absorption of digitoxin is thought to be essentially complete
    B. The usual daily oral maintenance dose of digitoxin in adults is 0.10 mg
    C. Digitoxin, like digoxin, is about 25 per cent bound to plasma proteins
    D. Excretion of digitoxin is split approximately equally between renal and hepatic clearance
    E. Clinical signs of digitalis toxicity may appear in patients who use digitoxin simultaneously with warfarin or clofibrate, because of displacement of the drug from its serum albumin binding site

151. Correct statements with respect to out-of-hospital resuscitation of sudden cardiac death patients include which of the following?

    A. The group of patients found to be in sustained VT at the time of first contact with medical personnel have the best prognosis
    B. Patients with bradyarrhythmias at first contact have a better prognosis than do patients with VF
    C. Early defibrillation is associated with improved survival compared with standard CPR
    D. Initiation of bystander CPR is associated with little change in long-term survival
    E. Initial defibrillation should be carried out with a shock of 200 joules

152. A 50-year-old woman visits the office complaining of episodes characterized by hot flushes, palpitations, sweats, and a sense of apprehension. Her blood pressure episodically reaches 210/100 mm Hg and in the interim periods is 150/85. Correct statements about this patient's condition include:

    A. 90 per cent of these patients have a solitary tumor in the adrenal cortex
    B. It is likely that a 24-hour urine assay for total metanephrines will be elevated
    C. Multiple adrenal tumors are more likely in

patients with type II multiple endocrine neoplasia (Sipple's syndrome)
    D. Abdominal ultrasound is the best noninvasive diagnostic test
    E. Urinary metanephrine secretion is increased following an intravenous pyelogram (IVP) with Renografin

153. True statements about cardiac physical findings in patients with congestive heart failure include which of the following?

    A. Heart failure due to restrictive cardiomyopathy is usually accompanied by signs of cardiomegaly
    B. Pulsus alternans occurs most commonly in heart failure due to concomitant mitral regurgitation
    C. Pulsus alternans results from variation of the stroke volume due to incomplete recovery of contracting myocardial cells
    D. A low-grade fever that is due to cutaneous vasoconstriction and impaired heat loss may occur in severe heart failure
    E. Cheyne-Stokes respiration is a cyclic respiratory pattern that results from a combination of a change in the sensitivity of the respiratory center and the presence of left ventricular failure

154. Correct statements regarding the association of oral contraceptive pills and hypertension include which of the following?

    A. The likelihood of developing hypertension is increased by significant alcohol consumption
    B. The incidence of hypertension is about 2.5 times greater in pill users than in nonusers
    C. The likelihood of developing hypertension is unaffected by the age of the user
    D. The mechanism for contraceptive-induced hypertension probably involves renin-aldosterone–mediated volume expansion
    E. Cigarette smoking more than doubles the cardiovascular complications associated with use of oral contraceptives

155. With respect to issues of patient compliance and adherence to antihypertensive therapy, true statements include which of the following?

    A. Use the fewest daily doses of drugs necessary
    B. Add only one drug at a time
    C. Attain normal BP (120/80) as quickly as possible
    D. Use home blood pressure readings
    E. Use nondrug therapies when possible

156. True statements with regard to distribution of blood flow and intravascular pressure in the upright lung include which of the following?

    1. Pulmonary artery pressure is greater than alveolar pressure at the lung apices
    2. Pulmonary venous pressure exceeds alveolar pressure at the lung bases
    3. Alveolar pressure increases from the lung base to the lung apex
    4. Pulmonary vascular redistribution occurs when there is a relative reduction in perfusion of the bases with a relative increase in apical perfusion

157. The presence of hypertension (BP >160/95) causes an increase in the age-adjusted morbidity when it is associated with which of the following disease processes?

    1. Congestive heart failure
    2. Coronary artery disease
    3. Atherothrombotic brain infarction
    4. Intermittent claudication

158. Clinical features suggestive of renovascular hypertension include which of the following?

    1. recent onset of hypertension, especially in younger patients
    2. rapidly progressive hypertension
    3. presence of an abdominal bruit, particularly lateral to the midline
    4. deterioration of renal function after initiation of therapy with a converting enzyme inhibitor

159. True statements with respect to the association of sudden cardiac death (SCD) and premature ventricular contractions (PVCs) include:

    1. PVCs in the absence of heart disease are, in general, prognostically benign
    2. In patients who have survived MI, more than 10 PVCs/hour are associated with an increased risk of SCD
    3. Left ventricular dysfunction after MI increases the risk of SCD associated with the presence of PVCs
    4. Treatment with antiarrhythmic drugs of increased numbers of PVCs after MI has been shown in most studies to decrease significantly the incidence of SCD

160. Features of the systemic lupus erythematosus (SLE)–like syndrome that may be induced by procainamide include:

    1. the development of antinuclear antibodies in 20 to 30 per cent of patients on chronic procainamide therapy
    2. the development of clinical symptoms of SLE in 20 to 30 per cent of patients on chronic procainamide therapy
    3. a similar occurrence of SLE syndrome due to the N-acetylprocainamide (NAPA) metabolite of the drug
    4. a response to steroids in some patients

161. A 32-year-old man who is a chronic intravenous drug abuser is admitted to the hospital in respiratory distress. Despite conservative therapy there is progressive deterioration of systemic oxygenation, and mechanical ventilation is instituted. During the next 24 hours further impairment of oxygenation occurs despite an inspired oxygen concentration (FIO_2) of 100 per cent. Therefore, positive end-expiratory pressure (PEEP) at 10 mm Hg is initiated. Possible complications secondary to PEEP in this setting may include:

    1. decreased cardiac output
    2. augmented venous return with right ventricular failure
    3. barotrauma with pneumothorax
    4. enhanced oxygen toxicity to pulmonary alveoli

162. True statements concerning the symptoms and signs of heart failure in the neonate and infant include which of the following?

    1. Excessive diaphoresis may be a manifestation of heart failure during the first year of life
    2. Atelectasis may be precipitated by obstruction of the airways from enlargement of the main pulmonary artery
    3. Hepatomegaly may be seen commonly in both left and right heart failure
    4. Ascites and peripheral edema are common sequelae of right heart failure

163. True statements with regard to events preceding sudden cardiac death (SCD) include which of the following?

    1. There is a high incidence of acute coronary thrombi or plaque fissuring or both

2. Unexpected circulatory failure is a rare cause of SCD
3. Ambulatory (Holter) monitor recordings obtained within an hour of SCD often show increasing frequency and complexity of ventricular ectopy
4. The overwhelming majority of patients with out-of-hospital SCD have evidence for new transmural myocardial infarction

164. Potential complications of diuretic therapy in heart failure include:

1. hypokalemia
2. hypermagnesemia
3. hyponatremia
4. hypernatremia

165. Patients with the electrocardiogram *shown below* could also exhibit:

1. a gradual increase in atrial rate with the administration of digitalis
2. an irregular atrial rate
3. precipitation of the arrhythmia by hypokalemia
4. an absence of underlying cardiac disease in 40 per cent of cases

166. Correct statements about patients with unexplained syncope or palpitations include which of the following?

1. A careful, accurately performed history and physical examination are the most important tests to perform in this population
2. In those patients with syncope of noncardiovascular causes, the 1- to 2-year mortality rate is less than 15 per cent
3. When a putative cause for unexplained syncope is found by electrophysiological study, subsequent therapy prevents recurrence of symptoms in about 80 per cent of patients
4. Electrophysiological induction of a sustained tachycardia in patients who do not develop spontaneous arrhythmia on noninvasive evaluations suggests that the induced rhythm is clinically significant and responsible for their symptoms

167. Lidocaine is a widely used pharmacological agent for the treatment of cardiac arrhythmias. Correct statements about lidocaine include:

1. Lidocaine has little effect on the electrophysiological properties of atrial myocardial cells or on conduction in accessory pathways
2. In the absence of severe left ventricular dysfunction, clinically significant adverse hemodynamic effects from lidocaine are rarely noted
3. The elimination half-life of lidocaine in patients after relatively uncomplicated myocardial infarction is two to four times that of normal subjects
4. Patients treated with an initial bolus of lidocaine followed by a maintenance infusion may experience transient excessive plasma concentrations of the drug 30 to 120 minutes after therapy is begun

168. Regulation of the intracellular concentration of Ca^{++} in myocardial cells is determined by which of the following mechanisms?

1. Phospholamban, a Ca^{++}-stimulated Mg^{2+}-ATPase, transports Ca^{++} into the sarcoplasmic reticulum (SR)
2. Voltage-dependent Ca^{++} channels increase Ca^{++} influx in response to membrane depolarization
3. A bidirectional Na^+-Ca^{++} exchange carrier transports Ca^{++} in exchange for Na^+
4. Receptor-operated channels in response to beta-adrenoceptor agonists increase Ca^{++} efflux

169. Which of the following statements concerning myocardial cell function in the failing heart are true?

1. In response to either pressure or volume overload, sarcomere length decreases
2. There is an increase in the maximal velocity of sarcomere shortening
3. There is a shift to the descending limb of the Frank-Starling curve
4. The depression of contractility is due to an intrinsic defect of cardiac muscle

170. For equivalent total and effective stroke volumes, left ventricular (LV) end-diastolic pressure and volume are greater in which of the following?

1. Mitral regurgitation as opposed to aortic regurgitation

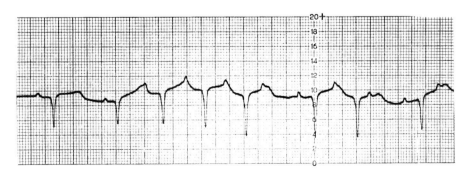

2. Aortic regurgitation as opposed to mitral regurgitation
3. Ventricular septal defect as opposed to patent ductus arteriosus
4. Patent ductus arteriosus as opposed to ventricular septal defect

---

171. In response to an excessive hemodynamic burden, the heart utilizes which of the following mechanisms to maintain cardiac output?

    1. The Frank-Starling mechanism
    2. Increased catecholamine release from adrenergic nerves and adrenal medulla
    3. Myocardial hypertrophy
    4. Decreased venous return

---

172. A 59-year-old woman with left ventricular dysfunction presents in mild congestive heart failure despite adhering to her regimen of digoxin and furosemide. You initiate outpatient therapy with oral captopril (12.5 mg). About 30 minutes after taking her first dose, while getting dressed, she has a syncopal event. Possible explanations include:

    1. an episode of tachyarrhythmia
    2. failure of baroreceptor-mediated increase in heart rate on standing up to dress
    3. abnormalities in regulation of peripheral vascular resistance
    4. decreased circulating renin levels with decreased angiotensin II levels

---

173. Which of the following hemodynamic parameters are associated with left ventricular failure?

    1. Acute inferior myocardial infarction with cardiac index 2 liters/min/m², left ventricular end-diastolic pressure (LVEDP) 5 mm Hg, BP 100/50 mm Hg
    2. Acute anterior myocardial infarction stabilized on dobutamine with cardiac index 2 liters/min/m², LVEDP 22 mm Hg, arterial pressure 100/50 mm Hg
    3. Breast cancer patient who has received 500 mg/m² of Adriamycin and now has a pericardial effusion with cardiac index 2 liters/min/m², LVEDP 10 mm Hg, arterial pressure 100/50 mm Hg
    4. Acute viral myocarditis with cardiac index 2 liters/min/m², LVEDP 30 mm Hg, arterial pressure 100/50 mm Hg

---

174. Under conditions of chronic pressure overload with a rise in wall stress such as occurs in aortic stenosis or hypertension, the LV

    1. exhibits a rise in end-diastolic pressure
    2. responds to positive inotropic agents with an increase in contractility
    3. undergoes hypertrophy by adding muscle fibers in parallel
    4. exhibits a fall in ejection fraction that always indicates a depression of contractile state

---

175. Prophylactic permanent pacing is indicated in which of the following asymptomatic patients with AV conduction disturbances?

    1. A man with acquired complete AV block
    2. A woman with RBBB and left anterior hemiblock
    3. A woman with Mobitz type II second-degree AV block
    4. A man with RBBB and first-degree AV block

---

176. The electrocardiogram illustrated *below* shows a pacemaker malfunction. The pacemaker is a VVI set at a rate of 70/min. True statements with respect to the malfunction include which of the following?

    1. There is pacing at an altered rate from initial programming
    2. There is intermittent undersensing
    3. There is intermittent oversensing
    4. There is intermittent loss of capture

---

177. Features suggestive of preeclampsia (as opposed to chronic hypertension) in a pregnant patient include which of the following?

    1. Younger age (<20 years)
    2. Proteinuria
    3. Primigravida status
    4. Systolic blood pressure <160 mm Hg

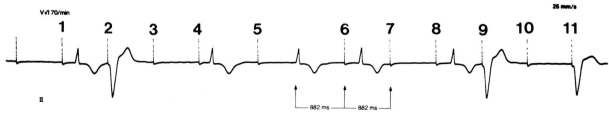

From Schuller, H. and Fahraeus, T.: Pacemaker Electrocardiograms: An Introduction to Practical Analysis. Sweden, Siemens-Elema, 1983, p. 77.

178. Clinical features of the Wolff-Parkinson-White (WPW) syndrome include:

   1. an absence of heart disease in most adults
   2. a decrease in the frequency of paroxysmal tachycardia with increasing age
   3. an association with Ebstein's anomaly
   4. a majority of tachycardias seen with this syndrome presenting as atrial fibrillation

179. True statements about the adverse effects of quinidine include which of the following?

   1. Quinidine may produce syncope in up to 2 per cent of patients
   2. The most common side effects of chronic oral quinidine therapy are central nervous system disturbances
   3. Potential therapies for quinidine-induced torsades de pointes include overdrive pacing and intravenous isoproterenol or magnesium
   4. The mechanism of thrombocytopenia due to quinidine is nonspecific bone marrow suppression

180. Clinical features of primary pulmonary hypertension include:

   1. a female predominance
   2. the occurrence of death an average of approximately 3 years after the onset of symptoms
   3. normal pulmonary function tests
   4. precordial chest pain

181. Which of the following physiological changes will exacerbate pulmonary edema?

   1. Increased pulmonary venous pressure
   2. Increased pulmonary capillary pressure secondary to increased pulmonary arterial pressure
   3. Rapid removal of unilateral pneumothorax
   4. Increased plasma oncotic pressure

182. Thiazide diuretics may cause many side effects, including which of the following?

   1. Hypomagnesemia
   2. Hyperuricemia
   3. Hyperlipidemia
   4. Hypercalcemia

DIRECTIONS: The group of questions below consists of lettered headings followed by a set of numbered items. For each numbered item select the ONE lettered heading with which it is MOST closely associated. Each lettered heading may be used ONCE, MORE THAN ONCE, OR NOT AT ALL.

For each rhythm disturbance, match the appropriate description.

   A. Sinus arrest
   B. Sinoatrial exit block
   C. Ventriculophasic sinus arrhythmia
   D. Wandering pacemaker
   E. Sinus arrhythmia

183. During complete AV block, P-P cycles that contain a QRS complex are shorter than P-P cycles without an intervening QRS complex

184. A pause in sinus rhythm for which the P-P interval does not equal a multiple of the sinus P-P interval

185. Both Wenckebach type I and type II forms of this arrhythmia are noted

186. Presumed to be secondary to augmented vagal tone, this arrhythmia is considered a normal phenomenon, particularly in the very young and the athlete

For each substance, match the appropriate description.

   A. Hydralazine
   B. Methyldopa
   C. Saralasin
   D. Ketanserin
   E. Enalapril

187. Inhibits juxtaglomerular apparatus secretion of renin

188. Requires metabolism to an active form

189. Competitively blocks angiotensin II action

190. Most likely to worsen renal function in renovascular hypertension

For each, match the appropriate description.

   A. Torsades de pointes
   B. Long QT syndrome
   C. Both
   D. Neither

191. In the appropriate clinical circumstance, no therapy is recommended

192. Provocative Valsalva maneuver may be useful

193. May be a congenital disorder

194. Cessation of phenothiazines may be part of appropriate therapy

---

For each statement or definition, match the appropriate physiological principle or reflex.

A. Bainbridge reflex
B. Force-frequency relation
C. Laplace's law
D. Anrep effect
E. Cushing reflex

195. Increased heart rate causes increased rate of force development and developed force

196. Ventricular wall stress is inversely related to wall thickness and directly related to the cross-sectional ventricular diameter

197. Abrupt increase in systolic BP causes increased cardiac contractility

198. Decreased cerebral blood flow causes bradycardia and an increase in peripheral vascular resistance

---

For each condition capable of precipitating high-output cardiac failure, match the appropriate phrase.

A. Hyperthyroidism
B. Beri-beri
C. Arteriovenous fistula
D. Carcinoid syndrome
E. Osler-Weber-Rendu syndrome

199. Branham's sign

200. Hepatomegaly and abdominal bruits

201. Means-Lerman scratch

202. Parasthesias and painful glossitis

For each disease state match the appropriate left ventricular volume data.

	END-DIASTOLIC VOLUME (ml/m²)	STROKE VOLUME (ml/m²)	MASS (gm/m²)
A.	70	45	92
B.	84	44	172
C.	193	92	200
D.	199	37	145
E.	70	40	80

203. Aortic valve stenosis with peak systolic gradient >30 mm Hg

204. Myocardial disease (primary dilated cardiomyopathy)

205. Aortic regurgitation with regurgitant flow >30 ml per beat

206. Mitral valve regurgitation with regurgitant flow >20 ml per beat

---

For each hormone, match the appropriate physiological response, especially as it pertains to the hypertensive state.

A. Ouabain-like natriuretic factor
B. Angiotensin II
C. Renin
D. Atrial natriuretic peptide (Atriopeptin)
E. Oxytocin

207. Increased adrenal glomerulosa cell synthesis of aldosterone

208. Inhibition of renal tubular cell Na^+, K^+-ATPase

209. Increased vascular smooth muscle cell cyclic GMP and vasorelaxation

210. Increased vascular smooth muscle cell Ca^{++} and vasoconstriction

---

For each pacemaker modality, match the appropriate function.

A. VAT
B. VDI
C. VVI
D. DVI
E. VDD

211. Senses ventricle, paces ventricle, inhibited by ventricular depolarization

212. Senses atrium, paces ventricle, triggered by atrial depolarization

213. Senses ventricle, paces atrium and ventricle, inhibited by ventricular depolarization

214. Senses ventricle and atrium, paces ventricle, inhibited by conducted atrial depolarization

---

For each definition regarding the cardiac action potential, match the appropriate physiologic description.

A. Phase 0, rapid depolarization
B. Phase 1, early rapid repolarization
C. Phase 2, plateau
D. Phase 3, final rapid repolarization
E. Phase 4, resting membrane potential; in diastolic repolarization

215. The phase determined primarily by intracellular potassium concentration.

216. The phase initiated by reduction of the membrane potential to threshold value.

217. The phase during which membrane conductance to all ions decreases to relatively low values.

218. The phase which is particularly well-defined in Purkinje fibers.

For each, match the appropriate substance.

    A. Leg cramps
    B. Hyperkalemia

    C. Rebound hypertension on discontinuation of therapy
    D. Positive antinuclear antibody test
    E. Hypermagnesemia

219. Amiloride

220. Methyldopa

221. Hydrochlorothiazide

222. Clonidine

DIRECTIONS: The group of questions below consists of four lettered headings followed by a set of numbered items. For each numbered item select

    A   if the item is associated with (A) *only*
    B   if the item is associated with (B) *only*
    C   if the item is associated with *both* (A) and (B)
    D   if the item is associated with *neither* (A) nor (B)

Each lettered heading may be used ONCE, MORE THAN ONCE, or NOT AT ALL.

For each drug, match the appropriate description.

    A. Alpha-receptor blocker
    B. Beta-receptor blocker
    C. Both
    D. Neither

223. Guanethidine

224. Prazosin

225. Labetalol

226. Clonidine

    A. Primary pulmonary hypertension
    B. Eisenmenger syndrome
    C. Both
    D. Neither

227. An occult ventricular septal defect may be present

228. An operative procedure may relieve the pulmonary hypertension

229. "Onion skinning" or intimal thickening of the smaller pulmonary arteries with fibrosis is frequently seen

230. "Plexiform lesions" of the muscular pulmonary arteries and arterioles are frequently seen

231. "Silent" mitral stenosis is part of the initial differential diagnosis

---

    A. Propranolol
    B. Bretylium tosylate
    C. Both
    D. Neither

232. May be useful in the treatment of ventricular arrhythmias associated with the prolonged Q-T syndrome

233. Elimination is primarily via a renal mechanism

234. Has proven useful in the treatment of victims of out-of-hospital ventricular fibrillation

235. May be useful in the therapy of digitalis-induced arrhythmias

---

    A. Relatively cardioselective
    B. Intrinsic sympathomimetic activity (ISA)
    C. Both
    D. Neither

236. Nadolol

237. Propranolol

238. Acebutolol

239. Pindolol

PART II: NORMAL AND ABNORMAL CIRCULATORY FUNCTION

CHAPTERS 13 THROUGH 29

ANSWERS

85-B *(Braunwald, pp. 683–685)*

The surface ECG is uninformative in patients with an accessory pathway that conducts unidirectionally from the ventricle to the atrium while sinus rhythm is present. However, when a PSVT occurs due to this mechanism, one clue to the possibility of concealed retrograde conduction over an accessory pathway may be the occurrence of a normal QRS complex and retrograde P waves that occur after completion of the QRS complex (either in the ST segment or early in the T wave).[1] In patients with apparent PSVT referred for electrophysiological study, the incidence of concealed accessory pathway participation in a reentry mechanism is estimated to be approximately 30 per cent. Most such accessory pathways are located between the LV and LA and participate in the tachycardia by retrograde conduction of an impulse conducted in an anterograde manner over the AV node–His bundle pathway, resulting in an AV-reciprocating tachycardia.

Treatment usually involves the use of agents that produce transient degrees of AV nodal block, such as verapamil, digitalis, and propranolol. Antiarrhythmic agents capable of prolonging activation time or refractory period in the accessory pathway may be useful in the prevention of such reciprocating tachycardias. The presence of AF in patients with a concealed accessory pathway may be approached in a manner identical to that of AF in patients without such a pathway because anterograde AV conduction in both instances occurs in an orthodromic manner (over the AV node). Under some circumstances, such as vagal or catecholamine stimulation, anterograde conduction down the accessory pathway may be provoked.[2]

REFERENCES

1. Ross, D.L., and Uther, J.B.: Diagnosis of concealed accessory pathways in supraventricular tachycardia. PACE 7:1069, 1984.
2. Przybylski, J., Chiale, P.A., Halpern, M.S., Nau, G.J., Elizari, M.V., and Rosenbaum, M.B.: Unmasking of ventricular pre-excitation by vagal stimulation or isoproterenol administration. Circulation 61:1030, 1980.

86-E *(Braunwald, pp. 434–436)*

Although impairment of ventricular emptying (systolic function) is the most common form of heart failure in hypertrophic cardiomyopathy, a defect in ventricular filling (diastolic function) may play a significant role in a variety of hypertrophic states. Diastolic function is worsened by increases in myocardial O_2 consumption, decreased O_2 delivery, increased heart rate or inotropic state, and loss of the atrial contribution to ventricular filling, the so-called atrial kick. Acute volume loads are handled poorly by "stiff" left ventricles, causing marked and rapid increases in diastolic pressure.[1]

REFERENCE

1. Lewis, B.S., and Gotsman, M.S.: Current concepts of left ventricular relaxation and compliance. Am. Heart J. 99:101, 1980.

87-B *(Braunwald, pp. 796–798)*

Pulmonary arterial hypertension due to increased resistance to pulmonary venous drainage may result from diseases affecting the LV or pericardium, left-sided valvular disease, and a variety of rare entities. The severity of pulmonary hypertension that develops depends in part on the performance capabilities of the RV. Systolic pressures of 80 to 100 mm Hg can be generated only by a hypertrophied RV that is normally perfused. If RV failure occurs with relatively low pulmonary vascular pressures, marked pulmonary hypertension cannot develop despite an increase in pulmonary vascular resistance.

In the human there is marked variability in pulmonary arterial vasoconstriction in response to pulmonary venous hypertension. While the precise mechanisms involved in elevating pulmonary vascular resistance are not well-defined, pulmonary blood volume is an identified determinant of pulmonary artery pressure in patients with increased resistance to pulmonary venous drainage. Pulmonary blood volume in turn is determined by the balance between flow into and out of the pulmonary vascular bed and is therefore influenced by both right and left ventricular output as well as by the relative distensibility of the pulmonary vasculture and the left side of the heart.

Regardless of the etiology, structural changes occur in the pulmonary vascular bed in response to chronic pulmonary venous hypertension. The anatomical changes that occur in the pulmonary arteries in pulmonary hypertension secondary to increased resistance to pulmonary venous drainage depend on whether the pulmonary venous hypertension is acquired or congenital. When it is congenital, the elastic tissue in the main pulmonary artery is of the fetal variety (long, uniform, unbranched, and parallel elastic fibers). In contrast, acquired pulmonary hypertension is characterized by elastic tissue in the pulmonary trunk of the adult variety (short, irregular, and branched elastic fibers). Small pulmonary arteries, arterioles, and venules undergo a variety of structural alterations, including medial hypertrophy, intimal fibrosis, and rarely necrotizing arteritis. However, vasodilatation and plexiform lesions are not seen in response to chronic pulmonary venous hypertension. Rather, these lesions characterize the "irreversible" forms of pulmonary arterial hypertension.

88-E (Braunwald, pp. 609–611)

Prolonged Holter monitoring of patients engaged in normal daily activity has proven extremely useful as a noninvasive method to document and quantitate underlying cardiac arrhythmias. While significant rhythm disturbances are relatively uncommon in healthy persons, a variety of arrhythmias including sinus bradycardia (with rates as low as 35 beats/min), sinus arrhythmia, sinoatrial exit block, Wenckebach second-degree AV block (especially during sleep), and junctional escape complexes may be seen in normal persons. In addition, the prevalence of arrhythmias in normal subjects increases with increasing age. Persons with ischemic heart disease, especially those recovering from acute myocardial infarction, exhibit PVCs when long-term recordings of the heart rhythm are obtained. The frequency of PVCs progresses over the first several weeks following infarction and decreases about 6 months after infarction. While controversy still exists regarding the significance of ventricular ectopy in this population, it is generally acknowledged that more complex forms and increased frequency of ventricular ectopy are correlated with an increased risk of sudden cardiac death.

Long-term ECG recordings have been useful for the detection of underlying rhythm disturbances in patients with hypertrophic cardiomyopathy[1] and mitral valve prolapse[2] as well as in patients who have unexplained syncope or transient cerebrovascular symptoms.[3] In both normal subjects and in patients with underlying rhythm disturbances, the cardiac rhythm may vary dramatically from one long-term recording period to the next.[4] Therefore, in order to help establish efficacy, it is important to show that an antiarrhythmic agent effects a large reduction in the frequency of ventricular ectopy.

REFERENCES

1. Maron, B.J., Savage, D.D., Wolfson, J.K., and Epstein, S.E.: Prognostic significance of 24-hour ambulatory electrocardiographic monitoring in patients with hypertrophic cardiomyopathy: A prospective study. Am. J. Cardiol. 48:252, 1981.
2. Mason, D.T., Lee, G., Chan, M.C., and DeMaria, A.N.: Arrhythmias in patients with mitral valve prolapse: Types, evaluation and therapy. Med. Clin. North Am. 68:1039, 1984.
3. Mikolich, J.R., Jacobs, W.C., and Fletcher, G.F.: Cardiac arrhythmias in patients with acute cerebrovascular accidents. JAMA 246:1314, 1981.
4. Pratt, C.M., Slymen, D.J., Wierman, A.M., Young, J.B., Francis, M.J., Seals, A.A., Quinones, M.A., and Roberts, R.: Analysis of the spontaneous variability of ventricular arrhythmias: Consecutive ambulatory electrocardiographic recordings of ventricular tachycardia. Am. J. Cardiol. 56:67, 1985.

89-C (Braunwald, p. 488)

A reduction in the physical activity of the patient with heart failure is one of the cornerstones of management of this syndrome. In patients with impaired cardiac reserve the usual recommendation is to tailor or adjust the degree of physical activity to the symptoms of the patient so as to allow activity up to the point at which the patient begins to become symptomatic. Such a practice may allow the continuation of employment for patients in functional class I or II. Even for patients with more severely symptomatic heart failure, part-time employment may still be feasible. Patients with acute heart failure, by contrast, should be rigidly restricted in their physical activities. In most instances, hospitalization of such patients to institute strict rest and other therapeutic measures as well as to facilitate the diagnostic search for a precipitant is desirable.

It should be emphasized that complete physical rest is *not* synonymous with complete *bed* rest. Patients are often more comfortable sitting in a chair, and this position may facilitate a reduction in venous return and cardiac preload due to venous pooling in the lower extremities. The risks of the immobilization that come with stricter rest include deep venous thrombosis and pulmonary embolism. Physician awareness of such problems is critical, and specific therapeutic interventions such as elastic stockings, leg exercises, and the use of anticoagulants should be considered in appropriate patients. Because patients with ejection fractions less than 20 per cent are at particularly high risk for both systemic and pulmonary embolization, long-term anticoagulation should be considered in such settings. As the patient improves, the restriction of physical activity may be relaxed in a gradual manner. It is advisable, however, to refrain from such liberalization of activity until frank clinical signs of heart failure, such as edema and pulmonary rales, have resolved.

90-B (Braunwald, pp. 746–750, 1635)

This child appears to have a disease that is familial and associated with sudden death. The prolonged Q-T interval syndrome is a functional abnormality that is associated with lethal arrhythmias. Two hereditary varieties have been reported: those with autosomal recessive inheritance and associated deafness (the Jervell and Lange-Nielsen syndrome) and those with autosomal dominant inheritance *without* deafness (the Romano-Ward syndrome). Since this patient was born with deafness it is likely that she has the Jervell and Lange-Nielsen syndrome. Although it is unclear which patients with prolonged Q-T intervals are most likely to develop ventricular arrhythmias, particularly torsades de pointes, patients at higher risk appear to be those characterized by deafness, female gender, and a history of syncope.[1]

A variety of other acquired causes of prolonged Q-T syndrome exist, including reactions to antiarrhythmic and psychotropic drugs, electrolyte abnormalities, hypothermia, central nervous system injury, and excessive weight loss associated with use of liquid protein diets.

The sudden infant death syndrome, by definition, occurs between birth and 6 months of age, more commonly in males. Although it is unclear whether or not the primary abnormality is neurological, cardiac, or pulmonary (sleep apnea), this syndrome has an incidence of close to 2 per 1000 live births.[2] The Lown-Ganong-Levine syndrome is a syndrome associated with a short P-R interval that appears to be caused by the presence of an anomalous pathway for conduction from the atria to the ventricle but is not associated with an increased incidence of sudden death. Barlow's syndrome, one of the eponyms for mitral valve prolapse, is associated with cardiac arrhythmias, but the incidence of sudden cardiac death is low.[3]

REFERENCES

1. Moss, A.J., Schwartz, P.J., Crampton, R.S., Locati, E., and Carleen, E.: The long Q-T syndrome: A prospective international study. Circulation 71:17, 1985.
2. Schwartz, P.J.: The quest for the mechanisms of the sudden infant death syndrome: Doubts and progress. Circulation 75:677, 1987.
3. Chesler, E., King, R.A., and Edwards, J.E.: The myxomatous mitral valve and sudden death. Circulation 67:632, 1983.

91-D   (Braunwald, pp. 802–804)

The term Eisenmenger *syndrome* was first used by Wood to describe patients with congenital cardiac lesions with severe pulmonary hypertension in whom a reversal of a left-to-right shunt had occurred. Patients described originally by Eisenmenger himself had ventricular septal defect as the specific cause of the shunt; therefore, such patients are diagnosed as having Eisenmenger *complex.*

The degree of reversibility of pulmonary vascular obstructive disease that exists in a given patient is determined primarily by the underlying pathology in the pulmonary vasculature. Heath and Edwards constructed a classification of structural change composed of six grades[1] that is widely used to describe the underlying pulmonary vascular pathology. Grade 1 is characterized by hypertrophy of the media of small muscular pulmonary arteries and arterioles; grade 2 by intimal cellular proliferation; and grade 3 by advanced medial thickening with hypertrophy and hyperplasia that, together with progressive intimal proliferation in concentric fibrosis, may begin to result in obliteration of arterioles and small arteries. These first three grades of the Heath-Edwards classification appear to represent a chronological progression and may be reversible.

Grade 4 is marked by the development of "plexiform" lesions; grade 5 by complex plexiform, angiomatous, and cavernous lesions as well as hyalinization of the intima; and grade 6 by the presence of necrotizing arteritis. Some evidence exists for the idea that grade 6 may appear before grades 4 and 5, but in any case grades 4 to 6 represent changes that are end-stage and that signify a particularly poor prognosis. The presence of anatomical changes in the pulmonary vasculature of grades 4 to 6 is generally considered to be a *contraindication* to surgical closure of any intracardiac communication because the irreversible nature of the pulmonary lesions merely increases the load on an already overburdened RV once the right-to-left communication is closed.

REFERENCE

1. Heath, D., and Edwards, J.E.: The pathology of hypertensive pulmonary vascular disease. A description of six grades of structural changes in the pulmonary arteries with special reference to congenital cardiac septal defects. Circulation 18:533, 1958.

92-E   (Braunwald, pp. 475–478)

The differentiation of pulmonary and cardiac causes of dyspnea may not always be straightforward. The sensation of dyspnea is a clinical expression of pulmonary venous and capillary congestion. The sudden onset of dyspnea and wheezing at night (PND) occurs as a result of the development of interstitial edema, which precipitates respiratory distress or cardiac asthma. Pulmonary edema, on the other hand, is a manifestation of alveolar edema caused by elevated left-sided cardiac pressures and the resultant transudation of fluid into the alveolar spaces. Since most bronchial capillaries drain via the pulmonary veins (which empty into the left atrium), bronchial and alveolar congestion tends to occur at the same time. When patients having COPD awaken at night with excessive sputum production, the condition may be relieved by coughing. Acute cardiac asthma (PND) usually occurs in patients with clinically *evident* heart disease. The presence of diaphoresis and "bubblier" airway sounds and the *more common* occurrence of cyanosis all help differentiate cardiac asthma from bronchial asthma.

93-C   (Braunwald, pp. 794–796)

A variety of substances are capable of exerting substantial effects upon the tone of the pulmonary vasculature. Acute hypoxia is a well-established cause of pulmonary vasoconstriction, and this mechanism in part allows for self-regulation of the ventilation-perfusion characteristics of the lung. In addition to the effects of alveolar oxygen tension upon pulmonary arteriolar tone, a decrease in oxygen tension in the mixed venous blood that flows through the small pulmonary arteries and arterioles may also lead to pulmonary arterial vasoconstriction.[1] Acidemia appears to lead to vasoconstriction as well; therefore, two of the most potent stimuli for *vasodilatation* in the systemic arteriolar bed lead to *vasoconstriction* of pulmonary arteries and arterioles.

While controversy exists concerning the effects of alpha-adrenoceptor agonists on the pulmonary vascular bed, beta-adrenoceptor stimulation with isoproterenol has been shown consistently to cause pulmonary vasodilatation. Acetylcholine is also a potent relaxant of pulmonary arteries and arterioles. In patients with elevated pulmonary vascular resistance with a major reversible component, this drug is capable of transiently lowering resistance. Histamine is a vasodilator in the systemic circulation but is primarily a vasoconstrictor in the pulmonary vascular bed. While serotonin is a potent pulmonary vasoconstrictor in animals, it has a little or no effect in humans. In patients with malignant carcinoid syndrome of the bowel and hepatic metastases, for example, large quantities of systemic serotonin release may lead to endocardial and valvular changes on the right side of the heart but do not lead to pulmonary hypertension.

REFERENCE

1. Silove, E.D., Inoue, T., and Grover, R.F.: Comparison of hypoxia, pH, and sympathomimetic drugs on bovine pulmonary vasculature. J. Appl. Physiol. 24:355, 1968.

94-C *(Braunwald, pp. 853–855)*

When a sudden rise in BP (typically diastolic BP > 140 mm Hg) causes acute damage to retinal vessels (hemorrhages, exudates, or papilledema), accelerated malignant hypertension is present. Hypertensive encephalopathy is frequently present and is manifested by headache, irritability, confusion, somnolence, stupor, focal neurological deficits, seizures, and eventually coma. Other clinical features include (1) renal insufficiency with proteinuria, hematuria, azotemia, and occasionally oliguric renal failure; (2) microangiopathic hemolytic anemia with red cell fragmentation and intravascular coagulation; (3) congestive heart failure; and (4) nausea and vomiting. The pathogenesis of hypertensive encephalopathy is thought to be failure of cerebral autoregulation with dilatation of cerebral arterioles leading to excessive cerebral blood flow and damage to the arteriolar wall with increased vascular permeability.[1]

REFERENCE

1. Kincaid-Smith, P.: Understanding malignant hypertension. Aust. N.Z. J. Med. *11*:64, 1981.

95-D *(Braunwald, pp. 844–847)*

Diabetics with mild chronic renal disease are particularly prone to develop the syndrome of hyporeninemic hypoaldosteronism because they are affected by a combination of low renin production and impaired insulin secretion, both of which increase the serum potassium concentration. Thus, supplemental potassium and potassium-sparing diuretics must be used with caution in such patients. Calcium channel blockers have also been reported to impair the adrenal secretion of aldosterone. Although tomatoes and bananas are rich sources of potassium, it would be unusual for a normal diet to cause such a marked rise in potassium. Urinary tract infections may increase potassium in the setting of worsened renal function (which was not observed in this patient). It is likely that either primary hypoaldosteronism or adrenal hypoplasia would have been detected by the finding of an elevated potassium concentration during the initial visit.[1]

REFERENCE

1. Gordon, R.D.: Syndrome of hypertension and hyperkalemia with normal glomerular filtration rate. Hypertension 8:93, 1986.

96-D *(Braunwald, pp. 530–531)*

Cardiac transplantation has been performed since 1967; a recent improvement in results is due to the potency and effectiveness of the immunosuppressant cyclosporine.[1] Important positive factors in considering a candidate for heart transplantation include psychological stability, a history of compliance with medical therapy, and younger age. Contraindications to cardiac transplantation include pulmonary hypertension or parenchymal pulmonary disease, insulin-dependent diabetes, coexistent liver or renal disease, psychological instability or substance abuse, active infection or duodenal ulcer, and clinically evident cerebral or vascular disease.

The transplanted heart is denervated but exhibits normal contractility and contractile reserve. It therefore responds to exercise by first increasing stroke volume, after which elevated levels of catecholamines lead to a reflex tachycardia. This mechanism allows near-normal circulatory response, excellent exercise tolerance, and successful rehabilitation in a large majority of long-term survivors. Acute rejection is monitored by right ventricular endomyocardial biopsy, which is carried out routinely at weekly intervals for the first 3 weeks postoperatively. The appearance of myocardial edema may be reflected in a fall in electrocardiographic QRS voltage; atrial arrhythmias and an S_3 gallop are other signs of rejection. Patients who survive for 3 months after transplantation have a greater than 80 per cent 2-year survival rate.

The difficulty in maintaining an adequate supply of donor hearts continues to be the limiting factor in the number of transplants performed. At present, over half the recipients of heart transplants have had coronary artery disease while many of the remainder have had idiopathic, rheumatic, or viral cardiomyopathies.[2]

REFERENCES

1. Uys, C.J., and Rose, A.G.: Pathologic findings in long-term cardiac transplants. Arch. Pathol. Lab. Med. *108*:112, 1984.
2. Lanza, R.P., Cooper, D.K.C., Boyd, S.T., and Barnard, C.N.: Comparison of patients with ischemic, myopathic, and rheumatic heart diseases as cardiac transplant recipients. Am. Heart J. *107*:8, 1984.

97-B *(Braunwald, pp. 642–644)*

Electrical cardioversion has proven to be an excellent method for termination of a variety of tachyarrhythmias, especially those presumed secondary to a reentry mechanism. In non-emergency situations, the procedure is well tolerated and may be performed on patients receiving digitalis therapy without stopping the digitalis prior to elective cardioversion, provided that no clinical evidence of digitalis toxicity exists.[1] Maintenance therapy with quinidine 1 to 2 days before electrical cardioversion in patients with atrial fibrillation produces reversion to sinus rhythm in 10 to 15 per cent and may help prevent recurrence of atrial fibrillation once sinus rhythm is restored in a number of these patients. The use of electrical cardioversion requires a clinical assessment of the likelihood of establishing and maintaining sinus rhythm and the potential risks of other forms of therapy. Emergent use of direct-current cardioversion is warranted for any tachycardia that produces congestive heart failure, angina, or hypotension and does not respond quickly to medical management. Rapid ventricular responses in patients with Wolff-Parkinson-White syndrome and atrial fibrillation may be best approached by using electrical cardioversion. Electrical cardioversion should be avoided, however, in patients with digitalis-induced tachyarrhythmias.

On occasion, the initial attempt at cardioversion will precipitate transient ventricular arrhythmias; these may be suppressed by administration of a bolus of lidocaine before subsequent cardioversion attempts.[2] Cardioversion restores sinus rhythm in over 70 to 95 per cent of patients, depending upon the underlying tachyarrhythmia present initially. In patients with chronic atrial fibrillation, however, the majority revert to atrial fibrillation within the first 12 months after cardioversion, limiting the effectiveness of cardioversion in the therapy of this disorder.

Complications from carefully performed direct-current cardioversion are uncommon, although occasionally even a properly synchronized shock may lead to ventricular fibrillation. Embolic episodes may occur in 1 to 3 per cent of patients converted to sinus rhythm and form the basis for the widespread clinical practice of prior anticoagulation for 1 to 2 weeks in patients at high risk for emboli and with no contraindications to anticoagulant therapy. However, few controlled studies regarding the use of anticoagulants in the prevention of cardioversion-induced embolic events have been published. While cardioversion of ventricular tachycardia may be achieved by a chest "thump," the thump cannot be timed well to the cardiac cycle and may, on rare occasions, precipitate ventricular flutter or fibrillation.[3] This technique must therefore be applied cautiously and only in emergency clinical settings.

REFERENCES

1. Mann, D.L., Maisel, A.S., Atwood, J.E., Engler, R.L., and Le-Winter, M.M.: Absence of cardioversion-induced ventricular arrhythmias in patients with therapeutic digoxin levels. J. Am. Coll. Cardiol. 5:882, 1985.
2. Waldecker, B., Brugada, P., Zehender, M., Stevenson, W., and Wellens, H.J.J.: Dysrhythmias after direct-current cardioversion. Am. J. Cardiol. 57:120, 1986.
3. Cotoi, S.: Precordial thump and termination of cardiac reentrant tachyarrhythmias. Am. Heart J. 101:675, 1981.

98-D   (*Braunwald, p. 431*)

Isotonic exercise resembles volume overload and causes a predominant increase in left ventricular (LV) end-diastolic volume, while isometric exercise resembles pressure overload and causes a predominant increase in wall thickness. However, both types of exercise increase LV wall thickness, mass, and stroke volume with little change in ejection fraction or resting cardiac output.[1] Furthermore, these changes are physiological adaptations that disappear when the increased exercise demands are reduced.

REFERENCE

1. Huston, T.P., Puffer, J.C., and Rodney, W.M.: The athletic heart syndrome. N. Engl. J. Med. 313:24, 1985.

99-C   (*Braunwald, pp. 549–553*)

Many medical and surgical conditions are associated with a chest x-ray pattern consistent with pulmonary edema as shown in the accompanying x-ray. The physical examination of this hypothetical patient was essentially normal, without dramatic chest examination findings, jugular venous distention, or a third heart sound. This suggests that in this patient the edema was primarily caused not by an alteration in the Starling forces across pulmonary capillaries but rather by abnormal permeability of the alveolar capillary membrane. These conditions are lumped under the term adult respiratory distress syndrome (ARDS).[1, 2] Among the conditions that have been described in association with ARDS are infectious pneumonia, inhaled toxins, circulating foreign substances including bacterial endotoxins, aspiration of gastric contents, acute radiation pneumonitis, release of endogenous vasoactive substances such as histamine, disseminated intravascular coagulation, immunological events including hypersensitivity pneumonitis and leukoagglutinins, shock lung in association with nonthoracic trauma, and acute hemorrhage pancreatitis.

In the patient described there appear to be at least two pathological processes predisposing to ARDS—possible gram-negative septicemia due to a urinary tract infection, which would be common in a nursing home patient, as well as incipient disseminated intravascular coagulation manifested by the low platelet count and prolonged prothrombin time.

Although there are many theories proposed for the development of ARDS, a current model[3] is that chemotactic factors, either circulating or in the tissues, cause movement of polymorphonuclear leukocytes to the lung where the endothelium has been damaged and there is adherence of the polymorphonuclear leukocytes to the endothelium. This interaction results in the release of many vasoactive substances, including arachidonic acid metabolites, oxygen radicals, proteases, kinins, and histamines. These factors combine to cause an increase in alveolar capillary permeability as well as augmenting blood flow to the lung, the combination of which results in transudation of fluid and pulmonary edema. This theory is particularly attractive since chemotoxins can arrive from distal sources and inflict injury or can be derived from alveolar macrophages of the alveolar wall. This may explain the presence of ARDS in systemic illnesses such as gram-negative septicemia, hemorrhagic pancreatitis, and disseminated intravascular coagulation.

Furthermore, bronchoalveolar lavage fluid from patients with ARDS has shown a predominance of neutrophils, leukocyte elastase, and partially inactivated alpha-1 antitrypsin (an antiprotease normally present in the lung). However, at this time, clinical therapeutic modalities specifically targeted at the neutrophil interactions in the lung are not available.

REFERENCES

1. Jardin, F., Eveleight, M.C., Gurdjian, F., Delille, F., and Margairaz, A.: Venous admixture in human septic shock. Comparative effects of blood volume expansion, dopamine infusion and isoproterenol infusion on mismatching of ventilation and pulmonary blood flow in peritonitis. Circulation 60:155, 1979.
2. Vincent, J.L., Weil, M.H., Puri, V., and Carlson, R.W.: Circulatory

shock associated with purulent peritonitis. Am. J. Surg. *142*:262, 1981.
3. Repine, J.E., Bowman, C.M., and Tate, C.M.: Neutrophils and lung edema. Chest *81*(Suppl):5, 1982.

100-E   *(Braunwald, p. 732)*

In bipolar lead systems the positive and negative electrodes are in an intracardiac position about 2.5 cm apart while in unipolar systems only the cathode (negative) electrode is in the heart and a large area anode (positive) electrode, usually the metal housing of the pulse generator, is at a remote location. Since the tips of both types of electrodes are placed in intimate contact with the endocardium (or epicardium/myocardium), the thresholds for depolarization are similar. Although many 12-lead ECGS show larger depolarization spikes with unipolar electrodes, there is no statistical difference in signal amplitude generated by unipolar and bipolar electrodes. The amplitude of the pacemaker spike depends on the quality and settings of the ECG recorder and the pulse energy; the latter is the product of voltage and pulse duration.

However, there is a significant difference between unipolar and bipolar electrodes in terms of their susceptibility to electromagnetic interference (EMI) from power lines, radio and television transmitters, and skeletal muscle potentials. Because of the large separation between electrodes in the unipolar configuration, there is enhanced EMI detection. Thus, when myopotentials cause inappropriate triggering or inhibition of a pacemaker employing a unipolar electrode, switching to a bipolar lead system may solve the problem.

101-E   *(Braunwald, pp. 482–483)*

A variety of laboratory abnormalities may be noted in patients with congestive heart failure. Alterations in serum electrolyte values usually occur after patients have begun treatment or in more longstanding, severe cases of heart failure. Hyponatremia may be seen for a variety of reasons. Included among these are prolonged or rigid sodium restriction, intensive diuretic therapy, a decrease in the ability to excrete water from reductions in renal blood flow and glomerular filtration rate,[1] and elevations in the concentration of circulating vasopressin.[2] Hypokalemia may result from aggressive diuretic therapy. Conversely, hyperkalemia may occasionally occur in patients with severe heart failure who have marked reductions in glomerular filtration rate. Such patients may be particularly prone to hyperkalemia if they are also receiving potassium-sparing diuretics.

Congestive hepatomegaly due to backward failure and cardiac cirrhosis from longstanding heart failure is often accompanied by impaired hepatic function, which may be reflected in abnormal values of the liver enzymes.[3] In acute hepatic venous congestion, severe jaundice may result, with bilirubin levels as high as 15 to 20 mg/dl, dramatic elevations of serum SGOT levels, and prolongation of the prothrombin time. While the clinical and laboratory profile of such an event may resemble viral hepatitis, the diagnosis of hepatic congestion due to heart failure is confirmed by the rapid normalization of these hepatic laboratory values with successful treatment of heart failure. It should be noted that in patients with longstanding heart failure and secondary severe hepatic damage, albumin synthesis may be impaired. Rarely, more severe sequelae may occur including hepatic hypoglycemia, fulminant hepatic failure, and even hepatic coma.

The size and shape of the cardiac silhouette on the chest roentgenogram are two features of particular clinical relevance in the patient with congestive heart failure. Increases in cardiothoracic ratio and heart volume on the plain chest x-ray film are specific but not sensitive indicators of elevated left ventricular end-diastolic volume. Elevations in pulmonary capillary pressure are reflected in the appearance of the vasculature on the plain chest film. With minimal elevations (i.e., approximately 13 to 17 mm Hg), early equalization in the size of the vessels in the apices and bases is first discernible. It is not until greater pressure elevations occur (approximately 18 to 20 mm Hg) that actual pulmonary vascular redistribution occurs. When pressure exceeds 20 to 25 mm Hg, frank interstitial pulmonary edema is usually observed.

REFERENCES

1. Hricik, D.E., and Kassirer, J.P.: How to interpret azotemia in cardiac failure. J. Cardiovasc. Med. 8:397, 1983.
2. Szatalowicz, V.L., Arnold, P.E., Chaimovitz, C., Bichet, D., Beri, T., and Schrier, R.W.: Radioimmunoassay of plasma arginine vasopressin in hyponatremic patients with congestive heart failure. N. Engl. J. Med. 305:263, 1981.
3. Kaplan, M.M.: Liver dysfunction secondary to congestive heart failure. Prac. Cardiol. 6:39, 1980.

102-C   *(Braunwald, pp. 865–868)*

Many patients with mild hypertension (diastolic BP < 95 mm Hg) may benefit significantly from nondrug therapy. In several studies weight loss has resulted in significant decreases in BP; in one study an average of 8 kg weight reduction was associated with a 13 mm Hg decrease in diastolic BP.[1] The effectiveness of decreasing sodium intake depends on the severity of pretreatment hypertension, with patients who have systolic BP > 190 registering 20 mm Hg decreases and those with systolic BP of 160 mm Hg averaging 10 mm Hg decreases.[2] Furthermore, activation of counterregulatory mechanisms such as the renin-angiotensin system limits the overall effect of lowering sodium intake. Daily *isotonic* (but not isometric) exercise is associated with a 5 to 10 mm Hg reduction in BP, as well as decreased cardiovascular mortality.[3] Although increased vascular smooth muscle calcium may represent a common pathway for hypertension, paradoxically, hypertensive patients have a lower calcium intake and higher urinary calcium excretion than normotensive individuals.[4] Furthermore, about half of hypertensives have lowering of their BP acutely in response to supplemental calcium.[5] Thus, reduction of dietary calcium is unlikely to be beneficial. Alcohol consumption of about 1 oz per day is associated with decreased cardiac mortality, but excessive alcohol intake exerts a pressor effect, so that alcohol abuse is a common cause of reversible hypertension.[6]

REFERENCES

1. MacMahon, S.W., MacDonald, G.J., Bernstein, L., Andrews, G., and Blacket, R.B.: Comparison of weight reduction with metoprolol in treatment of hypertension in young overweight patients. Lancet 1:1233, 1985.
2. MacGregor, G.A.: Sodium is more important than calcium in essential hypertension. Hypertension 7:628, 1985.
3. Jennings, G., Nelson, L., Nestel, P., Esler, M., Korner, P., Burton, D., and Bazelmans, J.: The effects of changes in physical activity on major cardiovascular risk factors, hemodynamics, sympathetic function and glucose utilization in man: A controlled study of four levels of activity. Circulation 73:30, 1986.
4. McCarron, D.A.: Is calcium more important than sodium in the pathogenesis of essential hypertension? Hypertension 7:607, 1985.
5. McCarron, D.A., and Morris, C.D.: Blood pressure response to oral calcium in persons with mild to moderate hypertension. Ann. Intern. Med. 103:825, 1985.
6. Jackson, R., Stewart, A., Beaglehole, R., and Scragg, R.: Alcohol consumption and blood pressure. Am. J. Epidemiol. 122:1037, 1985.

103-E   (Braunwald, pp. 630–631)

Procainamide is widely used to treat both supraventricular and ventricular arrhythmias. In electrophysiological studies, the intravenous response to procainamide predicts the response to the drug when given orally.[1] These studies have proven to be useful for evaluating the efficacy of this agent in appropriate patients. In patients with acute myocardial infarction, plasma concentrations of procainamide required to suppress PVCs may be less than the concentrations required to prevent spontaneous episodes of sustained ventricular tachycardia.[2] Procainamide may be used in the conversion of atrial fibrillation to sinus rhythm; however, as with quinidine, the prior use of digitalis, propranolol, or verapamil to slow atrial rate is recommended. This is because accelerated conduction through the AV node due to procainamide use, without prior slowing of the atrial rate, may lead to 1:1 conduction and an increase in the ventricular rate. Procainamide may block conduction in the accessory pathway of patients with WPW syndrome and thus may be useful in the treatment of tachyarrhythmias in these patients.

Multiple noncardiac side effects of procainamide have been reported, including skin rashes, myalgias, digital vasculitis, Raynaud's phenomenon, gastrointestinal side effects, and central nervous system toxicity. Higher doses of the drug may depress myocardial contractility and diminish myocardial performance, with resultant hypotension. In the presence of sinus node disease, procainamide tends to prolong the corrected sinus node recovery time and may therefore worsen symptoms in patients with the bradycardia-tachycardia syndrome.[3]

REFERENCES

1. Marchlinski, F.E., Buxton, A.E., Vassallo, J.A., Waxman, H.L., Cassidy, D.M., Doherty, J.U., and Josephson, M.E.: Comparative electrophysiologic effects of intravenous and oral procainamide in patients with sustained ventricular arrhythmias. J. Am. Coll. Cardiol. 4:1247, 1984.
2. Myerburg, R.J., Kessler, K.M., Kiem, I., Pefkaros, K.C., Conde, C.A., Cooper, D., and Castellanos, A.: Relationship between plasma levels of procainamide, suppression of premature ventric-

ular complexes and prevention of recurrent ventricular tachycardia. Circulation 64:280, 1981.
3. Goldberg, D., Reiffel, J.A., Davis, J.C., Gang, E., Livelli, F., Bigger, J.T., Jr.: Electrophysiologic effects of procainamide on sinus node function in patients with and without sinus disease. Am. Heart J. 103:75, 1982.

104-E   (Braunwald, p. 449)

The four determinants of ventricular performance or cardiac output are (1) heart rate, which can also affect contractility (see Braunwald, p. 413); (2) preload, which is closely related to left ventricular end-diastolic volume; (3) afterload, which is closely related to aortic impedance, i.e., the sum of the external factors that oppose ventricular ejection; and (4) contractility, which is a fundamental property of cardiac muscle and reflects the level of activation of cross-bridge formation. The oxygen-carrying capacity of blood, under normal conditions, is not rate-limiting for cardiac performance. Anemia raises cardiac output, presumably by reducing afterload (secondary to vasodilation) and increasing preload.

105-D   (Braunwald, p. 609)

Exercise testing has proven to be a useful diagnostic tool in the evaluation of patients with a history of cardiac arrhythmias. About one-third of normal subjects develop ventricular ectopy in response to exercise testing. A reading of up to six beats of nonsustained ventricular tachycardia, which does not indicate any increased risk of cardiovascular morbidity or mortality, may occur in such subjects.[1] Similarly, supraventricular premature beats are more common during exercise and do not necessarily suggest the presence of underlying heart disease. Patients with coronary artery disease develop PVCs at lower heart rates than do normal subjects, and they may demonstrate such ventricular ectopy more frequently during the early recovery period. Controversy still exists about whether exercise-induced ventricular arrhythmias in patients with coronary artery disease predict a higher cardiovascular risk.

Exercise testing is useful and relatively safe in patients who have had previously identified serious ventricular arrhythmias, with only a small percentage of patients requiring immediate intervention for induced arrhythmias during the exercise testing protocol.[2] While stress testing is more sensitive than the standard 12-lead resting ECG for the detection of ventricular ectopy, it is not as sensitive as prolonged ambulatory monitoring. However, the use of the combination of ambulatory monitoring and stress testing to uncover arrhythmias may be a prudent course in selected patients, because each technique may identify arrhythmias that the other technique fails to uncover.

REFERENCES

1. Fleg, J.L., and Lakatta, E.G.: Prevalence and prognosis of exercise-induced nonsustained ventricular tachycardia in apparently healthy volunteers. Am. J. Cardiol. 54:762, 1984.
2. Young, D.Z., Lampert, S., Graboys, T.B., and Lown, B.: Safety of maximal exercise testing in patients at high risk for ventricular arrhythmias. Circulation 70:184, 1984.

106-D *(Braunwald, pp. 842–843)*

Although renovascular disease is the second most common cause of secondary hypertension (after chronic renal disease), it is still quite rare.[1] The most common cause (60 per cent of cases) of renovascular hypertension is atherosclerosis affecting the proximal 2 centimeters of the renal artery and occurring most commonly in elderly males.[2] Nonatherosclerotic renal artery stenoses involve all layers of the vessel, most frequently the media. In children and young adults intimal and fibromuscular hyperplasia is common. Among blacks renovascular hypertension is less common than in Caucasians, although chronic renal disease is more common.[3] The greatest prevalence of renovascular disease (20 per cent) occurs in patients with severe hypertension.[4]

REFERENCES

1. Rudnick, K.J.: Hypertension in family practice. Can. Med. Assoc. J. 3:492, 1977.
2. Novick, A.C.: The case for surgical therapy. In Narins, R.G. (ed.): Controversies in Nephrology and Hypertension. New York, Churchill Livingstone, 1984, p. 181.
3. Keith, T.A., III: Renovascular hypertension in black patients. Hypertension 4:438, 1982.
4. Davis, B.A., Crook, M.E., Vestal, R.E., and Oates, J.A.: Prevalence of renovascular hypertension in patients with grade III or IV hypertensive retinopathy. N. Engl. J. Med. 301:1273, 1979.

107-B *(Braunwald, pp. 611–614)*

Invasive electrophysiological (EP) studies have proven to be safe and useful in the diagnostic evaluation of patients with underlying disturbances of cardiac rhythm and conduction. In patients with an intraventricular conduction disturbance, EP study may be used to evaluate the length of the H-V interval. H-V intervals greater than 55 msec are associated with organic heart disease, a greater likelihood of developing trifascicular block, and higher mortality. In patients with intraventricular conduction defects and syncope or presyncope, ventricular tachyarrhythmias are often found to be responsible.[1]

The technique of overdrive suppression may be used to evaluate sinus node function. The SNRT is measured by subtracting the spontaneous sinus node cycle length before pacing from the length of the first spontaneous sinus response after termination of pacing. Normal values are generally less than 525 msec, and prolongation of SNRTs has been found in patients suspected of having sinus node dysfunction. Since many patients with impaired sinus node function also exhibit abnormal AV conduction, it is important also to evaluate AV nodal and His-Purkinje function in this population.[2]

In patients with tachycardias, EP studies may be used to differentiate between supraventricular tachycardia with aberrant intraventricular conduction and a ventricular origin of the tachycardia. Supraventricular tachycardia is recognized electrophysiologically by the presence of an H-V interval equal to or greater than that recorded during normal sinus rhythm (see Braunwald, Fig. 20–35, p. 613). In contrast, only two situations result in an H-V interval that is measured as consistently shorter than normal: ventricular tachycardia when retrograde activation of the His bundle from a complex originating in the ventricle leads to a short H-V interval, and atrioventricular conduction that occurs over an accessory pathway.[3] Localizing the site of origin and the pathway involved in the maintenance of tachycardia due to Wolff-Parkinson-White syndrome or its variants by endocardial mapping has proven to be an important part of the preoperative evaluation of patients considered for ablative surgery. Patients with this syndrome who are at risk for the development of serious supraventricular or ventricular tachycardias or sudden cardiac death may be first identified by EP testing.[4]

REFERENCES

1. Dhingra, R.C., Palileo, E., Strasberg, B., Swiryn, S., Bauernfeind, R.A., Wyndham, C.R., and Rosen, K.M.: Significance of the HV interval in 517 patients with chronic bifascicular block. Circulation 64:1265, 1981.
2. Gomes, J.A., Hariman, R.I., and Chowdry, I.A.: New application of direct sinus node recordings in man: Assessment of sinus node recovery time. Circulation 70:663, 1984.
3. Miles, W.M., Prystowsky, E.N., Heger, J.J., Zipes, D.P.: Evaluation of the patient with a wide QRS tachycardia. Med. Clin. North Am. 68:1015, 1984.
4. Gallagher, J.J.: Accessory pathway tachycardia: Techniques of electrophysiologic study and mechanisms. Circulation 75:III-31, 1987.

108-D *(Braunwald, pp. 845–846)*

Primary aldosteronism is rare in unselected hypertensive patients but should be considered in hypertensive patients with hypokalemia.[1] Although solitary benign tumors are the most common etiology, up to 25 per cent of patients may have bilateral adrenal hyperplasia.[2] Typically, patients with excessive aldosterone have urinary potassium excretion > 30 mEq/day. Hypertensive patients with hypokalemia and low urine potassium may have gastrointestinal losses or may have had prior diuretic therapy. In primary aldosteronism plasma renin activity is low owing to feedback inhibition by high levels of circulating aldosterone. A high renin state with urinary potassium > 30 mEq/day suggests renovascular hypertension, or a salt-wasting renal disease. If renin and aldosterone are both low, and elevated urinary potassium coexists with hypokalemia, ingestion of exogenous mineralocorticoids such as licorice (glycyrrhizinic acid) should be considered.[3]

REFERENCES

1. Bravo, E.L., Tarazi, R.C., Dustan, H.P., Fouad, F.M., Textor, S.C., Gifford, R.W., and Vidt, D.G.: The changing clinical spectrum of primary aldosteronism. Am. J. Med. 74:641, 1983.
2. Banks, W.B., Kastin, A.J., Biglieri, E.D., and Ruiz, A.E.: Primary adrenal hyperplasia: A new subset of primary hyperaldosteronism. J. Clin. Endocrinol. Metab. 58:783, 1984.
3. Coreda, J.M., Trono, D., and Schifferli, J.: Liquorice intoxication caused by alcohol-free pastis. Lancet 12:1442, 1983.

109-E *(Braunwald, pp. 432–434)*

Myocardial hypertrophy appears to develop in a manner that maintains systolic stress within normal limits.

When the primary stimulus is pressure overload, the increase in systolic wall stress leads to addition of new myofibrils in parallel, wall thickening, and concentric hypertrophy. When the primary stimulus is volume overload, there initially is increased diastolic wall stress with addition of new myofibrils in series and ventricular dilatation, which results in a small increase in systolic stress (by the Laplace relationship) and a small increase in wall thickness. Thus, in states of volume overload, chamber enlargement (eccentric hypertrophy) predominates, while in pressure overload, wall thickness (concentric hypertrophy) predominates.

110-C (Braunwald, pp. 500–501; Marcus, F.I.: Pharmacokinetic interactions between digoxin and other drugs. J. Am. Coll. Cardiol. 5:82A, 1985.)

A variety of clinically important interactions occur between digoxin and other pharmacological agents. For instance, a number of drugs may enhance or inhibit the absorption of digoxin from the gut lumen. Cholestyramine, neomycin, and occasionally nonabsorbable antacids and kaopectate may interfere with the gastrointestinal absorption of digoxin. In contrast, certain antibiotics—notably erythromycin—may lead to an increased bioavailability of digoxin. This increase in bioavailability results from the increased intestinal metabolism of digoxin by specific intestinal flora that have emerged because of the presence of the antibiotic. Interventions that may be helpful in patients receiving erythromycin along with digoxin include measuring the serum digoxin concentration, decreasing the digoxin dose upon initiating antibiotic therapy, and using a solution or capsule form of digoxin.

In addition to the well-known interaction between quinidine and digoxin, other cardiovascular agents are capable of reducing digoxin clearance and increasing serum levels of the drug. Verapamil has been demonstrated to increase serum digoxin concentration by decreasing the volume of distribution of digoxin as well as its clearance.[1] Amiodarone leads to a decrease in both renal and nonrenal clearance of digoxin resulting in an increase in digoxin concentrations of 70 to 100 per cent. Therefore, the use of any of these agents concomitantly with digitalis requires monitoring of the serum digoxin concentration and a reduction of the dosage of digitalis by approximately 50 per cent. Nifedipine, procainamide, and disopyramide do not appear to alter serum digoxin levels. Potassium loss by diuretics may enhance the cardiac toxicity of glycosides.

REFERENCE

1. Antman, E.M., and Smith, T.W.: Drug interactions with digitalis glycosides. In Smith, T.W. (ed.): Digitalis Glycosides. Orlando, Grune and Stratton, 1985, pp. 65–81.

111-A (Braunwald, pp. 849–852)

Diagnosis of susceptibility to pregnancy-associated hypertension is performed by the "rollover" test at the 28th week. This test involves measuring BP first in the left lateral recumbent position and then in the supine position. A rise in the diastolic BP of > 20 mm Hg within 2 to 5 minutes is considered positive.[1] Patients with a positive test should be told to restrict their activity. Neither diuretics nor sodium restriction is an effective therapy.[2] Because pregnancy-induced hypertension is usually associated with decreased uteroplacental flow, reduction in intravascular volume is contraindicated. Methyldopa is useful in the chronic management of hypertension, while hydralazine is often chosen for acute parenteral use.[3] Beta blockers, especially metoprolol, have also been shown to be safe and effective antihypertensive therapy.[4]

REFERENCES

1. Oney, T., and Kaulhausen, H.: The value of angiotensin sensitivity test in the early diagnosis of hypertensive disorders in pregnancy. Am. J. Obstet. Gynecol. 142:17, 1982.
2. Collins, R., Yusuf, S., and Peto, R.: Overview of randomized trials of diuretics in pregnancy. Br. Med. J. 290:17, 1985.
3. Cockburn, J., Ounsted, M., Moar, V.A., and Redman, C.W.B.: Final report of study on hypertension during pregnancy. The effects of specific treatment on the growth and development of the children. Lancet 1:647, 1982.
4. Wichman, K., Ryden, G., and Karlberg, B.E.: A placebo controlled trial of metoprolol in the treatment of hypertension in pregnancy. Scand. J. Clin. Lab. Invest. 44 (Suppl 169):90, 1984.

112-D (Braunwald, pp. 721–727; see also Answer to Question 211, p. 87, this book.)

This athletic man would be treated best with a pacemaker that could respond to a variety of physiological demands. Although the universal pacemaker (DDD) in general is best able to meet this demand, in this particular patient the presence of frequent and rapid PSVTs is a relative contraindication since the DDD pacemaker senses the atrial rate and paces the ventricle subject to upper rate limits. By setting the limits low enough to prevent symptomatic tachycardia when the patient suffers PSVT episodes, the ability to increase heart rate appropriately during exercise would be compromised.

The DDD pacemaker actually combines the features of the AAI, VDD, and DVI pacemakers, acting as an atrial demand pacemaker (AAI) during sinus bradycardia with normal AV conduction, as an atrial synchronous pacemaker (VDD) during normal sinus rhythm with AV conduction delay, and as an AV sequential pacemaker (DVI) during sinus bradycardia with prolonged AV conduction. All three of these pacemaker modalities would be less than optimal in this patient; the VDD would be subject to the same rate control problems as those of the DDD during PSVT, and the DVI cannot respond with physiological alterations in heart rate.

Although the VVI pacemaker would not provide AV synchronous contraction, a rate-responsive VVI pacemaker would allow the patient's heart rate to increase with exercise in response to a physiological parameter other than the atrial rate. However, the VVI, unlike the DDD, would not respond to PSVT under nonphysiological conditions.

Among the currently developed rate-responsive pacemakers are designs that vary pacing rate in response to changes in the sensed mechanical activity of the body, changes in respiratory rate, or changes in the Q-T interval.[1] In patients without myocardial disease, rate increase is of greater importance for increasing cardiac output with exercise than is AV synchrony.[2]

REFERENCES

1. Beyersdorf, F., Kreuzer, J., Happ, J., Zegelman, M., and Satter, P.: Increase in cardiac output with rate-responsive pacemaker. Ann. Thorac. Surg. 42:201, 1986.
2. Kristensson, B., Arnman, K., and Ryden, L.: The hemodynamic importance of atrioventricular synchrony and rate increase at rest and during exercise. Eur. Heart J. 6:773, 1985.

113-D (Braunwald, pp. 504–507)

Digitalis toxicity is an extremely common adverse drug reaction encountered in clinical practice and may occur in between 5 and 15 per cent of hospitalized patients receiving these drugs. While a variety of clinical manifestations may occur with digitalis toxicity, gastrointestinal symptoms, neurological symptoms, and cardiac rhythm disturbances are among the most frequent.[1] Early digitalis intoxication may be manifested by anorexia, which then may be followed by nausea and vomiting resulting from central nervous system mechanisms.[2] A variety of neurological symptoms may result from excess digitalis. These include visual symptoms such as scotomas, halos, and changes in color perception, as well as headache, fatigue, malaise, neuralgic pain, disorientation, delirium, and even seizures. With both gastrointestinal and neurological symptoms it may be difficult to determine whether digitalis excess is the causative factor or whether the associated illness leads to these disturbances.

Cardiac toxicity from digitalis may be manifested by essentially any known rhythm disturbance.[3] Among the most common of these are atrioventricular junctional escape rhythms, ventricular bigeminy or trigeminy, nonparoxysmal junctional tachycardia, unifocal or multifocal ectopic ventricular beats, and ventricular tachycardia. Rhythms that combine features of increased automaticity of ectopic pacemakers with impaired conduction, such as PAT with block, strongly suggest digitalis toxicity (see also Question and Answer 165, pp. 47 and 78, this book). However, PAT with block may frequently result from underlying heart disease rather than digitalis excess.[4] A demonstration of a reversion to normal rhythm when the drug is withheld may at times help clarify this dilemma. Other less common manifestations of digitalis toxicity include allergic skin lesions, sexual dysfunction, and occasionally gynecomastia.[5]

REFERENCES

1. Wellens, H.J.J.: The electrocardiogram in digitalis intoxication. In Yu, P.N., and Goodwin, J.F. (eds.): Progress in Cardiology. Vol. 5. Philadelphia, Lea and Febiger, 1976, p. 271.
2. Borison, H.L., and Wang, S.C.: Physiology and pharmacology of vomiting. Pharmacol. Rev. 5:193, 1953.
3. Friedman, P.L., and Antman, E.M.: Electrocardiographic manifestations of digitalis toxicity. In Smith, T.W. (ed.): Digitalis Glycosides. Orlando, Grune and Stratton, 1985, pp. 241–275.
4. Storstein, O., and Rasmussen, K.: Digitalis and atrial tachycardia with block. Br. Heart J. 36:171, 1974.

5. LeWinn, E.B.: Gynecomastia during digitalis therapy: Report of eight additional cases with liver-function studies. N. Engl. J. Med. 248:316, 1953.

114-B (Braunwald, pp. 801–802)

While pulmonary hypertension is a common sequela of chronic bronchitis and emphysema, the extent of destruction of alveoli and the resultant decrease in alveolar surface area is *not* closely correlated with the degree of pulmonary hypertension. Current views suggest that hypoxia-induced vasoconstriction probably plays a major role in producing pulmonary hypertension in patients with these diseases.[1] However, decreased cross-sectional area of the pulmonary vascular bed secondary to parenchymal disease may contribute to secondary pulmonary hypertension in a variety of disorders. Progressive interstitial pulmonary fibrosis due to progressive systemic sclerosis causes large reductions in the cross-sectional area of the pulmonary vascular bed due to obliteration of alveolar capillaries and many small pulmonary arteries and arterioles.[2]

In the CREST syndrome (calcinosis, Raynaud's phenomenon, esophageal dysmotility, sclerodactyly, and telangiectasia), marked pulmonary arterial hypertension and elevations of pulmonary vascular resistance have been reported.[3] Such patients may demonstrate dramatic reductions in RV function due to systolic overload of the RV. Diffuse lymphatic spread of carcinoma may cause pulmonary hypertension and right heart failure; frank obstruction of the major pulmonary arteries may occur secondary to invasion by a tumor, usually a sarcoma. In addition, microemboli from tumor may lead to thrombotic and fibrotic reactions in the pulmonary vasculature. These in turn cause frank vascular obstruction and secondary pulmonary hypertension.

REFERENCES

1. Abraham, A.S., Cole, R.B., Green, I.D., Hedworth-Whitty, R.B., Clarke, S.W., and Bishop, J.M.: Factors contributing to the reversible pulmonary hypertension in patients with acute respiratory failure studied by serial observation during recovery. Circ. Res. 24:51, 1969.
2. Harris, P., and Heath, D.: The Human Pulmonary Circulation. 3rd ed. New York, Churchill Livingstone, 1986, 702 pp.
3. Salerni, R., Rodnan, G.P., Leon, D.F., and Shaver, J.A.: Pulmonary hypertension in the CREST syndrome variant of progressive systemic sclerosis (scleroderma). Ann. Intern. Med. 86:394, 1977.

115-D (Braunwald, pp. 519–523)

A number of vasodilator agents have been used to treat congestive heart failure; among these, intravenous sodium nitroprusside is probably the most widely used for the treatment of acute heart failure. Sodium nitroprusside is a short-acting, balanced dilator with direct relaxing effects on vascular smooth muscle in both arteries and veins. The most important adverse effect of the agent, hypotension, is thus an extension of its therapeutic actions. The drug is particularly useful in patients with severe hypertension and accompanying left ventricular failure or heart failure associated with regurgitant valvular lesions.

A variety of formulations of nitrates have all found applications in the treatment of congestive heart failure. Sublingual nitroglycerin has been shown to initiate a rapid decrease in LV filling pressure. In patients in whom LV filling pressure is elevated to ≥ 20 mm Hg, a decline to approximately 12 mm in 5 to 10 minutes was noted in one study.[1] The effect is maximal in 8 to 10 minutes and persists for up to 30 minutes.

Hydralazine is an orally effective agent that acts directly on arteriolar smooth muscle. Patients with marked cardiomegaly and elevations of systemic vascular resistance appear to respond most favorably to this agent.[2] An important recent multicenter trial, the VHEFT study,[3] demonstrated that 300 mg of hydralazine daily combined with isosorbide dinitrate resulted in improved survival compared with placebo or prazosin in patients with heart failure. This is the first demonstration of a beneficial effect of vasodilator agents on survival.

In many patients with congestive heart failure, the renin-angiotensin-aldosterone system is highly active. Angiotensin-converting enzyme (ACE) inhibitors have found wide application in the management of heart failure in recent years. These agents usually diminish both left and right ventricular filling pressures and lead to a rise in cardiac output. However, they have little or no effect on heart rate or arterial blood pressure.[4] In addition to improving hemodynamics in response to other therapeutic agents, ACE inhibitors often enhance the sense of well-being in patients with congestive heart failure.

REFERENCES

1. Williams, D.O., Amsterdam, E.A., and Mason, D.T.: Hemodynamic effects of nitroglycerin in acute myocardial infarction. Decrease in ventricular preload at the expense of cardiac output. Circulation 51:421, 1975.
2. Packer, M., Meller, J., Medina, N., Gorlin, R., and Herman, M.V.: Importance of left ventricular chamber size in determining the response to hydralazine in severe chronic heart failure. N. Engl. J. Med. 303:250, 1980.
3. Cohn, J.N., Archibald, D.G., Ziesche, S., Franciosa, J.A., Harston, W.E., Tristani, F.E., Dunkman, W.B., Jacobs, W., Francis, G.S., Flohr, K.H., Goldman, S., Cobb, F.R., Shah, P.M., Saunders, R., Fletcher, R.D., Loeb, H.S., Hughes, V.C., and Baker, B.: Effect of vasodilator therapy on mortality in chronic congestive heart failure. Results of a Veterans Administration Cooperative Study. N. Engl. J. Med. 314:1547, 1986.
4. Creager, M.A., Halperin, J.L., Bernard, D.B., Faxon, D.P., Melidossian, C.D., Gavras, H., and Ryan, T.J.: Acute regional circulatory and renal hemodynamic effects of converting enzyme inhibition in patients with congestive heart failure. Circulation 64:483, 1981.

116-A   (Braunwald, pp. 31; 50; 481)

Protodiastolic (S_3) gallop sounds are more commonly heard from the left ventricle but may be heard from the right ventricle as well. These sounds occur between 0.13 and 0.16 second after the second heart sound and may be a normal finding in healthy children and young adults. A protodiastolic gallop sound originating from the left ventricle is best heard at the apex with the patient in the left lateral decubitus position, whereas those originating from the right ventricle are best heard along the left sternal border in the fourth or fifth interspace with the patient supine. Left ventricular gallops are more commonly palpable than right ventricular gallops.

In general, the presence of an S_3 gallop sound is an excellent sign of heart failure provided that certain causes have been excluded. Specifically, an S_3 gallop may be heard in healthy children or young adults and in patients with mitral or tricuspid regurgitation or with left-to-right shunts. In these conditions, the presence of the S_3 gallop does not signify the presence of heart failure. In patients with mitral regurgitation, for example, the protodiastolic sound is generated by the excessive flow of blood into the ventricle in early diastole. In heart failure the etiology of the protodiastolic gallop sound is thought to be the sharp deceleration of ventricular inflow that occurs immediately after the early filling phase of diastole. The simultaneous closure of the mitral valve and a decrease in ventricular compliance may also contribute to the genesis of this protodiastolic sound.

117-C   (Braunwald, pp. 750–755)

Although it is difficult to estimate the percentage of all sudden deaths that are due to cardiac causes, in the Framingham study 13 per cent of all deaths observed during a 26-year period were classified as sudden cardiac death (defined as death within an hour of the onset of symptoms).[1] In contrast, when sudden deaths were defined as deaths occurring within 24 hours of symptoms, the percentage of all natural deaths falling into the sudden death category increased to 32. Recent prospective studies demonstrated that approximately 50 per cent of all coronary heart disease deaths are sudden and unexpected, occurring shortly (within 1 hour) after the onset of symptoms. In the prospective combined Albany-Framingham study, sudden death (defined as death within 1 hour of observed collapse) was analyzed for a population of men between 45 and 74 years of age who died.[2] During a 16-year follow-up there were a total of 234 coronary deaths per 1000 population observed, of which 109 (47 per cent) were sudden and unexpected. It is estimated that in the United States the total number of sudden cardiac deaths ranges from 200,000 to nearly 400,000 yearly. Using a value of approximately 300,000 sudden cardiac deaths annually, this would represent approximately 50 per cent of all cardiovascular deaths in the United States.

REFERENCES

1. Schatzkin, A., Cuppies, L.A., Heeren, T., Morelock, S., Mucatel, M., and Kannel, W.B.: The epidemiology of sudden unexpected death: Risk factors for men and women in the Framingham Heart Study. Am. Heart J. 107:1300, 1984.
2. Kannel, W.B., Doyle, J.T., McNamara, P.M., Quickenton, P., and Gordon, T.: Precursors of sudden coronary death: Factors related to the incidence of sudden death. Circulation 51:606, 1975.

118-C   (Braunwald, pp. 490–491)

The beneficial effects of digitalis in congestive heart failure derive in part from the positive inotropic effect on the myocardium that the drug displays. This inotropic action of digitalis has been demonstrated in both normal and failing heart muscle. Experimental studies of the velocity of contraction of heart muscle at varying loads have demonstrated an augmentation of the velocity of muscle shortening at any given load by digitalis. The absolute increase in tension development induced by digitalis in normal myocardium is at least as great as that induced in failing myocardium. However, because the failing myocardium has a lower peak tension, the *relative* augmentation of tension in failing myocardium may be greater.

It should be noted that administration of cardiac glycosides in normal subjects results in little or no change in cardiac output. It has been demonstrated that digitalis augments the contractile state of the nonfailing myocardial tissue, but compensatory adjustments in preload, afterload, and heart rate prevent any obvious increase in cardiac output in the normal heart.[1]

A number of studies using both noninvasive and invasive techniques have demonstrated sustained improvement in cardiac performance in patients with chronic congestive heart failure. Both patient selection and the degree of ventricular dysfunction help determine whether or not a clinical response will be achieved. In general, studies of patients with depressed left ventricular ejection fractions and an audible S[3] gallop sound have demonstrated a benefit from digoxin therapy.[2] The role of digitalis therapy in minimally symptomatic or treated patients with congestive heart failure is less well defined.[3, 4]

REFERENCES

1. Braunwald, E.: Effects of digitalis on the normal and the failing heart. J. Am. Coll. Cardiol. 5:51A, 1985.
2. Lee, D.C.S., Johnson, R.A., Bigham, J.B., Leahy, M., Dinsmore, R.E., Gorol, A.H., Newell, J.B., Strauss, H.W., and Haber, E.: Heart failure in outpatients. A randomized trial of digoxin versus placebo. N. Engl. J. Med. 306:699, 1982.
3. Fleg, J.L., Gottlieb, S.H., and Lakatta, E.G.: Is digoxin really important in treatment of compensated heart failure? Am. J. Med. 73:244, 1982
4. Gheoreghiade, M., and Beller, G.A.: Effects of discontinuing maintenance digoxin therapy in patients with ischemic heart disease and congestive heart failure in sinus rhythm. Am. J. Cardiol. 51:1243, 1983.

119-C   *(Braunwald, pp. 625–628)*

Lidocaine has found wide clinical application in the treatment of ventricular arrhythmias due to the ease and rapidity of parenteral administration of the drug and a low incidence of complications and side effects. The drug, however, is generally ineffective against arrhythmias of supraventricular origin. In addition, in patients with the Wolff-Parkinson-White syndrome with a short effective refractory period of the accessory pathway, lidocaine has no significant effect and may even accelerate the ventricular response during atrial fibrillation.[1]

Lidocaine has been used clinically primarily in patients with acute myocardial infarction or recurrent ventricular tachyarrhythmias. In one study, patients resuscitated from out-of-hospital ventricular fibrillation and studied in a randomized, blinded fashion were noted to have comparable responses to lidocaine and bretylium for prevention of recurrent episodes of ventricular tachyarrhythmias.[2] The use of lidocaine in a prophylactic manner to prevent ventricular arrhythmias in patients hospitalized with acute myocardial infarction remains a controversial issue.[3] Thus, the choice of patients appropriate for prophylactic lidocaine therapy is primarily a clinical one, with factors such as age, the presence of hepatic dysfunction, and the elapsed time since the onset of chest pain all contributing to the decision to employ this agent.

REFERENCES

1. Akhtar, M., Filbert, C.K., and Shenasa, M.: Effect of lidocaine on atrioventricular response via the accessory pathway in patients with Wolff-Parkinson-White syndrome. Circulation 63:435, 1981.
2. Haynes, R.E., Chinn, T.L., Copass, M.K., and Cobb, L.A.: Comparison of bretylium tosylate and lidocaine in management of out-of-hospital ventricular fibrillation: A randomized clinical trial. Am. J. Cardiol. 48:353, 1981.
3. DeSilva, R.A., Hennekens, C.H., Lown, B., and Casscells, W.: Lignocaine prophylaxis in acute myocardial infarction: An evaluation of randomized trials. Lancet 2:855, 1981.

120-C   *(Braunwald, pp. 672–674)*

Atrial fibrillation (AF) is characterized by total disorganization of atrial depolarizations without effective atrial contractions. This disorganization results in the absence of P waves on the ECG and an irregular ventricular response between 100 and 160 beats/min (in the untreated patient with normal AV conduction). When the ventricular rate is quite rapid or quite slow, an apparent regularization of the ventricular response may occur. Although intermittent AF may occur in patients without cardiac disease, the chronic form of the arrhythmia is usually associated with underlying heart disease. AF is commonly found in populations with hypertensive cardiovascular disease, rheumatic heart disease, and atrial septal defect, as well as with cardiomyopathies and coronary artery disease, and after cardiac surgery.[1] In patients without obvious cardiovascular disease and paroxysms of AF, no increase in mortality rates has been noted. However, the development of chronic AF in patients with known cardiovascular disease results in a doubling of overall mortality.[2]

In individuals with "lone" AF (without obvious heart disease), no increase in the risk of cardiac events is noted, but a significant increase in the frequency of stroke has been documented.[3] AF may develop in the periinfarction setting as well as in the year following MI. Patients developing AF at the time of an acute MI tend to be older and to have a higher pulmonary capillary wedge pressure. Those developing AF in the first year following MI in general have a more severe infarction, a higher total mortality, and a greater frequency of ventricular tachyarrhythmias and right bundle branch block.[4]

Physical findings in patients with AF may include a slight variation in the intensity of S[1], an *absence* of *a* waves in the jugular venous pulse, and an irregularly irregular ventricular rhythm. As the ventricular rate increases, a pulse *deficit* may appear. During this, the apical rate is notably faster than the rate palpated at the wrist because some early ventricular depolarizations are not associated with normal opening of the aortic valve.

REFERENCES

1. Ormerod, O.J., McGregor, C.G., Stone, D.L., Wisbey, C., and Petch, M.D.: Arrhythmias after coronary bypass surgery. Br. Heart J. *51*:618, 1984.
2. Kannel, W.B., Abbott, R.D., Savage, D.D., and McNamara, P.M.: Epidemiologic features of chronic atrial fibrillation. The Framingham study. N. Engl. J. Med. *306*:1018, 1982.
3. Brand, F.N., Abbott, R.D., Kannel, W.B., and Wolf, P.F.: Characteristics and prognosis of lone atrial fibrillation. 30-year follow-up in the Framingham study. JAMA *254*:3449, 1985.
4. Hunt, D., Sloman, G., and Penington, C.: Effects of atrial fibrillation on prognosis of acute myocardial infarction. Br. Heart J. *40*:303, 1978.

121-A   (Braunwald, p. 2242)

In an unselected general practice the overwhelming majority of patients with hypertension have essential hypertension as shown in many studies.[1, 2] This is true even in a series in which patients with pressures above 175/110 mm Hg were studied.[3] Chronic renal disease is the second most common cause of hypertension; the third most common cause, renovascular disease, is rare (≤ 1 per cent). Other forms of secondary hypertension such as coarctation of the aorta, pheochromocytoma, Cushing's disease, and primary aldosteronism have an incidence much less than 1 per cent.

REFERENCES

1. Rudnick, K.V., Sackett, D.L., et al.: Hypertension in family practice. Can. Med. Assoc. J. *3*:492, 1977.
2. Danielson, M., and Dammstrom, B.: The prevalence of secondary and curable hypertension. Acta Med. Scand. *209*:451, 1981.
3. Berglund, G., et al.: Prevalence of primary and secondary hypertension. Studies in a random population sample. Br. Med. J. *2*:554, 1976.

122-E   (Braunwald, pp. 563–566)

Circulatory shock is characterized by a marked reduction in blood flow to vital organs. In general, cerebral and coronary blood flow are protected at the expense of splanchnic and renal perfusion. While coronary and cerebral blood flow are protected, if the process of shock continues, clinical signs of hypoperfusion of these organs will appear. A decrease in mental alertness may then be noted and electrocardiographic abnormalities including ischemic ST and T wave changes may appear, even in patients with clinically normal hearts.[1] Perfusion of the kidneys, the gastrointestinal tract, and the lungs is less well protected than coronary and cerebral blood flows. In patients with septic shock, pulmonary arteriovenous shunts may appear, and further ventilation/perfusion mismatch may develop as therapeutic agents are used in attempts to reverse the condition.[2]

The pathophysiology of circulatory shock may vary on the basis of the underlying etiology. In addition, age and sex differences may contribute to the pathophysiology of the syndrome. Circulatory shock during the first 3 months of life is frequently associated with bacteremia due to gram-negative bacilli. During the syndrome of shock, large increases in sympathetic activity lead to arterial vasoconstriction and to an even larger increase in post-capillary venular constriction. This results in an increase in capillary hydrostatic pressure and a net loss of plasma water, with resultant decreases in intravascular volume and hemoconcentration.

REFERENCES

1. Terradellas, J.B., Bellot, J.F., Saris, A.B., Gil, C.L., Torrallardona, A.T., and Garriga, J.R.: Acute and transient ST-segment elevation during bacterial shock in seven patients without apparent heart disease. Chest *81*:444, 1982.
2. Jardin, F., Eveleigh, M.C., Gurdjian, F., Delille, F., and Margairaz, A.: Venous admixture in human septic shock. Comparative effects of blood volume expansion, dopamine infusion and isoproterenol infusion on mismatching of ventilation and pulmonary blood flow in peritonitis. Circulation *60*:155, 1979.

123-C   (Braunwald, pp. 628–630; see also Answer to Question 179, pp. 81–82, this book.)

Quinidine is an alkaloid that is isolated from the bark of the cinchona tree. The agent suppresses automaticity in normal Purkinje fibers by decreasing the slope of phase IV diastolic depolarization and shifting resting threshold voltage toward zero. Quinidine is capable of exerting a significant anticholinergic effect[1] as well as an alpha-adrenoceptor blocking effect that may lead to reflex sympathetic stimulation. Therefore, quinidine decreases peripheral vascular resistance and may lead to significant hypotension in certain clinical settings. Both the liver and the kidneys clear quinidine, with hepatic metabolism being the more important. The elimination half-life of quinidine is 5 to 8 hours after oral administration, but drugs that induce hepatic enzymes, such as phenobarbital and phenytoin, may shorten this half-life.

Quinidine may be used in the treatment and prevention of a variety of supraventricular and ventricular arrhythmias. AV-nodal reentry tachycardias are inhibited by quinidine, in part by depression of conduction in the retrograde fast pathway.[2] In patients with the Wolff-Parkinson-White syndrome, quinidine may prevent reciprocating tachycardias and slow the ventricular response to atrial flutter or fibrillation by prolonging the effective refractory period of the accessory pathway. While quinidine may be useful in the termination or subsequent suppression of atrial fibrillation or flutter, because of the vagolytic effect of the drug on AV-nodal conduction quinidine may occasionally convert a 2:1 AV response in atrial flutter to a 1:1 response, unless the atrial rate is slowed prior to the administration of quinidine by another agent such as propranolol or verapamil. Because it crosses the placenta, quinidine has been found useful in the treatment of fetal arrhythmias.[3]

REFERENCES

1. Mirro, M.J., Manalan, A.S., Failey, J.C., and Watanabe, A.M.: Anticholinergic effects of disopyramide and quinidine on guinea pig myocardium: Mediation by direct muscarinic receptor blockade. Circ. Res. *47*:855, 1980.
2. Wu, D., Hung, J.S., Kuo, C.T., Hsu, K.S., and Shieh, W.B.: Effects of quinidine on atrioventricular nodal reentrant paroxysmal tachycardia. Circulation *64*:823, 1981.

3. Guntheroth, W.G., Cyr, D.R., Mack, L.A., Benedetti, T., Lenke, R.R., and Petty, C.N.: Hydrops from reciprocating atrioventricular tachycardia in 27-week fetus requiring quinidine for conversion. Obstet. Gynecol. 66(Suppl. 3):29S, 1985.

124-B *(Braunwald, p. 480)*

While edema is a common and important physical finding in congestive heart failure, its presence does not correlate well with the level of systemic venous pressure. The excess volume of extracellular fluid volume is a more important determinant of edema. Thus, in adults, a minimum of 5 liters of excess extracellular fluid volume must usually accumulate before peripheral edema is manifested. In patients with chronic LV failure and a low cardiac output, peripheral edema may develop in the presence of normal or minimally elevated systemic venous pressure because of a gradual but persistent accumulation of extracellular fluid volume.

Edema generally accumulates in dependent portions of the body such as the ankles or feet of ambulatory patients or the sacrum of bedridden patients. As heart failure progresses, edema becomes more severe and may become massive and generalized (anasarca). In rare instances, especially when edema develops suddenly and severely, frank rupture of the skin with extravasation of fluid may result. Edema is usually more marked on the paralyzed side of patients with hemiplegia; unilateral edema may also result from unilateral venous obstruction.

125-B *(Braunwald, pp. 781–782)*

Anemia is one of the most common conditions that is associated with a sustained increase in cardiac output. While an increase in cardiac output occurs consistently when the hematocrit falls below 25 per cent, the occurrence of heart failure at this level of anemia usually implies the presence of underlying heart disease. In patients with severe anemia (hematocrit less than 15 per cent) clinical evidence of heart failure may occur even in the absence of underlying heart disease. In addition, patients with sickle cell anemia may develop signs of heart failure at less severe levels of anemia for a variety of reasons, including impaired systemic cardiac oxygenation due to microthrombi and a loss of the hemodynamic benefits of reduced viscosity, which is not seen in this particular form of anemia.[1,2]

The rate of development of anemia plays an important role in determining whether increases in cardiac output occur to any significant degree. When anemia is secondary to rapid blood loss, maintenance of blood volume is not possible and a clinical picture of hypovolemic shock ensues. However, when anemia develops more slowly, cardiac output is augmented primarily through an increase in stroke volume that is associated with cardiac dilatation and hypertrophy. Heart rate usually remains in the normal range. The augmentation of cardiac output that occurs during exercise in patients with anemia tends to be excessive.[3] Such a response may occur in patients with only mild anemia who have normal resting cardiac output.[4]

REFERENCES

1. Varat, M.A., Adolph, R.J., and Fowler, N.O.: Cardiovascular effects of anemia. Am. Heart J. 83:415, 1972.
2. Denenberg, B.S., Criner, G., Jones, R., and Spann, J.F.: Cardiac function in sickle cell anemia. Am. J. Cardiol. 51:1674, 1983.
3. Sproule, B.J., Mitchell, J.H., and Miller, W.F.: Cardiopulmonary physiological responses to heavy exercise in patients with anemia. J. Clin. Invest. 39:378, 1960.
4. Graettinger, J.S., Parsons, R.L., and Campbell, J.A.: A correlation of clinical and hemodynamic studies in patients with mild and severe anemia with and without congestive failure. Ann. Intern. Med. 58:617, 1963.

126-C *(Braunwald, pp. 507–513)*

The loop diuretics, including ethacrynic acid, furosemide, bumetanide, and piretanide, are capable of inducing a vigorous natriuresis by blocking the sodium transport system in the ascending limb of Henle's loop. Each of these drugs is secreted into the renal tubular lumen by the organic acid secretory pathway; therefore, their pharmacological actions may be delayed or diminished by exogenous competitive inhibitors of this pathway such as probenecid and indomethacin. The absorption of loop diuretics is highly variable even among normal subjects; furosemide, for instance, has an average bioavailability of 60 per cent.[1] This may be markedly diminished when the drug is given with meals. In addition, the presence of heart failure may lead to delayed intestinal absorption and delivery of the drug to its tubular site of action. Nonsteroidal antiinflammatory drugs, including aspirin, may blunt the natriuretic response to all the diuretics. This occurs by prevention of the prostaglandin-induced rise in renal blood flow associated with the natriuretic response to these agents. Finally, all the loop diuretics may cause changes in systemic hemodynamics before the initiation of diuresis.

REFERENCE

1. Grahnen, A., Hammarlund, M., and Lundquist, T.: Implications of intraindividual variability in bioavailability studies of furosemide. Eur. J. Clin. Pharmacol. 27:595, 1984.

127-E *(Braunwald, p. 473)*

In patients with low-output heart failure, the ability of the heart to deliver O_2 to metabolizing tissues is compromised and the arterial–mixed venous O_2 difference is thus abnormally widened. In high-output heart failure, the mixed venous O_2 saturation is elevated by the admixture of blood that has been shunted away from the metabolizing tissues due to the condition that has caused the high-output state. The arterial–mixed venous O_2 difference is therefore normal or even reduced in high-output heart failure. However, regardless of the *absolute* level of the arterial–mixed venous O_2 difference, it still exceeds the value that existed before the development of high-output heart failure. Cardiac output is lower than it had been before the development of heart failure. Thus, although a patient with high-output heart failure from thyrotoxicosis may have an absolute cardiac output that is within the normal range, it is a value that is abnormally low for this individual, being less than the cardiac output measured when the patient was hyperthyroid but not in heart failure.

128-C   (Braunwald, pp. 636–637)

The calcium antagonist verapamil prolongs conduction time through the AV node by blocking the slow inward (calcium) current in cardiac fibers. Because the drug interferes with excitation-contraction, it inhibits contraction of vascular smooth muscle and leads to dilatation of coronary and peripheral vascular beds. In addition, verapamil exerts a direct negative inotropic action on isolated cardiac muscle. In patients with impaired left ventricular function, verapamil may exert accentuated hemodynamic depressant effects, especially if administered simultaneously with a beta blocker. Within 3 to 5 minutes after intravenous injection of verapamil, mean arterial pressure decreases and left ventricular end-diastolic pressure rises. The resultant reduction of afterload due to the agent's vasodilatory effects minimizes its negative inotropic action so that the net result is little or no change in the cardiac index.

Intravenous verapamil is the treatment of choice for terminating sustained sinus-nodal or AV-nodal reentry tachycardias, as well as reciprocating tachycardias associated with Wolff-Parkinson-White syndrome when one of the reentrant pathways is the AV node. However, reflex sympathetic stimulation induced by verapamil may increase the ventricular response over the accessory pathway to atrial fibrillation in patients with the Wolff-Parkinson-White syndrome;[1] therefore, the drug is contraindicated in this situation. Verapamil is able to terminate between 60 and 80 per cent of paroxysmal supraventricular tachycardias within several minutes.[2]

In patients with atrial fibrillation, verapamil decreases the ventricular response by increasing the effective refractory period of the AV node and may convert a small percentage of episodes to sinus rhythm, especially if the atrial flutter or fibrillation is of recent onset.[3] However, in patients with chronic atrial fibrillation, quinidine appears to be more effective than verapamil in the establishment and maintenance of sinus rhythm.[4]

Side effects in patients on verapamil are more likely if preexisting LV dysfunction or beta blocker therapy is present. In addition, hemodynamic collapse has been noted in response to verapamil in infants. Therefore, the drug should be used extremely cautiously in patients less than 1 year of age. Contraindications to the use of verapamil include marked sinus node dysfunction, second- or third-degree AV block, and hypotension, as well as the clinical conditions just mentioned. In patients taking digoxin, verapamil may increase the serum digitalis level by decreasing excretion of digoxin. Appropriate caution is warranted.

REFERENCES

1. Gulamhusein, S., Ko, P., Carruthers, S.G., and Klein, G.J.: Acceleration of the ventricular response during atrial fibrillation in the Wolff-Parkinson-White syndrome after verapamil. Circulation 65:348, 1982.
2. Rikenberger, R.L., Prystowsky, E.N., Heger, J.J., Troup, P.J.,

Jackman, W.M., and Zipes, D.P.: Effects of intravenous and chronic oral verapamil administration in patients with supraventricular tachyarrhythmias. Circulation 62:996, 1980.
3. Waxman, H.L., Myerburg, R.J., Appel, R., and Sung, R.J.: Verapamil for control of ventricular rate in paroxysmal supraventricular tachycardia and atrial fibrillation or flutter: A double-blind randomized cross-over study. Ann. Intern. Med. 94:1, 1981.
4. Kates, R.E., Keefe, D.L., Schwartz, J., Harapats, S., Hirsten, E.B., Harrison, D.C.: Verapamil disposition kinetics in chronic atrial fibrillation. Clin. Pharmacol. Ther. 30:44, 1981.

129-D   (Braunwald, pp. 479–482)

A variety of physical findings appear in patients with heart failure. Elevation of systemic venous pressure for long periods of time may produce several signs in patients, including protrusion of the eyes and severe tricuspid regurgitation. This may result in a visible systolic pulsation of the eyes.[1] In attempts to compensate and support the circulation in the presence of reduced cardiac output, increased activity of the adrenergic activity system is noted in patients with heart failure. This adrenergic activity is responsible for peripheral vasoconstriction, which leads to both pallor and coldness of the extremities as well as cyanosis of the digits in severe cases.

In patients with right heart failure the resting jugular venous pressure may not appear abnormal but may be seen to be elevated when the abdomen is compressed by palpation over the liver. This sign is known as abdominojugular reflux. Since a positive test usually reflects both hepatic congestion and failure of the right side of the heart to transport the increased venous return of this condition appropriately, a positive test may be helpful in differentiating hepatomegaly due to heart failure from other causes.

If hepatomegaly occurs rapidly with a relatively acute onset of heart failure, stretching of the liver capsule occurs; this may lead to tenderness in the right upper quadrant. However, in chronic heart failure, this tenderness is less likely to be present, although the liver itself usually remains large. Accumulation of ascitic fluid in the peritoneal cavity may occur in patients with increased hepatic venous pressure. The ascitic fluid has an elevated protein content relative to a pure transudate, suggesting that increased capillary permeability plays a role in this process. Longstanding, severe heart failure may be accompanied by a protein-losing enteropathy caused by visceral congestion.[2] The resultant reduction in plasma oncotic pressure may exacerbate the underlying tendency to form ascites.

REFERENCES

1. Earnest, D.L., and Hurst, J.W.: Exophthalmos, stare and increase in intraocular pressure and systolic protrusion of the eyeballs due to congestive heart failure. Am. J. Cardiol. 26:351, 1970.
2. Strober, W., Cohen, L.S., Waldmann, T.A., and Braunwald, E.: Tricuspid regurgitation: A newly recognized cause of protein-losing enteropathy, lymphocytopenia, and immunologic deficiency. Am. J. Med. 44:842, 1968.

130-A   (Braunwald, pp. 631–632; Tables 21–2 and 21–3, pp. 626–627)

Disopyramide has been approved for oral but not intravenous administration in the United States, primarily to treat patients with ventricular arrhythmias. The drug has been shown to terminate and prevent recurrent episodes of paroxysmal supraventricular tachycardia due to AV-nodal reentry mechanisms as well. In studies of intravenous disopyramide, a number of hemodynamic effects have been noted, including reductions of arterial pressure and cardiac index and increases in atrial pressures and total peripheral resistance.[1] Disopyramide may reduce contractility in subjects with normal ventricles and may lead to profound depression of ventricular function in patients with preexisting abnormal ventricular function.[2]

Oral administration of disopyramide leads to peak blood levels in 1 to 2 hours, with a mean elimination half-life of 8 to 9 hours in healthy volunteers but a somewhat lower half-life in patients with heart failure or ventricular arrhythmias. Doses of the drug are generally 100 to 200 mg orally every 6 hours with a total dose ranging between 400 to 1200 mg/day.

Disopyramide has been used effectively to reduce the frequency of premature ventricular complexes and prevent recurrent tachycardia. It has been administered in combination with mexiletine to treat patients with recurrent ventricular tachycardia and/or ventricular fibrillation.[3] The most common side effects of disopyramide result from the drug's antiparasympathetic properties and include urinary retention or hesitancy, blurred vision, closed-angle glaucoma, dry mouth, and constipation. In addition, the drug has been shown to produce Q-T prolongation and ventricular tachyarrhythmias secondary to torsades de pointes.[4] Disopyramide is capable of creating 1:1 conduction during atrial flutter due to a direct vagolytic effect.[5]

REFERENCES

1. Leach, A.J., Brown, J.E., and Armstrong, P.W.: Cardiac depression by intravenous disopyramide in patients with left ventricular dysfunction. Am. J. Med. 68:839, 1980.
2. Podrid, P.J., Schoeneberger, A., and Lown, B.: Congestive heart failure caused by disopyramide. N. Engl. J. Med. 302:614, 1980.
3. Breithardt, G., Seipel, L., and Abendroth, R.R.: Comparison of the antiarrhythmic efficacy of disopyramide and mexiletine against stimulus-induced ventricular tachycardia. J. Cardiovasc. Pharmacol. 3:1026, 1981.
4. Tzivoni, D., Keren, A., Stern, S., and Gottlieb, S.: Disopyramide-induced torsades de pointes. Arch. Intern. Med. 141:946, 1981.
5. Robertson, C.E., and Miller, H.C.: Extreme tachycardia complicating the use of disopyramide in atrial flutter. Br. Heart J. 44:602, 1980.

131   A-Y, B-Y, C-N, D-Y, E-N (*Braunwald, pp. 842–844*)

The Cooperative Study on Renovascular Hypertension[1] delineated two major forms of renovascular disease—atherosclerosis and fibromuscular hyperplasia. Atherosclerotic patients were older, had higher systolic BP, and had greater target organ damage. Patients with fibromuscular hyperplasia were younger, were more often female, had no family history of hypertension, and had less evidence of target organ damage.

REFERENCE

1. Simon, N., Franklin, S.S., Bleifer, K.W., and Maxwell, M.H.P.: Clinical characteristics of renovascular hypertension JAMA 220:1209, 1972.

132   A-Y, B-N, C-Y, D-Y, E-Y (*Braunwald, p. 475; Braunwald, E., and Frahm, C.J.: Studies on Starling's law of the heart. IV. Observations on hemodynamic function of the left atrium in man. Circulation 24:633, 1961.*)

All of the statements describe mechanisms whereby cardiac arrhythmias can precipitate and intensify heart failure. Tachyarrhythmias may lead to ischemia as noted, which in turn may raise left atrial pressure by impairing both normal cardiac relaxation and normal systolic function. In addition, by *reducing* ventricular filling time, underlying abnormalities of ventricular filling (e.g., mitral stenosis) or compliance (e.g., hypertension with diastolic dysfunction) may lead to elevated left atrial pressures. In patients with underlying heart disease, compensatory mechanisms may lead to a hemodynamic equilibrium in which stroke volume is maximized. In such instances, onset of bradycardia may precipitate heart failure by resulting in a net fall in cardiac output. In many arrhythmias, dissociation between atrial and ventricular contraction occurs, with loss of the atrial contribution to diastolic ventricular filling, decreased cardiac output, and elevation in atrial pressure. Finally, abnormal intraventricular conduction may precipitate heart failure by causing a loss of the normal synchronicity of ventricular contraction and a resultant impairment of myocardial performance.

133   A-Y, B-N, C-Y, D-Y, E-N (*Braunwald, pp. 506–507*)

Successful treatment of digitalis intoxication begins with maintaining a high level of suspicion regarding any rhythm disturbance that appears in a patient using digitalis preparations. Both lidocaine and phenytoin have been found to be useful in the treatment of arrhythmias due to digitalis toxicity. Both have been shown to have little negative effect on sinoatrial rate, atrial conduction, or atrioventricular conduction. In the appropriate clinical setting, these agents may be administered intravenously to control digitalis-induced arrhythmias. In contrast, quinidine may actually intensify digitalis intoxication by raising serum digoxin levels and should be avoided in patients suspected of digitalis intoxication. Occasionally, direct-current countershock must be used when other methods have failed and a life-threatening rhythm disturbance is present. However, countershock is in general inadvisable in the presence of digitalis intoxication because it may precipitate severe arrhythmias. The risk of arrhythmias due to countershock is decreased when lower energy levels are used[1] and may be much less if no digitalis-induced rhythm disturbance is present in a patient.[2]

The use of cardiac glycoside-specific antibodies and their Fab fragments as a specific, effective treatment of severe digitalis toxicity has emerged in recent years.[3] Fab fragments have been demonstrated to be particularly effective in situations of excessive digitalis dosage due to accident or suicidal intent, and they have been approved by the U.S. Food and Drug Administration.

REFERENCES

1. Citrin, D., Stevenson, I.H., and O'Malley, K.: Massive digoxin overdose: Observations on hyperkalemia and plasma digoxin levels. Scott. Med. J. 17:275, 1972.
2. Ditchey, R.V., and Karliner, J.S.: Safety of electrical cardioversion in patients without digitalis toxicity. Ann. Intern. Med. 95:676, 1981.
3. Wenger, T.L., Butler, V.P., Haber, E., and Smith, T.W.: Treatment of 63 severely digitalis-toxic patients with digoxin-specific antibody fragments. J. Am. Coll. Cardiol. 5:118A, 1985.

134   A-Y, B-Y, C-Y, D-N, E-N (Braunwald, p. 564)

A variety of alterations occur in myocardial function when the syndrome of circulatory shock occurs. Decreases in coronary perfusion pressure are minimized at first by peripheral vasoconstriction and the resultant maintenance of diastolic aortic blood pressure. However, as the syndrome progresses and coronary pressure and flow are reduced, there is a significant reduction in endocardial blood flow.[1] A number of investigators have noted myocardial depression during shock states effected in part by circulating humoral factors. Reductions in LV ejection fraction and dilatation of the ventricles appears to occur in the absence of reductions in coronary perfusion pressure or flow. The precise substance or substances responsible for myocardial depression in circulatory shock have not been clearly identified, but their presence has been confirmed, especially in septic shock.[2]

The oxygen requirements of the myocardium are increased in shock because of the large increase in adrenergic activity as well as the aforementioned increase in afterload due to peripheral arterial vasoconstriction.[3] During the shock state the risks of digitalis toxicity and arrhythmia are increased because there is a decrease in myocardial clearance of this agent.[4] Therefore, in patients with shock who are taking digitalis, further reductions in cardiac output may be precipitated by the development of cardiac arrhythmias.

REFERENCES

1. Carlson, E.L., Selinger, S.L., Utley, J., and Hoffman, J.I.E.: Intramyocardial distribution of blood flow in hemorrhagic shock in anesthetized dogs. Am. J. Physiol. 230:41, 1976.
2. Parrillo, J.E., Burch, C., Shelhamer, J.H., Parker, M.M., Natanson, C., and Schuette, W.: A circulating myocardial depressant substance in humans with septic shock. J. Clin. Invest. 76:1539, 1976.
3. Udhoji, V.N., and Weil, M.H.: Circulatory effects of angiotensin, levarterenol and metaraminol in the treatment of shock. N. Engl. J. Med. 270:501, 1964.
4. Lloyd, B.L., and Taylor, R.R.: Augmentation of myocardial digoxin concentration in hemorrhagic shock. Circulation 51:718, 1975.

135   A-Y, B-N, C-Y, D-Y, E-Y (Braunwald, pp. 823–828)

The degree of risk from hypertension can be categorized taking into account: (1) the level of blood pressure; (2) the histological nature of the hypertension based on end-organ damage; and (3) coexisting risks including hypercholesterolemia, cigarette smoking, and diabetes[1, 2] as well as race[3] and sex. Thus, males and blacks have increased morbidity from hypertension independent of other risk factors. Although low plasma renin activity (PRA) was initially reported as indicative of a benign prognosis, subsequent studies have not verified this finding.[4]

REFERENCES

1. Castelli, W.P., and Anderson, K.: A population at risk. Prevalence of high cholesterol levels in hypertensive patients in the Framingham Study. Am. J. Med. 80(Suppl 2A):23, 1986.
2. MacMahon, S.W., and Macdonald, G.J.: Antihypertensive treatment and plasma lipoprotein levels: The association in data from a population study. Am. J. Med. 80(Suppl 2A):40, 1986.
3. Sugimoto, T., and Rosansky, S.J.: The incidence of treated end stage renal disease in the Eastern United States: 1973–1979. Am. J. Public Health 74:14, 1984.
4. Kaplan, N.M.: The prognostic implications of plasma renin in essential hypertension. JAMA 231:167, 1975.

136   A-N, B-N, C-Y, D-Y, E-N (Braunwald, pp. 632–633; Table 21–1, pp. 622–623)

Diphenylhydantoin (phenytoin) was developed and originally used to treat seizure disorders and was only subsequently noted to have activity against ventricular tachycardia in animal studies. The drug has found limited usage in the treatment of arrhythmias, primarily because of erratic pharmacokinetics and a relatively small number of clinically useful effects (see below). Phenytoin is absorbed erratically after oral administration and plasma concentrations peak 8 to 12 hours after an oral dose. The elimination half-life of the drug is about 24 hours and metabolism occurs primarily by hydroxylation in the liver. In the presence of liver disease or when phenytoin is administered along with drugs such as phenylbutazone, isoniazide, and phenothiazines that may compete with phenytoin for hepatic enzymes, the half-life of phenytoin may be markedly altered. In addition, the hepatic enzyme system that metabolizes phenytoin becomes saturated at plasma concentrations (10 to 20 µg/ml). Phenytoin elimination after reaching this point follows zero-order kinetics, so that only a fixed amount of drug is eliminated per unit of time. This may result in sudden or unexpected toxicity due to disproportionately large changes in plasma concentrations of phenytoin following small increases in drug dosage. Therapeutic plasma concentrations of phenytoin may be achieved rapidly by administration of 100 mg of the drug every 5 minutes intravenously until the arrhythmia is controlled, up to a maximum of 1 gm. In general, 700 to 1000 mg given intravenously will control the arrhythmia being treated.

Diphenylhydantoin has been particularly useful in the treatment of atrial and ventricular arrhythmias caused by digitalis toxicity. However, phenytoin is much less effective in treating ventricular arrhythmias in patients with ischemic heart disease[1] or in treating atrial arrhythmias due to causes other than digitalis toxicity. The most common side effects of phenytoin include central nervous system toxicity manifested as nystagmus, ataxia, drowsiness, and stupor. Gastrointestinal effects that are also commonly seen include nausea, epigastric pain, and anorexia.

REFERENCE

1. Peter, T., Ross, D., Duffield, A., Luxton, M., Harper, R., Hunt, D., and Sloman, G.: Effect on survival after myocardial infarction of long-term treatment with phenytoin. Br. Heart J. 40:1356, 1978.

137 A-Y, B-N, C-Y, D-Y, E-Y *(Braunwald, pp. 630–631)*

Procainamide is useful in the treatment of both supraventricular and ventricular arrhythmias in a manner analogous to quinidine. Oral administration of the drug achieves peak plasma concentrations in approximately 1 hour, although absorption may be reduced in the first week following myocardial infarction. The bioavailability of procainamide is approximately 80 per cent following oral administration, with an overall elimination half-life of 3 to 5 hours; the majority of the drug is eliminated unchanged in the urine. Procainamide may be given by intravenous, oral, or intramuscular routes, the last of which shows excellent absorption, with close to 100 per cent bioavailability. Oral administration of the drug is on an every 3 to 4 hour basis except for the prolonged-release form of procainamide. This is given every 6 hours and provides a steady-state plasma level similar to that for the short-acting form of the agent when given in an equal total daily dose. Several intravenous regimens exist for the acute administration of procainamide, and constant-rate intravenous infusion of procainamide for temporary maintenance therapy can be given in doses of 2 to 6 mg/min. With any form of procainamide, the total daily dosage is usually in the 2 to 6 gm range.

138 A-Y, B-N, C-Y, D-Y, E-Y *(Braunwald, pp. 697–698)*

Ventricular arrhythmias including VT have been identified in association with a variety of clinical states. Arrhythmogenic RV dysplasia, a localized cardiomyopathy with hypokinetic areas involving the wall of the RV, may be associated with VT. The characteristics of this VT include a left bundle branch block contour, often with right-axis deviation, and with T waves that are inverted over the right precordial leads.[1] This entity may be uncovered as an important cause of ventricular arrhythmia in children and young adults with apparently normal hearts. The disease shows a male predominance and is best identified by echocardiography or RV angiography.[2] Both dilated and hypertrophic cardiomyopathies may be associated with VT and an increased risk of sudden death. Of patients with hypertrophic cardiomyopathy, up to one-third may experience sudden death within 10 years of the diagnosis. Amiodarone has been reported to prevent sudden death in some of these patients.[3]
Patients with depressed LV ejection fraction and dilated cardiomyopathy are at an increased risk of sudden death when 24-hour ambulatory monitoring reveals ventricular couplets or tachycardia.[4] Electrophysiological testing may be useful in such patients to identify a tendency toward developing sustained VT. In patients who have undergone repair of tetralogy of Fallot, sustained VT may emerge some years after the operation, perhaps due to reentry at the site of the previous operation in the RV outflow tract.[5] Use of phenytoin, propranolol, mexiletene, or amiodarone may decrease the occurrence of sudden death in this population. Although patients with mitral valve prolapse frequently display ventricular arrhythmias, a causal relationship between mitral valve prolapse and the underlying ventricular ectopy has not been clearly established. In general, prognosis for most patients with mitral valve prolapse is quite good and no clear correlation between sudden death and underlying ventricular ectopy has yet been discovered.

REFERENCES

1. Fontaine, G., Frank, R., Tonet, J.L., Guiraudon, G., Cabrol, C., Chomette, G., and Grosgogeat, Y.: Arrhythmogenic right ventricular dysplasia: A clinical model for the study of chronic ventricular tachycardia. Jpn. Circ. J. 48:515, 1984.
2. Marcus, F.I., Fontaine, G.H., Guiraudon, G., Frank, R., Laurenceau, J.L., Malergue, C., and Grosgogeat, Y.: Right ventricular dysplasia: A report of 24 adult cases. Circulation 65:384, 1982.
3. McKenna, W.J., Oakley, C.M., Krikler, D.M., and Goodwin, J.F.: Improved survival with amiodarone in patients with hypertrophic cardiomyopathy and ventricular tachycardia. Br. Heart J. 53:412, 1985.
4. Meinertz, T., Hofmann, T., Kasper, W., Treese, N., Bechtold, H., Stienen, U., Pop, T., Leitner, E.V., Andresen, D., and Meyer, J.: Significance of ventricular arrhythmias in idiopathic dilated cardiomyopathy. Am. J. Cardiol. 53:902, 1984.
5. Harken, A.H., Horowitz, L.N., and Josephson, M.E.: Surgical correction of recurrent sustained ventricular tachycardia on complete repair of tetralogy of Fallot. J. Thorac. Cardiovasc. Surg. 80:779, 1980.

139 A-N, B-Y, C-N, D-N, E-Y *(Braunwald, pp. 876–877)*

Minoxidil, like hydralazine, is a potent vasodilator with relative selectivity for smooth muscle in precapillary arterial vessels. As a result peripheral resistance falls with reflex sympathetic stimulation, leading to increased venous return, heart rate, and contractility as well as fluid retention. These reflex changes are the source of many side effects, which can be controlled by coadministration of a beta blocker and diuretic. Minoxidil is currently used most often in patients with severe hypertension and renal insufficiency because of its preservation of renal function.[1] Its other side effects include hirsutism and pericardial effusion in 3 per cent of patients. Unlike with hydralazine, a lupus-like syndrome is rarely observed with minoxidil.

REFERENCE

1. Hagstam, K., Lundgren, R., and Wieslander, J.: Clinical evidence of long-term treatment with minoxidil in severe arterial hypertension. Scand. J. Urol. Nephrol. 16:57, 1982.

140   A-Y, B-Y, C-N, D-N, E-N (*Braunwald, pp. 637–639*; Mason, J.W.: Amiodarone. N. Engl. J. Med. *316:*455, 1987.)

Amiodarone was originally introduced as a smooth muscle relaxant and coronary vasodilator for the treatment of angina. Oral administration of the drug in ordinary doses does not depress left ventricular ejection fraction; however, the intravenous form of amiodarone may exert some negative inotropic action and must be given cautiously to patients with depressed ejection fractions.[1] The use of amiodarone clinically is complex, in part due to the slow and variable achievement of plasma concentrations of the drug capable of suppressing arrhythmias. The onset of action following oral administration ranges from 2 days to 1 to 3 weeks. The elimination half-life of amiodarone is biphasic, with an initial 50 per cent reduction in plasma concentration in the first 2 weeks after stopping therapy and a subsequent terminal half-life of between 26 and 107 days. To achieve steady-state amiodarone concentrations without an initial loading dose takes approximately 9 months. In addition, marked interpatient variability of the pharmacokinetics described above complicates therapy with this agent.

Although optimal dosing of amiodarone has not been clearly defined, the usual approach begins with daily doses of 800 to 1600 mg, tapering over 1 to 2 weeks to an eventual maintenance dose of 400 mg per day.

Amiodarone has been used to suppress a wide variety of both supraventricular and ventricular tachyarrhythmias. In general, the drug's efficacy is equal to or greater than that of other antiarrhythmic agents and is in the range of 60 to 80 per cent for most supraventricular tachyarrhythmias and 40 to 60 per cent for ventricular tachyarrhythmias.[2] However, because of amiodarone's long half-life, its interactions with other antiarrhythmic drugs, and an extensive list of side effects, therapy with this agent is usually a late or last resort. Side effects from amiodarone occur in approximately 75 per cent of patients maintained on 400 mg/day. Discontinuation of the drug is required in up to 20 per cent of patients.[3]

The most serious noncardiac side effect of amiodarone is its pulmonary toxicity, which occurs in between 5 to 15 per cent of patients after 1 year of treatment and is an absolute contraindication for continuation of the drug. The toxicity is marked by dyspnea and nonproductive cough as well as fever, with a positive gallium scan and radiographic evidence of pulmonary infiltrates often noted. The mortality due to this pulmonary process approaches 10 per cent, especially in patients with unrecognized pulmonary involvement that is allowed to continue. All patients on amiodarone therapy should therefore be monitored with chest x-rays at 3-month intervals during the first year and then twice annually.

Amiodarone blocks the conversion of thyroxine (T_4) to triiodothyronine (T_3). This effect results in a slight increase in T_4, reverse T_3, and TSH with clinical hypothyroidism appearing in 2 to 4 per cent of patients.[4] In 1 to 2 per cent of patients, hyperthyroidism may appear and is characterized by an increase in T_3 levels.

Cardiac side-effects of amiodarone occur in 2 to 3 per cent of patients and include symptomatic bradycardias, aggravation of ventricular tachyarrhythmias, and worsening of congestive heart failure. Because amiodarone interacts with a number of other cardiac drugs, including warfarin and digoxin, reductions in these agents are routinely made when amiodarone therapy is initiated. Serum levels of such drugs require close observation.

REFERENCES

1. Kosinski, E.J., Albin, J.B., Young, E., Lewis, S.M., and Leland, O.S., Jr.: Hemodynamic effects of intravenous amiodarone. J. Am. Coll. Cardiol. *4:*565, 1984.
2. Zipes, D.P., Prystowsky, E.N., and Heger, J.J.: Amiodarone: Electrophysiologic actions, pharmacokinetics and clinical effects. J. Am. Coll. Cardiol. *3:*1059, 1984.
3. Raeder, E.A., Podrid, P.J., and Lown, B.: Side effects and complications of amiodarone therapy. Am. Heart J. *109:*975, 1985.
4. Borowski, G.D., Garofano, C.D., Rose, L.I., Spielman, S.R., Rotmensch, H.R., Greenspan, A.M., and Horowitz, L.N.: Effect of long-term amiodarone therapy on thyroid hormone levels and thyroid function. Am. J. Med. *78:*443, 1985.

141   A-Y, B-Y, C-Y, D-N, E-N (*Braunwald, p. 940*)

A number of unusual conditions including cor triatriatum may lead to obstruction of pulmonary venous drainage and secondary pulmonary hypertension. Cor triatriatum is a malformation in which partitioning of the left atrium creates two atrial subchambers, a posterior subchamber that receives pulmonary venous inflow, and an anterior subchamber that subsequently leads to the mitral orifice. When the opening in the partition between the posterior and anterior subchambers is small, severe pulmonary venous and subsequent pulmonary arterial hypertension may result.[1] The resultant elevation in pulmonary venous pressures leads to a reactive pulmonary arterial hypertension. A substantial component of the pulmonary hypertension resides in the pulmonary arteriolar bed. Pressure in the anterior subchamber of the left atrium distal to the site of pulmonary venous obstruction is often normal.

Diagnosis of cor triatriatum may be made by echocardiography and definitively by cardiac catheterization. Operative correction of this disorder may be curative.

REFERENCE

1. Magidson, A.: Cor triatriatum. Severe pulmonary arterial hypertension and pulmonary venous hypertension in a child. Am. J. Cardiol. *9:*603, 1962.

142   A-N, B-N, C-N, D-N, E-Y (*Braunwald, pp. 703–705*)

Type I second-degree AV block is characterized by progressive P-R prolongation culminating in a nonconducted P wave while Type II second-degree AV block is characterized by a constant P-R interval prior to a blocked P wave (see Braunwald, Figs. 22–42 through 22–44, pp. 703 to 704). Clinically, Type I AV block with a normal QRS complex is a generally benign rhythm. However, in older age groups Type I AV block has been associated with a more serious, symptomatic presentation.[1] Type I second-degree AV block in acute myocardial infarction usually accompanies inferior infarction, especially if an RV infarction is present. When higher degrees of AV block such as Type II second-degree block occur in patients with acute inferior myocardial infarction, an association is seen with greater myocardial damage and a higher mortality rate.[2]

The surface ECG allows a reasonably reliable differentiation of the site of block in instances of second-degree AV block. Type I AV block with a normal QRS complex almost always occurs at the level of the AV node proximal to the His bundle. In contrast, Type II AV block, especially when it occurs in association with bundle branch block, may be localized to the His-Purkinje system. Type I AV block in a patient with a bundle branch block may be due to block either in the AV node or more distally in the His-Purkinje system. In patients with 2:1 AV block it is difficult to distinguish between Type I and Type II forms of second-degree block. However, if the QRS complex is normal, Mobitz Type I is the more likely diagnosis and longer rhythm strips may reveal transition from 2:1 to, for example, 3:2 block with typical P-R interval prolongation prior to block.

REFERENCES

1. Shaw, D.B., Kekwick, C.A., Veale, D., Gowers, J., and Whistance, T.: Survival in second degree atrioventricular block. Br. Heart J. 53:587, 1985.
2. Strasberg, R., Pinchas, A., Arditti, A., Lewin, R.F., Sclarovsky, S., Hellman, C., Zafir, N., and Agmon, J.: Left and right ventricular function in inferior acute myocardial infarction and significance of advanced atrioventricular block. Am. J. Cardiol. 54:985, 1984.

143 A-Y, B-Y, C-Y, D-Y, E-N (*Braunwald, pp. 387–390*)

The contractile apparatus of cardiac tissue consists of partially overlapping rod-like filaments that are fixed in length both at rest and during contraction. The thicker filaments, which are composed of myosin molecules, are created by an orderly aggregation of approximately 300 longitudinally stacked molecules from myosin proteins held parallel and in register by a centrally located connection termed the "M" line. The structure formed by these aggregates can form cross bridges and interact with actin filaments. Myosin by itself has the ability to split the ATP, which is due to its activity as an ATPase, inhibited by magnesium and activated by calcium. When myosin combines with actin it becomes enzymatically much more active in its ability to split ATP. Myosin can be separated into three isoenzyme components—V_1, V_2, and V_3, which have different heavy chain compositions. It has been shown that hypertrophied heart muscle has a greater proportion of the V_3 isoenzyme. The thin filament, which is a double alpha helix, contains two strands of actin. These actin molecules interact with myosin to form actomyosin, which is the primary contractile protein of the cardiac cell.

The proteins that regulate the activity of actomyosin are called troponin and tropomyosin. Tropomyosin is a rod-like protein forming a continuing strand through the center of the thin filament. Troponin consists of three separate proteins and is located at intervals along the thin filament. Troponin can be separated into three components: (1) troponin C, a calcium-sensitizing factor that binds calcium; (2) troponin I, an inhibitory factor that inhibits magnesium-stimulated ATPase of actomyosin; and (3) troponin T, which serves to allow attachment of the troponin complex to actin and tropomyosin.[1]

Under normal conditions when intracellular calcium is low, troponin C has no effect on the ability of troponin I to inhibit actin-myosin binding. However, calcium can rise in the cell with a depolarization, during which the calcium concentration *increases* from 10^{-7} M to 10^{-5} M. When this occurs, troponin C binds calcium and inhibits the binding of troponin I to actin, which triggers the interaction between actin and myosin. The formation of actomyosin results in hydrolysis of ATP by myosin. The actin rods are drawn toward the center of the sarcomere. Once such a stroke is completed another ATP is bound and attaches to the actin site and the cycle is repeated, the myyosin head attaching to a different actin monomer. Thus, shortening of cardiac muscle involves a relative change in the position of the two sets of filaments; actin filaments are displaced by the force-generating process at many cross-bridge sites and pulled in toward the center of the sarcomere. The force that is developed is related to the quantity of calcium that is bound to troponin C, which in turn is related to the intracellular calcium concentration. Finally, removal of calcium from troponin results in relaxation.[2]

REFERENCES

1. Ebashi, S.: Regulatory mechanism of muscle contraction with special reference to Ca-troponin-tropomyosin system. Essays Biochem. 10:1, 1974.
2. Winegrad, S.: Regulation of cardiac contractile proteins. Circ. Res. 55:565, 1984.

144 A-Y, B-Y, C-Y, D-N, E-Y (*Braunwald, pp. 426–427*)

Although many of the compensatory adjustments made in response to decreased cardiac output such as salt and water retention cause or intensify pulmonary and peripheral edema, they are all directed at maintenance of cardiac output and arterial pressure to preserve perfusion of the coronary and cerebral beds. The primacy of coronary and cerebral perfusion is revealed by the redistribution of blood flow away from other tissues. Furthermore, in heart failure there is significant venoconstriction, probably mediated by venous compression due to increased tissue pressure, by increased concentrations of circulating vasoconstrictors, and by neural (adrenergic) stimulation. Finally, there is a *decline* in the affinity of hemoglobin for O_2 due to an increase in 2,3-diphosphoglycerate,[1] which facilitates O_2 delivery to the tissues.

REFERENCE

1. Woodson, R.D., Torrance, J.D., Shappell, S.D., and Lenfant, C.: The effect of cardiac disease on hemoglobin-oxygen binding. J. Clin. Invest. 49:1349, 1970.

145   A-Y, B-Y, C-Y, D-N, E-Y (*Braunwald, pp. 555–556*)

The initial treatment of acute pulmonary edema is multifaceted. Important measures include the following:

1. Administration of oxygen to improve oxygenation of arterial blood.

2. Placing the patient in a sitting position to improve oxygenation and diminish venous return.

3. Administration of morphine sulfate to diminish patient distress and to diminish central sympathetic output responsible for venous and arterial constriction. This peripheral vasoconstriction increases venous return and elevates blood pressure, actions that are detrimental in this setting.

4. Administration of a diuretic, such as furosemide, preferably in an intravenous form. The fact that even before diuresis occurs there is an improvement in respiratory function suggests that the initial effect of furosemide is not on renal function but on venous dilation.[1]

5. Reduction of preload. This can be accomplished by applying rotating tourniquets, by sitting, and by administration of furosemide and nitrates.

6. Use of vasodilators. As in this patient, cardiogenic pulmonary edema frequently is a consequence of elevations of arterial and left ventricular end-diastolic pressures and systemic vascular resistance. Therefore, vasodilators would be appropriate initial therapy. In this patient nitroglycerin would be of particular value since it is likely that myocardial ischemia may be present. It should be noted that administration of vasodilators is contraindicated, while administration of a positive inotropic agent may be useful in patients with pulmonary edema who are hypotensive.

7. Phlebotomy, which in the past has been advocated as an appropriate intervention, is not widely used because it is time-consuming and also cumbersome in an acutely ill patient.

8. Administration of digitalis is frequently a useful means of slowing heart rate and improving ventricular function. However, in patients such as the one described, who are known to be taking digoxin chronically, the issue of digitalis toxicity must be raised. In particular, this patient presents with a narrow complex junctional tachycardia, which may be seen in digitalis intoxication. Other findings suggestive of digitalis intoxication include nausea, vomiting, paroxysmal atrial tachycardia with atrioventricular block, frequent premature ventricular contractions, ventricular tachycardia, and hyperkalemia.

9. Use of aminophylline. This drug is particularly useful when bronchospasm complicates pulmonary edema because it dilates bronchioles and is also a mild positive inotropic agent. However, in patients with severe congestive heart failure metabolism of theophylline is impaired and careful monitoring of blood levels is critical to avoid intoxication.

REFERENCE

1. Wilson, J.R., Reichek, N., Dunkman, W.B., and Goldberg, S.: Effect of diuresis on the performance of the failing left ventricle in man. Am. J. Med. 70:234, 1981.

146   A-Y, B-Y, C-N, D-N, E-N (*Braunwald, pp. 734–737; see also* Answer to Question 211, p. 87, this book.)

Most dual chamber pacemakers operate with unipolar leads, as in this case. The metal capsule of the generator then serves as the indifferent electrode. This can result in oversensing, in which skeletal muscle potentials generated by contraction of the major pectoralis muscles result in inappropriate inhibition (AAI, VVI, DVI, DDI, VDD, or DDD) or triggering (AAT, VVT, VDD, VAT, or DDD) of stimuli. Whether sensing of myopotentials in the VVD or DDD mode occurs via the atrial or via the ventricular amplifier depends on the configuration, amplitude, and timing of the interference signals. In the illustrated example the occurrence of total inhibition during arm movements indicates sensing via the ventricular amplifier.

The first two PQRST complexes show appropriate dual chamber atrial and ventricular sensing and pacing at a rate of 70/min. There is no evidence for lack of capture (all pacing stimuli cause myocardial depolarizations) or undersensing (since there are no native atrial or ventricular complexes).

After the third PQRST complex there is a four-second period during which no pacemaker activity is observed. This complete lack of pacemaker activity indicates that the ventricular lead has sensed the erratic electrical activity generated by the arm and chest muscles and has been inappropriately inhibited.

In cases of suspected oversensing, placing the pacemaker in an asynchronous mode (with application of a magnet) will abolish the symptoms caused by pacemaker malfunction and aid in the diagnosis. Conversion of the lead system to bipolar function frequently eliminates sensing of myopotentials.

147   A-Y, B-Y, C-N, D-N, E-Y (*Braunwald, pp. 495–496*)

Digoxin has become the most widely used digitalis glycoside preparation in clinical practice. An understanding of digoxin pharmacokinetics is important in avoiding the serious side effects that may result from the drug's narrow toxic:therapeutic ratio. In patients with normal renal function, about one-third of body stores are lost daily via renal excretion with a resultant half-life of about 36 to 48 hours. The excretion of digoxin is proportional to glomerular filtration rate and therefore creatinine clearance. When patients use digitalis on a daily basis, a steady state is achieved in which daily excretion via the renal route is matched by the daily dosage intake. For patients not previously taking digitalis, initiating a daily maintenance dose of digitalis without a loading dose leads to this steady-state after approximately four to five half-lives, or about 7 days in subjects with normal renal function.[1] Digoxin is highly bound to tissue, making it resistant to removal from the body by dialysis, exchange transfusion, and cardiopulmonary bypass.[2] Studies of digoxin metabolism in obesity[3] reveal that serum digoxin levels and pharmacokinetics remain essentially unchanged before and after dramatic weight loss in massively obese subjects. This implies that lean body mass should be used as a basis for the calculation of digoxin dosage.

In the late 1970s the clinically important interaction between digoxin and quinidine was described.[4] Investigators noted that initiation of quinidine therapy in patients taking digoxin resulted in an approximate doubling of the serum digoxin concentration and that this increase was not uncommonly associated with the rhythm disturbances of digoxin toxicity. Subsequent reports have identified interactions between digoxin and other drugs used in cardiovascular therapy, notably verapamil and amiodarone.

REFERENCES

1. Marcus, F.L., Burkhalter, L., Cuccia, C., Pallovich, J., and Kapadia, G.G.: Administration of tritiated digoxin with and without a loading dose: A metabolic study. Circulation 34:865, 1966.
2. Coltart, D.J., Chamberlain, D.A., Howard, M.R., Kettlewell, M.G., Mercer, J.L., and Smith, T.W.: The effect of cardiopulmonary bypass on plasma digoxin concentrations. Br. Heart J. 33:334, 1971.
3. Ewy, G.A., Groves, B.M., Ball, M.F., Nimmol, L., Jackson, B., and Marcus, F.: Digoxin metabolism in obesity. Circulation 44:810, 1971.
4. Leahey, E.B., Jr., Reiffel, J.A., Drusin, R.E., Heissenbuttel, R.H., Lovejoy, W.P., and Bigger, J.T., Jr.: Interaction between quinidine and digoxin. JAMA 240:533, 1978.

148   A-Y, B-Y, C-Y, D-Y, E-Y (*Braunwald, pp. 457–462*)

Accurate assessment of myocardial contractility is hampered by the fact that most measurements of left ventricular function are affected by preload and afterload. Generation of ventricular pressure-volume curves[1] over a range of afterloads yields a unique line relating end-systolic pressure to volume which is independent of load. The slope of this line defines contractility. At constant levels of preload (left ventricular end-diastolic pressure or end-diastolic dimensions) and afterload (left ventricular end-systolic pressure) ejection phase indices, such as ejection fraction and fractional shortening, vary directly with contractility. However, in mitral and aortic regurgitation, in which the volume overload is accompanied by reductions in afterload, the ejection fractions are inappropriately elevated.[2]

REFERENCES

1. Pouleur, H., Rousseau, M.F., Van Eyll, C., Van Mechelen, H., Brasseur, L.A., and Charlier, A.A.: Assessment of left ventricular contractility from late systolic stress-volume relations. Circulation 65:1204, 1982.
2. Carabello, B.A., Nolan, S.P., and McGuire, L.B.: Assessment of preoperative left ventricular function in patients with mitral regurgitation: Value of the end-systolic wall stress-end-systolic volume ratio. Circulation 64:1212, 1981.

149   A-N, B-N, C-Y, D-Y, E-N (*Braunwald, pp. 717–720; 1266*)

Although the indications for prophylactic temporary pacing in acute MI are controversial, certain broad guidelines have been agreed upon. Patients who develop Type II second- or third-degree AV block or bifascicular block of recent onset should be paced. Patients with isolated first-degree AV block or Mobitz Type I second-degree AV block usually have a transient conduction disturbance, and can be managed conservatively. Mobitz Type II second-degree AV block usually occurs in the setting of an anterior MI, is caused by block in the His-Purkinje system, and may progress to complete AV block.[1] Although the major influence on patient mortality is the severity of myocardial damage, patients who develop Mobitz Type II second-degree or complete AV block (even without heart failure) do have a higher mortality than that noted for patients without conduction disturbance[2] and should be paced. Patients with new bifascicular block—including alternating RBBB and LBBB, RBBB with right or left axis deviation, and LBBB with P-R prolongation—also appear to be at increased risk for developing high-degree AV block[3] and should be paced. On the other hand, patients with preexisting RBBB or LBBB with or without axis deviation do not need temporary pacing.

REFERENCES

1. Dhingra, R., Denes, P., Wu, D., Chulquimia, R., and Rosen, K.: The significance of second degree atrioventricular block and bundle branch block. Observations regarding site and type of block. Circulation 49:638, 1974.
2. Hindman, M., Wagner, G., JaRo, M., Atkins, J., Scheinman, M., DeSanctis, R., Hutter, H., Yeatman, L., Rubenfire, M., Pujura, C., Rubin, M., and Mars, J.: The clinical significance of bundle branch block complicating acute myocardial infarction. I. Clinical characteristics, hospital mortality, and one year follow-up. Circulation 58:679, 1978.
3. Hollander, G., Nadiminti, V., Lichstein, E., Greengart, A., and Sanders, M.: Bundle branch block in acute myocardial infarction. Am. Heart J. 105:738, 1983.

150   A-Y, B-Y, C-N, D-N, E-N (*Braunwald, pp. 496–497*)

Digitoxin is absorbed from the gastrointestinal tract in a passive, essentially complete manner. The drug subsequently binds avidly to human serum albumin and at clinically relevant concentrations is approximately 97 per cent albumin bound, unlike digoxin, which is only about 23 per cent bound to plasma proteins. The half-life of digitoxin in plasma is in the range of 4 to 6 days. Gradual digitalization with administration of a daily maintenance dose of digitoxin (0.10 mg) without a prior loading dose results in establishment of a steady-state drug concentration in 3 to 4 weeks.

Digitoxin is the least polar and most slowly excreted of the cardiac glycosides in common use. The drug undergoes extensive metabolism principally in the liver, with only minor renal clearance. Digitoxin undergoes enterohepatic cycling. This cycle can be interrupted by cholestyramine and other resins that bind the drug in the lumen of the gastrointestinal system. While this has been demonstrated to modestly accelerate excretion of digitoxin in human subjects,[1] the approach has not been systematically applied in patients with digitoxin intoxication. Despite digitoxin's avidity for serum albumin binding sites, it can be displaced from these by high concentrations of other drugs that are bound to serum protein, including warfarin, clofibrate, phenylbutazone, and tolbutamide. However, studies indicate that this displacement is probably *not* of clinical relevance at usual plasma concentrations of digitoxin.[2]

REFERENCES

1. Caldwell, J.H., Bush, C.A., and Greenberger, N.J.: Interruption of the enterohepatic circulation of digitoxin by cholestyramine. II. Effect on metabolic disposition of tritium-labeled digitoxin and cardiac systolic intervals in man. J. Clin. Invest. 50:2638, 1971.
2. Solomon, H.M., and Abrams, W.B.: Interactions between digitoxin and other drugs in man. Am. Heart J. 83:277, 1972.

151   A-Y, B-N, C-Y, D-N, E-Y   *(Braunwald, pp. 757–759)*

Since the initiation of out-of-hospital cardiac arrest intervention, including CPR and emergency medical technician–initiated therapy, there has been a significant improvement in the initial and eventual discharge survival of patients with SCD. In the early 1970's only about 12 per cent of patients with SCD survived until discharge but by the early 1980's this had increased to 30 per cent or more.[1] Among the important prognostic indicators of eventual discharge is the initial arrhythmia presentation. Although the subgroup of patients who present with sustained VT at the time of first contact is the smallest, these patients have by far the best prognosis. In one study, approximately 88 per cent were successfully resuscitated and admitted to the hospital alive, and of these approximately 67 per cent were discharged alive.[2] Patients who present with bradyarrhythmia or asystole upon initial contact have the worst prognosis; in a study carried out in Miami only 9 per cent of such patients were admitted to the hospital alive and none was discharged.[2] Patients with VF have a prognosis that is intermediate between those with VT and bradyarrhythmias. In general, approximately 40 per cent of patients with VF have been successfully resuscitated and admitted to the hospital alive and 23 per cent were ultimately discharged alive.

The second element of prehospital care that appears to contribute to the outcome is the role of bystander CPR by laypersons awaiting the arrival of emergency rescue personnel. Although there is no significant difference in early survival as determined by admission to the hospital alive with or without bystander intervention, almost twice as many victims of prehospital cardiac arrest were ultimately discharged alive when they had bystander CPR (43 per cent) than when such support was not provided (22 per cent).[3] Finally, upon initial arrival of rescue personnel, immediate defibrillation with 200 joules should be attempted on all patients, except those with bradyarrhythmia. This dose is effective in virtually all patients weighing less than 90 kg.

REFERENCES

1. Cobb, L.A., and Hallstrom, A.P.: Community-based cardiopulmonary resuscitation: What have we learned? Ann. NY Acad. Sci. 382:330, 1982.
2. Myerburg, R.J., Conde, C.A., Sung, R.J., Mayorga-Cortes, A.,

   Mallon, S.M., Sheps, D.S., Appel, R.A., and Castellanos, A.: Clinical, electrophysiologic, and hemodynamic profile of patients resuscitated from prehospital cardiac arrest. Am. J. Med. 68:568, 1980.
3. Eisenburg, M.S., et al: Treatment of out-of-hospital cardiac arrests with rapid defibrillation by emergency medical technicians. N. Engl. J. Med. 302:1379, 1980.

152   A-N, B-Y, C-Y, D-N, E-N   *(Braunwald, pp. 847–848)*

This patient presents with the classic symptoms of epinephrine excess as would be found in association with a pheochromocytoma. About 90 per cent of pheochromocytomas arise in the adrenal *medulla*, while 10 per cent are bilateral and another 10 per cent are malignant. Multiple adrenal tumors are common in patients with familial pheochromocytoma and in association with multiple endocrine neoplasia Type II, medullary carcinoma of the thyroid (Sipple's syndrome), or mucosal ganglioneuromas (Type III). If the predominant substance released is epinephrine (formed only in the adrenal medulla), the symptoms include systolic hypertension, tachycardia, sweating, flushing, and apprehension. If norepinephrine is primarily secreted, as is the case for some adrenal medullary tumors and most extraadrenal tumors, symptoms include both systolic and diastolic hypertension (increased vasoconstriction) and, less frequently, tachycardia, palpitations, and anxiety.

The easiest and most reliable test for tumor localization is abdominal CT scan, while laboratory confirmation is typically made by measurement of urinary metanephrines or vanillylmandelic acid.[1] Interference with urinary secretion of metabolites is common, with *increases* in patients taking sympathomimetic drugs, monoamine oxidase inhibitors, or labetalol[2] and *decreases* after administration of x-ray contrast media containing methylglucamine (e.g., Renografin, Hypaque).

REFERENCES

1. Manu, P., and Hunge, L.A.: Biochemical screening for pheochromocytoma: Superiority of urinary metanephrines measurements. Am. J. Epidemiol. 120:788, 1984.
2. Bouloux, P.M.G., and Perrett, D.: Interference of labetalol metabolites in the determination of plasma catecholamines by HPLC with electrochemical detection. Clin. Chim. Acta 150:111, 1985.

153   A-N, B-N, C-Y, D-Y, E-Y   *(Braunwald, pp. 480–482)*

While cardiomegaly is a nonspecific, common finding in chronic heart failure which is seen in the majority of patients, there are several notable situations in which its presence is an exception. In circumstances in which heart failure develops before the heart has had a chance to enlarge, cardiomegaly is often absent. Such circumstances include the sudden development of arrhythmias, rupture of a valve or valve apparatus, and acute myocardial infarction. In addition, heart failure due to chronic constrictive pericarditis or restrictive cardiomyopathy is usually not associated with cardiomegaly.

Pulsus alternans is characterized by a regular rhythm with alternation of strong and weak contractions in which the weak beat is equally spaced from or slightly closer to the preceding strong beat. It usually occurs in patients who have a protodiastolic gallop sound, who have advanced myocardial disease, and who have not yet received treatment. Pulsus alternans most commonly occurs in heart failure caused by increased resistance to left ventricular ejection such as in systemic hypertension or AS. It is also seen in coronary atherosclerosis and dilated cardiomyopathies. The mechanism of pulsus alternans is thought to be a depletion in the number of contracting myocardial cells in alternating cardiac cycles, caused by incomplete recovery, which results in an alternation in stroke volume.[1]

The presence of fever in congestive heart failure should always alert the physician to the possibility of underlying infection, pulmonary infarction, or infective endocarditis. In severe heart failure, low-grade fever may be seen as a consequence of cutaneous vasoconstriction and impairment of heat loss due to the marked elevation of adrenergic nervous system activity.

The mechanism of Cheyne-Stokes respirations in congestive heart failure results from the complex interaction between left ventricular failure and the sensitivity of the medullary respiratory center. Left ventricular dysfunction leads to a prolongation of the circulation time from the lung to the brain and results in a sluggish response of the respiratory center. During apnea, arterial PO_2 falls and PCO_2 rises. This combination excites the depressed respiratory center and leads to hyperventilation, a reduction of PCO_2, and another period of apnea. While the principal cause of Cheyne-Stokes respiration is cerebral lesions as in stroke or cerebral arteriosclerosis, the alterations in circulation time mentioned are capable of exaggerating and making more clinically evident a Cheyne-Stokes pattern of respiration.

REFERENCE

1. Gleason, W.B., and Braunwald, E.: Studies on Starling's law of the heart. VI. Relationships between left ventricular end-diastolic volume and stroke volume in man with observations on the mechanisms of pulsus alternans. Circulation 25:841, 1962.

154   A-Y, B-Y, C-N, D-Y, E-Y   *(Braunwald, pp. 837–839)*

The use of oral contraceptive pills may be the most common cause of secondary hypertension, resulting in a 5 per cent incidence of hypertension over 5 years of use.[1] The likelihood of developing hypertension is increased by alcohol consumption, age > 35 years, and obesity and is probably related to the estrogen content of the agent.[2] The excess annual death rate attributable to oral contraceptive use among nonsmokers is 1 per 77,000 while for women 35 to 44 who smoke, this rate is 1 per 2000. Since estrogen increases the hepatic production of renin substrate, one possible mechanism for hypertension induced by oral contraceptives is activation of the renin-angiotensin system with sodium retention and volume expansion.

REFERENCES

1. Royal College of General Practitioners' Oral Contraception Study: Further analyses of mortality in oral contraceptive users. Lancet 1:541, 1981.
2. Tsai, C.C., Williamson, O., Kirkland, B.H., Braun, J.O., and Lam, C.F.: Low-dose oral contraception and blood pressure in women with a past history of elevated blood pressure. Am. J. Obstet Gynecol. 151:28, 1985.

155   A-Y, B-Y, C-N, D-Y, E-Y   *(Braunwald, pp. 868–869)*

Since hypertension is usually a lifelong disease, the importance of patient compliance cannot be overestimated. Therefore, the patient should be well educated about the disease and its treatment, have readily available health personnel to contact, and be involved in nondrug therapy such as exercise and diet. Pharmacological treatment should ideally be simple, inexpensive, and devoid of side effects. It is important that a stepwise approach to initiation of drugs and increases in dosage be undertaken. Rapid escalation of drugs in an effort to lower BP to normal frequently makes the patient fatigued, weak, and dizzy. These symptoms may be related to chronic alterations in autoregulation of cerebral blood flow in hypertensive patients, such that normal blood flow is maintained at a mean BP of about 60 mm Hg in normotensive and 110 mm Hg in hypertensive individuals.[1] Thus, rapid lowering of BP may cause cerebral ischemia in the hypertensive patient. Home BP readings are useful since many patients have artificially elevated BP when seen in the office because of anxiety. Home BP readings also frequently involve the spouse, which further improves patient compliance.

REFERENCE

1. Strandgaard, S., and Paulson, O.B.: Cerebral autoregulation. Stroke 15:413, 1984.

156-C   *(2 and 4 are correct)*   *(Braunwald, pp. 547–548)*

There is a gravity-dependent distribution of blood in the lungs. Since blood is more dense than gas-containing lung tissue, effects of gravity are much greater on the distribution of blood flow than on the distribution of tissue forces in the lung. Thus, from apex to base the effect of perfusion pressure on the pulmonary circulation increases by 1 cm H_2O per cm of vertical distance, whereas the pleural pressure increases by only 0.25 cm H_2O per cm of vertical distance.[1] Pulmonary capillaries are exposed to alveolar pressure that does not vary from apex to base. However, pulmonary arteries and veins are exposed to pleural pressure that does vary from apex to base.

On the basis of these concepts, the upright lung can be divided into three zones. In zone 1 (at the apex), pulmonary arterial pressure is less than alveolar pressure so that there is essentially no flow. In zone 2, arterial pressure exceeds alveolar pressure, which in turn exceeds venous pressure. Here, the pressure which controls blood flow is determined by the difference between upstream (arterial) and chamber (alveolar) pressures. It is in this zone that large increases in blood flow occur as the lung is studied from apex to base. In zone 3, venous pressure exceeds alveolar pressure, which results in distention of the capillaries. Mean intravascular pressures are greatest in this zone so that small elevations in venous pressure can cause edema formation most rapidly in this zone. It is only in this zone that calculations of pulmonary vascular resistance and measurement of pulmonary capillary wedge pressure have relevance. Furthermore, it is in this zone that elevation of pulmonary capillary wedge pressure causes vascular redistribution.

True vascular redistribution reflects a relative reduction of perfusion of the bases with a relative increase in apical perfusion. This phenomenon is probably due to compression of vessels at the lung bases as a result of greater formation of edema. This leads to hypoxemia, pulmonary arteriolar vasoconstriction, and increased pressure, which in turn cause blood flow redistribution to more apical segments.

REFERENCE

1. West, J.B.: Ventilation Blood Flow and Gas Exchange. Oxford, Blackwell Scientific Publications, 1970.

157-E   (All are correct)   *(Braunwald, p. 819)*

From data based on the Framingham Heart Study,[1] the risk for all four types of cardiovascular disease was increased more than twofold. Furthermore, patients with borderline hypertension (pressures between 140/90 and 160/95) also had significantly increased cardiovascular morbidity (averaging 50 per cent higher than that for normotensive patients). The risk of cardiovascular morbidity was proportional to the elevation in blood pressure, had a greater effect in men than women, and caused the greatest increase in risk for atherothrombotic brain infarction.

REFERENCE

1. Castelli, W.P., and Anderson, K.: Population at risk: Prevalence of high cholesterol levels in hypertensive patients in the Framingham Study. Am. J. Med. 80(Suppl. 2A):23, 1986.

158-E   (All are correct)   *(Braunwald, pp. 842–844)*

The presence of certain clinical features should alert the clinician to screen for renovascular hypertension. The four most typical features are recent onset of hypertension, rapid progression, lack of response to therapy, and presence of an abdominal bruit. Although abdominal bruits may be secondary to renal artery or abdominal aortic disease, bruits confined to systole and loudest in the midepigastrium are likely to reflect abdominal aortic atherosclerosis. Patients with renovascular disease are likely to have a greater acute increase in their plasma renin levels after receiving a converting enzyme inhibitor than that seen in patients with essential hypertension.[1] This rise in renin may correlate with deterioration in chronic renal function secondary to inhibition of the renin-angiotensin system.

REFERENCE

1. Muller, F.B., Sealey, J.E., Case, D.B., Atlas, S.A., Pickering, T.G., Pecker, M.S., Prebisz, J.J., and Laragh, J.H.: The captopril test for identifying renovascular disease in hypertensive patients. Am. J. Med. 80:633, 1986.

159-A   (1, 2, and 3 are correct)   *(Braunwald, pp. 749–754)*

Most forms of PVCs are prognostically benign in patients who have no known heart disease.[1] However, in patients who have had a prior MI, the occurrence of PVCs—particularly if they are frequent and of certain forms—is associated with a high risk of sudden cardiac death.[2] Although there is a great deal of controversy over which classification system and which kinds of PVCs are most frequently associated with SCD, in general increased frequency (usually defined as $\geq$ 10 PVCs per hour), certain forms of PVCs (multiform, bigeminy, short-coupling intervals [R-on-T phenomenon]), and runs of three or more ectopic beats are associated with increased risk of SCD.

LV dysfunction has been shown to be a major factor for increased risk in association with PVCs following MI.[3] Furthermore, it appears that the increased risk of SCD following MI persists for at least up to 3 years following MI as long as frequent and complex forms of PVCs are present. Unfortunately, the efficacy of antiarrhythmic therapy in the treatment of PVCs after MI has not been well documented. As of this writing it is probably reasonable to treat patients after MI with antiarrhythmic therapy. However, definitive clinical studies documenting the efficacy of antiarrhythmic therapy in these patients are not yet available.[4, 5]

REFERENCES

1. Kennedy, H.L., Whitlock, J.A., Sprague, M.K., Kennedy, L.J., Buckingham, T.A., and Goldberg, R.J.: Long-term follow-up of asymptomatic healthy subjects with frequent and complex ventricular ectopy. N. Engl. J. Med. 312:193, 1985.
2. Ruberman, W., Weinblatt, E., Goldberg, J.D., Frank, C.W., and Shapiro, S.: Ventricular premature beats and mortality after myocardial infarction. N. Engl. J. Med. 297:750, 1977.
3. Bigger, J.T., Fleiss, J.L., Kleiger, R., Miller, J.P., Rolnitzky, L.M., and the Multicenter Post-Infarction Research Group: The relationships among ventricular arrhythmias, left ventricular dysfunction and mortality in the 2 years after myocardial infarction. Circulation 69:250, 1984.
4. Graboys, T.B., Lown, B., Podrid, P.J., and DeSilva, R.: Long-term survival of patients with malignant ventricular arrhythmias treated with antiarrhythmic drugs. Am. J. Cardiol. 50:437, 1982.
5. Myerburg, R.J., Saman, L., Luceri, R., Kessler, K.M., Kayden, D., and Castellanos, A.: Antiarrhythmic drug therapy after myocardial infarction. In Kulbertus, H.E., and Wellens, H.J.J. (eds.): The First Year After Myocardial Infarction. Mt. Kisco, NY, Futura Publishing Co., 1983, pp. 321–339.

160-C   (2 and 4 are correct)   *(Braunwald, text and Table 21–4, p. 631)*

The systemic lupus erythematosus (SLE)-like syndrome induced by procainamide therapy occurs in approximately 20 to 30 per cent of patients taking the drug on a chronic basis despite the development of antinuclear antibodies in between 60 and 70 per cent of all patients receiving this drug. The syndrome, which is reversible when procainamide therapy is stopped, is characterized by a variety of symptoms including arthralgias, pleuro-pericarditis, fever, hepatomegaly, and less commonly a hemorrhagic pericardial effusion with tamponade. Formation of NAPA, which occurs by acetylation of the aromatic amino group on procainamide, appears to prevent the development of the SLE-like syndrome, implicating this amino group in the pathophysiology of the syndrome.[1] It is not necessary to discontinue the drug upon the development of positive serological tests. However, the development of symptoms or a positive anti-DNA antibody is a contraindication to procainamide therapy, except in patients whose life-threatening arrhythmia is controlled only by procainamide. In this latter group, the concomitant use of steroids may eliminate the clinical manifestations of the SLE-like syndrome.

REFERENCE

1. Kluger, J., Drayer, D.E., Reidenberg, M.M., and Lahita, R.: Acetylprocainamide therapy in patients with previous procainamide-induced lupus syndrome. Ann. Intern. Med. 95:18, 1981.

161-B (1 and 3 are correct) (*Braunwald, p. 557*)

In the case of respiratory failure in which hypoxemia is present without hypercapnia, the role of mechanical ventilation is to increase the mean lung volume during the respiratory cycle; this opens more alveoli for gas exchange. If hypoxemia is not corrected by mechanical ventilation, increasing concentrations of inspired O_2 are required, as in this case. When the FIO_2 exceeds 60 per cent for more than 24 hours, pulmonary alveolar damage due to O_2 toxicity develops. Therefore, positive end-expiratory pressure (PEEP) is utilized because it allows equivalent levels of arterial oxygenation at lower concentrations of FIO_2 by increasing end-expiratory lung volume.

Several common complications of PEEP should be considered. The first is that the high intrathoracic pressure and increased lung volumes which occur impede venous return and prevent appropriate functioning of the right ventricle, with resulting reductions in cardiac output. This is manifested by the development of cool extremities and decreased urine output. Therefore, it is important to monitor cardiac function with a Swan-Ganz catheter and/or thermodilution techniques upon institution of PEEP. The appropriate PEEP setting is achieved when the pulmonary capillary wedge pressure is minimized while cardiac output is maintained.

The predominant mechanism for decreased cardiac output secondary to PEEP is believed to be increased intrathoracic pressure with impaired venous return. This causes inadequate right ventricular output, which results in decreased left ventricular output. Displacement of the interventricular septum toward the left ventricle impairs left ventricular diastolic filling directly. Barotrauma, another complication of mechanical ventilation, is worsened by PEEP. The development of pneumomediastinum, pneumothorax, and subcutaneous emphysema is not uncommon during PEEP.

162-A (1, 2, and 3 are correct) (*Braunwald, p. 474*)

The clinical expression of congestive heart failure in neonates and infants is somewhat different from that in adults or older children. Growth retardation, feeding difficulties, tachypnea, and excessive sweating may all be manifestations of heart failure in the first year of life. Other common signs of heart failure in this group include repeated pulmonary infections, tachycardia, and tachypnea (from the reduction in tidal volume precipitated by interstitial edema), nasal flaring and rib retraction with breathing, and poor peripheral perfusion with cool limbs. Left atrial or pulmonary artery enlargement may actually impinge on adjacent airways, leading to emphysematous expansion of the left lung or even atelectasis. While hepatomegaly is seen frequently in either right or left heart failure, the ascites and peripheral edema that are often seen in adults with heart failure are much less common in infants. Interestingly, facial edema is more common than peripheral edema in this age group. A further physical finding of systemic venous congestion is the prominence of veins on the dorsum of the hands. This may be a valuable clue in an infant, in whom jugular venous distention is not easily observed because of a short neck.

163-A (1, 2, and 3 are correct) (*Braunwald, pp. 755–756*)

Studies of in-hospital mortality due to acute myocardial infarction have shown a significant reduction in mortality since the advent of coronary care units. This has been postulated to be due to the rapid and appropriate management of potentially lethal arrhythmias in this setting. Because of these findings, the extrapolation was made in the 1960's that sudden cardiac death in the out-of-hospital setting was also due to acute myocardial infarction. However, recent studies have demonstrated that only a minority of survivors of out-of-hospital ventricular fibrillation had evidence for a new transmural myocardial infarction.[1] Instead, these studies have indicated that in the majority of such patients, transient events such as acute ischemia and/or thrombosis were responsible for the cardiac arrest.

It has become clear that arrhythmias are the dominant cause for out-of-hospital sudden cardiac death. Hinkle[2] classified cardiac deaths among 142 subjects who died during a follow-up of 5 to 10 years as either arrhythmic death or circulatory failure death. Of all cardiac deaths that occurred less than 1 hour after the onset of the terminal illness, 93 per cent were due to arrhythmias. In addition, 90 per cent of all deaths due to heart disease were initiated by arrhythmic events rather than circulatory failure. Furthermore, when Holter monitors have been fortuitously applied prior to SCD, a pattern of progressive increase in the frequency of both heart rate and ventricular ectopy and the severity of ectopy, including R-on-T phenomenon, has been documented.[3] Finally, Davies and Thomas[4] found that 95 of 100 subjects who died suddenly (less than 6 hours after onset of symptoms) had acute coronary thrombi, plaque fissuring, or both. It is noteworthy that in only 44 per cent of these patients did the largest thrombus occlude 51 per cent or more of the cross section of the involved artery, and only 18 per cent of the patients had more than a 75 per cent occlusion. This suggests that, in addition to the purely mechanical obstruction, a vasomotor (coronary spasm) component may have been involved in the generation of the ventricular arrhythmias leading to SCD.

REFERENCES

1. Baum, R.S., Alvarez, H., and Cobb, L.A.: Survival after resuscitation from out-of-hospital ventricular fibrillation. Circulation 50:1231, 1974.
2. Hinkle, L.E.: The immediate antecedents of sudden death. Acta Med. Scand. 210:207, 1981.
3. Pratt, C.M., Francis, M.J., Luck, J.C., Wyndham, C.R., Miller, R.R., and Quinones, M.A.: Analysis of ambulatory electrocardiograms in 15 patients during spontaneous ventricular fibrillation with special reference to preceding arrhythmic events. J. Am. Coll. Cardiol. 2:789, 1983.
4. Davies, M.J., and Thomas, A.: Thrombosis and acute coronary artery lesions in sudden cardiac ischemic death. N. Engl. J. Med. 310:1137, 1984.

164-B   (1 and 3 are correct)   (Braunwald, pp. 515–516)

Diuretic therapy causes profound effects on the renal handling of most electrolytes, including potassium, sodium, and magnesium.[1] While the role of oral potassium supplementation in diuretic-induced hypokalemia is controversial,[2] certain patients remain at higher risk for hypokalemic complications and should receive such supplementation. Patients with congestive heart failure are at increased risk for development of malignant ventricular arrhythmias and also often receive digitalis therapy. In such patients it is prudent to administer supplemental potassium or a potassium-sparing diuretic to maintain a serum potassium level greater than 3.5 mEq/liter. However, in other patients, such as those in whom hypokalemia has not emerged with diuretic therapy or in patients with reduced renal function, potassium supplementation may be inadvisable or even hazardous.

Hyponatremia is a common complication of diuretic therapy with all of the diuretics currently used to treat heart failure. Hyponatremia is more prevalent in patients in whom diuretic therapy is relatively ineffective or in patients who have worsening myocardial failure, and it is thus correlated with cardiovascular mortality.[3] Mild hyponatremia may respond to fluid restriction.

Hypomagnesemia may also occur with either loop or thiazide diuretics and is caused by renal magnesium wasting. Chronic diuretic therapy usually leads to depletion of total body magnesium stores. The clinician thus needs to remain aware of the potential need for magnesium supplementation.

REFERENCES

1. Hollenberg, N.K.: Potassium, magnesium, and cardiovascular morbidity. Am. J. Med. 80(4A):1, 1986.
2. Papademetrius, V.: Diuretics, hypokalemia and cardiac arrhythmias: A critical analysis. Am. Heart J. 111:1217, 1986.
3. Lee, W.H., and Packer, M.: Prognostic importance of serum sodium concentration and its modification by converting enzyme inhibition in patients with severe chronic heart failure. Circulation 73:257, 1986.

165-A   (1, 2, and 3 are correct)   (Braunwald, pp. 674–675)

The electrocardiogram illustrated shows atrial tachycardia with block (or paroxysmal atrial tachycardia with block; PAT with block). In this condition an atrial rate of 130 to 200 beats/min with a ventricular response less than or equal to the atrial rate is noted. Digitalis toxicity accounts for this rhythm in 50 to 75 per cent of cases, and in such instances the atrial rate may show a gradual increase as digitalis dosing is continued. Commonly other signs of digitalis excess are present, including frequent premature ventricular complexes and noncardiac signs of digitalis toxicity.

In nearly half of all patients with PAT with block, the atrial rate is irregular and demonstrates a characteristic isoelectric interval between each P wave, in contrast to the morphology of atrial flutter waves. Most instances of PAT with block occur in patients with significant organic heart disease. Etiologies other than digitalis toxicity include ischemic heart disease, MI, and cor pulmonale. In patients taking digitalis, potassium depletion may precipitate the arrhythmia, and the oral administration of potassium and the withholding of digitalis often will allow reversion to normal sinus rhythm. Because PAT with block is seen primarily in patients with serious underlying heart disease, its onset may lead to significant clinical deterioration. Thus it must be carefully sought in cardiac patients receiving digitalis treatment.

166-E   (1, 2, 3, and 4 are correct)   (Braunwald, pp. 614)

A careful, accurate history and thorough physical examination are most important in the evaluation of syncope of unknown cause.[1] In patients with syncope of unknown cause, the overall 1-year mortality approaches 6 per cent. In patients with noncardiovascular causes, 1-year mortality is between 1 and 12 per cent, but in those with identified cardiovascular causes, mortality approaches 20 to 30 per cent.[2] The three most common arrhythmic causes of syncope are sinus node dysfunction, tachyarrhythmias, and AV block. While electrophysiological (EP) studies have proven useful for identifying each of these disturbances, of the three, tachyarrhythmias are most reliably initiated in the electrophysiology laboratory.

When an abnormality is found on EP testing that may explain syncope, subsequent therapy directed at this abnormality prevents recurrence of syncope in about 80 per cent of patients.[3] However, the ability of EP testing to uncover a cause for syncope varies widely and is lowest in patients with no recognizable structural heart disease. The induction of a sustained supraventricular or monomorphic ventricular tachycardia in patients who have not displayed spontaneous development of such tachycardias on noninvasive evaluation is relatively uncommon but highly suggestive that the induced tachyarrhythmia is clinically relevant.

REFERENCES

1. Lipsitz, L.A.: Syncope in the elderly. Ann. Intern. Med. 90:92, 1983.
2. Kapoor, W.N., Karpf, M., Wieland, S., Peterson, J.R., and Levey,

G.S.: A prospective evaluation and followup of patients with syncope. N. Engl. J. Med. 309:197, 1983.
3. DiMarco, J.P., Garan, H., and Ruskin, J.N.: Approach to the patient with recurrent syncope of unknown causes. Mod. Concepts Cardiovasc. Dis. 52:11, 1983.

167-A (1, 2, and 3 are correct) *(Braunwald, pp. 625–628)*

Lidocaine has proven to be an extremely effective agent in the therapy of ventricular arrhythmias of diverse etiologies. The drug has a fairly wide toxic:therapeutic ratio, with a low incidence of hemodynamic complications that are rarely seen unless left ventricular function is severely impaired. While lidocaine reduces the action potential duration and the effective refractory period of Purkinje fibers and ventricular muscle, it has little effect on atrial fibers and does not affect conduction in accessory pathways.

Metabolism of lidocaine is largely hepatic and thus depends on hepatic blood flow. The elimination half-life of the substance averages 1 to 2 hours in normal subjects but is more than 4 hours in patients after relatively uncomplicated MI and is 10 hours or longer in patients who sustain MI complicated by cardiac failure or cardiogenic shock. In addition, hepatic disease or decreased hepatic blood flow, as in congestive heart failure, decreases the rate of lidocaine metabolism. Thus, there are a variety of clinical situations requiring that maintenance doses of lidocaine be reduced by one-third to one-half of normal. Patients treated with an initial bolus of lidocaine followed by a maintenance infusion may experience transient *subtherapeutic* plasma concentrations at 30 to 120 minutes after therapy is begun.[1] Therefore, a second bolus of lidocaine of approximately one-half the initial dose 20 to 40 minutes following onset of therapy is recommended.

REFERENCE

1. Nattel, S., and Zipes, D.P.: Clinical pharmacology of old and new antiarrhythmic drugs. Cardiovasc. Res. *11*:221, 1980.

168-A (1, 2, and 3 are correct) *(Braunwald, pp. 389–394)*

Since the classic experiments of Ringer in 1882, it has been appreciated that cardiac contraction depends on the presence of intracellular Ca^{++}. In fact, the magnitude of cardiac contraction has been shown to be proportional to the intracellular Ca^{++} concentration. It has also been observed that depolarization of the plasma membrane associated with the upstroke of the action potential opens voltage-dependent channels that bring Ca^{++} into the cell. Ca^{++} that passes into the cell through these channels does not actually appear to activate the contractile system directly but rather is stored in membrane sites within the cells, specifically the T system and the sarcoplasmic reticulum (SR). The Ca^{++} that actually activates the contractile system appears to be stored in the cisternae of the SR and released upon membrane depolarization. This process is termed Ca^{++}-induced Ca^{++} release. According to this concept, the depolarization of the cell membrane causes release of Ca^{++} from the terminal cisternae of the SR into the cytoplasm. Ca^{++} binding by troponin results in activation of the contractile elements, and relaxation is brought about by the active uptake of Ca^{++} into another area of the SR. There it is stored only to be released during the subsequent contraction.

Several mechanisms have been identified for regulation of intracellular Ca^{++} concentration in cardiac cells.[2] Included in these are: (1) Inward movement of Ca^{++} along its concentration gradient across the sarcolemma via Ca^{++} channels to generate the "slow" inward current. Beta-adrenergic agonists increase myocardial contractility in part by increasing Ca^{++} *influx* into cardiac cells by opening receptor-activated channels. (2) A bidirectional Na^+-Ca^{++} exchange system that mediates movement of Ca^{++} across the sarcolemma along a concentration gradient provided by Na^+. In general, Ca^{++} is pumped out in exchange for Na^+. However, when cardiac glycosides inhibit the Na^+, K^+-ATPase with elevation of intracellular Na^+, then Ca^{++} may enter the cell, bringing about a positive inotropic effect.[3] (3) A sarcolemmal Ca^{++}-ATPase that extrudes Ca^{++} from the cell. (4) A Ca^{++}-stimulated magnesium-ATPase in the membrane of the SR which transports Ca^{++} into the SR. (5) Uptake of Ca^{++} in other structures such as mitochondria. (6) A buffering of intracellular Ca^{++} by proteins such as calmodulin, troponin C, and the myosin light chains.

REFERENCES

1. Fabiato, A.: Stimulated calcium current can both cause calcium loading in and trigger calcium release from the sarcoplasmic reticulum of a skinned canine cardiac Purkinje cell. J. Gen. Physiol. 85:291, 1985.
2. Braunwald, E.: Mechanisms of actions of calcium channel blocking agents. N. Engl. J. Med. 307:1618, 1982.
3. Mullins, L.J.: The role of Na-Ca exchange in heart. *In* Sperelakis, N (ed.): Physiology and Pathophysiology of the Heart. Boston, Martinus Nijhoff, 1984, p. 199.

169-D (4 is correct) *(Braunwald, pp. 427–429)*

Many studies have shown that the fundamental defect in cardiac contractility in the hypertrophied and failing ventricle is an intrinsic property of the muscle. Despite this depressed contractility, cardiac output in the basal state is often maintained. Compensatory mechanisms at the cellular level include (1) an *increase* in length of the sarcomeres so that the overlap between myofibrils is optimal (approximately 2.2 μm) and (2) an increase in muscle mass due to cellular hypertrophy. Often, however, there is clear evidence for myocardial dysfunction, reflected in a reduction in the maximal shortening velocity. Studies involving manipulation of left ventricular end-diastolic volume have shown that failing hearts function on the ascending limb of a depressed Starling curve rather than on the descending limb of a normal curve.[1]

REFERENCE

1. Spann, J.F., et al.: Contractile performance of the hypertrophied and chronically failing cat ventricle. Am. J. Physiol. 223:1150, 1972.

170-C (2 and 4 are correct) *(Braunwald, pp. 429–434)*

LV afterload, which reflects the impedance (resistance) to ejection, is a fundamental determinant of LV performance. In mitral regurgitation (MR) and ventricular septal defect (VSD), LV afterload is reduced because blood is ejected into low impedance reservoirs, the left atrium and right ventricle, respectively. In both aortic regurgitation and patent ductus arteriosus, there is a decrease in aortic impedance as documented by the fall in diastolic pressure. However, the decrease in impedance to ventricular ejection is considerably smaller than in VSD or MR. LV afterload remains the same, namely the high pressure aorta.[1] Furthermore, the myocardial oxygen requirements are much lower in MR and VSD, allowing for greater myocardial functional reserve at any given workload.[2]

REFERENCES

1. Urschel, C.W., Covell, J.W., Sonnenblick, E.H., Ross, J., Jr., and Braunwald, E.: Myocardial mechanics in aortic and mitral valvular regurgitation: The concept of instantaneous impedance as a determinant of the performance of the intact heart. J. Clin. Invest. 47:867, 1968.
2. Urschel, C.W., Covell, J.W., Graham, T.P., Clancy, R.L., Ross, J., Jr., Sonnenblick, E.H., and Braunwald, E.: Effects of acute valvular regurgitation on the oxygen consumption of the canine heart. Circ. Res. 23:33, 1968.

171-A (1, 2, and 3 are correct) *(Braunwald, pp. 426–427)*

The three fundamental mechanisms by which the left ventricle compensates for decreased contractile function or increased contractile burden are:

1. The Frank-Starling mechanism by which an increase in preload lengthens resting sarcomeres to enhance their performance via increased activation;

2. An increase in neurohumoral adrenergic responses which results in increased inotropy; and

3. Myocardial hypertrophy with or without chamber dilation.

Venous return in congestive heart failure is often maintained by coexisting venoconstriction.

172-A (1, 2, and 3 are correct) *(Braunwald, pp. 439–444)*

The importance of the adrenergic nervous system in heart failure is shown by the nearly universal worsening of symptoms upon administration of adrenoceptor blocking agents. On one hand there is an enhanced adrenoceptor state that may be responsible for vasoconstriction and that may cause cardiac arrhythmias. On the other hand, there is diminished adrenoceptor control in heart failure, including blunted increases in heart rate, vascular resistance, and arterial pressure during tilting.[1] In low–cardiac output states there also usually is activation of the renin-angiotensin-aldosterone axis with elevations of circulating renin and angiotensin II. Therefore, although administration of an angiotensin-converting enzyme inhibitor will benefit the patient by decreasing afterload, it may also increase the risks of development of orthostatic hypotensive events.

To avoid hypotensive episodes such as occurred in this patient, several precautions should be observed. First, patients with elevated blood urea nitrogen values, low blood pressure, and signs of volume depletion who are taking high diuretic doses should be considered at increased risk. In patients with heart failure captopril should be initiated under close supervision and in those at increased risk of hypotension, as outlined, it should be begun with a small dose (6.25 mg). If well tolerated, the dosage can be increased at weekly intervals, based on clinical response and blood pressure to a maximum of 50 mg t.i.d. Following the first dose and each upward adjustment of dosage, the patient should be particularly cautious when assuming the erect posture.

REFERENCE

1. Hubo, S.T., and Cody, R.J.: Circulatory aorto-regulation in chronic congestive heart failure. Responses to head-up tilt in 41 patients. Am. J. Cardiol. 52:512, 1983.

173-C (2 and 4 are correct) *(Braunwald, pp. 451–452)*

The utility of measuring both ventricular performance (cardiac index) and ventricular preload (LVEDP) is that the combination can distinguish patients with depressed ventricular performance due to depressed contractility (patients 2 and 4) from patients with hypovolemia and decreased preload (patients 1 and 3). In the intensive care unit differentiating patients with decreased preload from those with decreased LV contractility can be difficult. A diagnostic maneuver that may also be therapeutic is rapid infusion of 300 ml of normal saline over 15 to 30 min. This acutely increases preload and raises LVEDP. In patients with decreased cardiac output from hypovolemia an increase in cardiac output would be expected, but not in those with impaired LV contractility.

174-A (1, 2, and 3 are correct) *(Braunwald, pp. 458–464)*

The LV responds to an increased afterload by hypertrophy in an attempt to maintain wall stress constant. In a pressure-overload state, hypertrophy is concentric due to addition of muscle fibers in parallel. This is associated with a rise in end-diastolic pressure as the LV wall stiffens. Ultimately, ejection fraction may fall. However, this must be related to the existing level of afterload to determine whether this reduction reflects a true decrease in contractility—e.g., after aortic valve replacement, in many patients ejection fraction increases dramatically, reflecting primarily a reduction in afterload.

175-E (1 and 3 are correct) *(Braunwald, p. 720)*

Patients with symptomatic AV conduction disturbances such as third-degree (complete) AV block, sick sinus syndrome, and severe sinus bradycardia should receive permanent pacemakers.[1] However, prophylactic permanent pacing in the *asymptomatic* individual is a controversial issue. Most experts agree that patients with complete AV block and well-documented Mobitz Type II second-degree AV block commonly progress to symptomatic AV block and therefore should also be paced. In contrast, the prognosis for patients with chronic bundle branch block is largely determined by the nature of their underlying cardiac disease so that patients with isolated bundle branch block and normal cardiac function have a good prognosis. Although patients with chronic bifascicular block and a prolonged H-V interval develop AV block much more often than do patients with a normal H-V interval (4.5 versus 0.6 per cent), the absolute risk of complete heart block in these patients is still small; therefore, permanent pacing is not indicated.[2]

REFERENCES

1. Frye, R., Collins, J., DeSanctis, R., Dodge, H., Dreifus, L., Fisch, C., Gettes, L., Gillette, P., Parsonnet, V., Reeves, T.J., and Weinberg, S.: Guidelines for permanent cardiac pacemaker implantation. Report of the Joint American College of Cardiology/American Heart Association Task Force on Assessment of Cardiovascular Procedures Subcommittee on Pacemaker Implantation. J. Am. Coll. Cardiol. 4:434, 1984.
2. Dhingra, R., Palileo, E., Strasberg, B., Swiryn, S., Bauernfeind, R., Wyndham, C., and Rosen, K.: Significance of the HV interval in 517 patients with chronic bifascicular block. Circulation 64:1265, 1981.

176-C   (2 and 4 are correct)   (Braunwald, pp. 734–737)

The electrocardiogram illustrates a combination of intermittent failure to pace with loss of capture (pacer spikes 1, 3–8, and 10) and intermittent undersensing (pacer spike 7). Failure to pace occurs when the pacemaker fails to deliver a stimulus when one should occur or when it delivers a stimulus that fails to depolarize the myocardium at a time when the tissue is excitable. Failure to deliver a stimulus may be due to (1) improper lead connection to the generator, (2) broken lead wires, (3) failure of a component of the pulse generator, (4) power-source depletion, or (5) oversensing. Delivery of an ineffective stimulus with loss of capture may result from (1) lead dislodgement or an unstable tip, as in this case; (2) defective lead insulation or wire breakage; (3) increased stimulation threshold due to infarct, drugs, or fibrosis; and (4) inappropriate pacemaker stimulus strength.

Failure to sense may be due to lead dislodgement (the most common cause). Inadequate amplitude or wave slope of the intracardiac electrogram may be caused by fibrosis, infarct, drugs, electrolyte disturbances, inappropriate programming sensitivity, lead breakage or insulation defect, or component failure.

Oversensing occurs when a pacemaker senses signals other than the signals it is designed to detect. Common causes include sensed T waves if unusually large or delayed, sensed atrial activity, and sensed skeletal muscle potentials with inappropriate inhibition.

Pacing at an altered rate may be caused by oversensing with rate slowing due to inhibition or rate acceleration due to triggering; built-in rate reduction, which indicates power source depletion; and component failure.

177-E   (All are correct)   (Braunwald, pp. 849–852)

Pregnancy-induced hypertension is defined as hypertension developing after the 20th week of gestation. If proteinuria or edema accompanies the hypertension, preeclampsia is present. The development of convulsions heralds eclampsia. Indications of preeclampsia include age < 20, primigravid state, sudden weight gain (> 2 pounds/week) or edema, and increasing plasma uric acid. The absolute level of blood pressure is usually lower than in the chronic hypertensive, especially since blood pressure falls during the course of normal pregnancy.[1] However, the blood pressures of women who develop preeclampsia were found to be higher during the first half of pregnancy compared with those who remained normotensive throughout.[1]

REFERENCE

1. Mountquin, J.M., Rainville, C., Giroux, L., Raynauld, P., Amyot, G., Bilodeau, R., and Pelland, N.: A prospective study of blood pressure in pregnancy. Prediction of preeclampsia. Am. J. Obstet. Gynecol. 151:191, 1985.

178-B   (1 and 3 are correct)   (Braunwald, pp. 685–692)

Electrocardiographic evidence of the WPW syndrome is present in approximately 0.25 per cent of healthy individuals. Three basic features characterize the ECG abnormalities of the syndrome: the presence of a P-R interval less than 120 msec during sinus rhythm; a QRS duration greater than 120 msec with a slurred, slowly rising onset of the QRS in some leads (the delta wave); and secondary ST-T wave changes generally directed opposite to the major QRS vector.[1]

While the prevalence of WPW decreases with age, the frequency of paroxysmal tachycardia associated with the syndrome apparently increases with age. Most such tachycardias are reciprocating arrhythmias (80 per cent), with 15 to 30 per cent presenting as atrial fibrillation and 5 per cent as atrial flutter. Although most adults with the WPW syndrome have normal hearts, a number of cardiac defects are occasionally associated with this syndrome, including Ebstein's anomaly.[2] In patients with Ebstein's anomaly, multiple accessory pathways are often present and are located on the right side of the heart, with preexcitation localized to the atrialized ventricle. These patients often have reciprocating tachycardia with a long V-A interval and RBBB morphology of the QRS complex.

REFERENCES

1. Willems, J.L., Robles de Medina, E.O., Bernard, R., Coumel, P., Fisch, C., Krikler, D., Mazur, N.A., Meijler, F.L., Morgensen, L., Moret, P., Pisa, Z., Rautaharju, P.M., Surawicz, B., Watanabe, Y., and Wellens, H.J.J.: Criteria for intraventricular conduction disturbances and preexcitation. J. Am. Coll. Cardiol. 5:1261, 1985.
2. Smith, W.M., Gallagher, J.J., Kerr, C.R., Sealy, W.C., Kasell, J.H., Benson, D.W., Jr., Reiter, M.J., Sterba, R., and Grant, A.O.: The electrophysiologic basis and management of symptomatic recurrent tachycardia in patients with Ebstein's anomaly of the tricuspid valve. Am. J. Cardiol. 49:1223, 1982.

179-B   (1 and 3 are correct)   (Braunwald, pp. 628–630; see also Answer to Question 123, p. 64, this book.)

Gastrointestinal symptoms, which include nausea, vomiting, anorexia, diarrhea, and abdominal pain, are the most common side effects of chronic oral quinidine therapy. *Cinchonism* is the term used to describe the less common central nervous system toxic side effects of the drug. These are manifested as tinnitus, hearing loss, visual disturbances, and alterations in mental status including confusion, delirium, and even psychosis. Allergic reactions to the drug may occur and include rash or fever as well as an immune-mediated thrombocytopenia. This arises from the presence of antibodies to quinidine-platelet complexes capable of causing platelet agglutination and lysis. In between 0.5 and 2 per cent of patients, quinidine may produce syncope, which is usually the result of a self-terminating episode of polymorphic ventricular tachycardia with long Q-T interval as an antecedent, known as torsades de pointes.[1] Quinidine prolongs the Q-T interval in most patients, and relatively marked prolongation of this interval is a general characteristic of quinidine therapy. Therapy for quinidine syncope includes immediate discontinuation of the drug, the use of atrial or ventricular pacing to suppress the tachyarrhythmia, isoproterenol infusion to pharmacologically increase the heart rate, and the use of intravenous magnesium to suppress the rhythm.[2] In addition, concomitant hypokalemia must be corrected and other antiarrhythmic agents with similar mechanisms of action (such as disopyramide) must be avoided in patients with quinidine syncope.

REFERENCES

1. Roden, D.M., Woosley, R.L., and Primm, K.: Incidence and clinical features of the quinidine-associated long QT syndrome: Implications for patient care. Am. Heart J. *111*:1088, 1986.
2. Tzivoni, D., Keren, A., Cohen, A.M., Loebel, H., Zahair, I., Chenzbraun, A., and Stern, S.: Magnesium therapy for torsades de pointes. Am. J. Cardiol. 53:538, 1984.

180-E   (1, 2, 3, and 4 are correct)   *(Braunwald, pp. 809–810)*

Primary pulmonary hypertension (PPH) is found more commonly in females and presents at a mean age of 34 years. In the largest natural history study of PPH, reported from the Mayo Clinic,[1] the most common clinical features at the time of diagnosis included prominent second heart sounds (98 per cent); cardiomegaly and prominent central pulmonary arteries on chest x-ray (95 per cent); RV hypertrophy, right axis deviation, and P pulmonale on the ECG (95 per cent); and exertional dyspnea (75 per cent). Exertional dizziness or syncope was seen in approximately 30 per cent of the patients, and the average time from initial clinical manifestations to the time of diagnosis was approximately 2 years. Prognosis in this and in other series was poor, with approximately 20 per cent 5-year survival.

In the Mayo Clinic series (a nonrandomized study), patients receiving anticoagulants had a better survival rate than patients who did not receive these agents. Death in patients with PPH was most commonly due to right heart failure, with pneumonia and sudden death playing lesser roles. It should be noted that death related to cardiac catheterization is not uncommon, and this procedure must be carried out with caution in such patients. Patients with PPH may complain of precordial

chest pain that is probably due to either ischemia of the RV subendocardium and/or distention of the major pulmonary arteries.[2] This pain more commonly radiates to the neck but not characteristically to the arms, which helps distinguish it from angina pectoris. Exertional dyspnea, syncope, weakness, and later dyspnea at rest are among the more common symptoms of PPH.

Physical examination discloses evidence of pulmonary hypertension and RV pressure overload. The ECG in PPH usually displays right axis deviation, RV hypertrophy, and right atrial abnormality. Chest x-ray may show enlargement of the right pulmonary artery and its major branches, with marked tapering or pruning of peripheral arteries. Pulmonary function tests are usually normal. Perfusion lung scans in patients with PPH are usually either normal or indeterminate. It should be noted that performance of lung scanning may be dangerous late in the course of PPH due to impingement on the pulmonary vascular bed by the radioisotope-labeled particles used to perform the scan.

REFERENCES

1. Fuster, V., Steele, P.M., Edwards, W.D., Gersh, B.J., McGoon, M.D., and Frye, R.L.: Primary pulmonary hypertension: Natural history and the importance of thrombosis. Circulation 70:580, 1984.
2. Ross, R.S.: Right ventricular hypertension as a cause of precordial pain. Am. Heart J. *61*:134, 1961.

181-A   (1, 2, and 3 are correct)   *(Braunwald, pp. 548–549)*

In the lung there is normally a continuous exchange of liquid, colloid, and solutes between the vascular bed and interstitium. An imbalance of the forces resulting in net influx of liquids, colloids, and solutes from the vasculature to the interstitial space results in pulmonary edema. The classic Starling equation can be applied to the lung as well as to the systemic circulation, and it states that the net rate of transudation (flow of liquid from blood vessels to interstitial space) is equal to the hydrostatic force minus the colloid osmotic force. Thus, the classification of pulmonary edema can be made on the basis of whether there are imbalances of the Starling forces or alterations in alveolar capillary membrane permeability, lymphatic insufficiency, or other unknown mechanisms such as neurogenic pulmonary edema.

With regard to imbalance of the Starling forces, three major mechanisms exist: (1) increased pulmonary capillary pressure secondary to increased pulmonary venous pressure without left ventricular failure (as in mitral stenosis or with left ventricular failure as in acute MI) or increased pulmonary capillary pressure secondary to increased pulmonary arterial pressure as occurs in so-called overperfusion pulmonary edema, which exists experimentally (although questionably clinically); (2) decreased plasma oncotic pressure, as occurs with hypoalbuminemia secondary to nephrotic syndrome, hepatic disease, or protein-losing enteropathy; and (3) increased negative interstitial pressure as occurs with rapid removal of a pneumothorax with a large applied negative unilateral pressure. Theoretically, increased interstitial oncotic pressure could also generate pulmonary edema; however, no clinical example of this has been documented. Nonetheless, the appearance of increased concentrations of macromolecules in the liquid phase of the interstitium or in the alveoli probably does serve to perpetuate the process of edema formation. Increased plasma oncotic pressure would decrease the transudative forces and theoretically decrease flow from the blood vessel to lung.

182-E (All are correct) (*Braunwald, pp. 870–871*)

Although thiazide diuretics are an inexpensive and effective therapy, their role as the initial therapeutic choice for hypertension has been increasingly questioned because of side effects. The most common side effect is hypokalemia; serum potassium falls an average of 0.67 mmol/liter after institution of continuous daily thiazide therapy.[1] Hypomagnesemia is usually mild but may prevent the restoration of intracellular deficits of potassium.[2] Therefore, it should be corrected. Serum uric acid is elevated in one-third of untreated hypertensives and hyperuricemia appears in another third during diuretic therapy, probably due to increased proximal tubule reabsorption of uric acid. Hyperlipidemia is a particularly vexing problem associated with diuretics[3] because the rise in cholesterol may ultimately increase the incidence of coronary disease. Interestingly, there is a rise in serum calcium (usually < 0.5 mg/dl) probably as a consequence of increased calcium reabsorption in the proximal tubule induced by volume contraction.[4] Other rare side effects associated with diuretics include hyperglycemia and impotence.

REFERENCES

1. Morgan, D.B., and Davidson, C.: Hypokalemia and diuretics: An analysis of publications. Br. Med. J. *280*:905, 1980.
2. Whang, R., Flink, E.B., Dyckner, T., Wester, P.O., Aikawa, J.K., and Ryan, M.P.: Magnesium depletion as a cause of refractory potassium repletion. Arch. Intern. Med. *145*:1686, 1985.
3. Johnson, B.F., Saunders, R., Hickler, R., Marwaha, R., and Johnson, J.: The effects of thiazide diuretics upon plasma lipoproteins. J. Hypertension *4*:235, 1986.
4. Stier, C.T., Jr., and Itskovitz, H.D.: Renal calcium metabolism and diuretics. Annu. Rev. Pharmacol. Toxicol. *26*:101, 1986.

183-C, 184-A, 185-B, 186-D (*Braunwald, pp. 663–669*)

Ventriculophasic sinus arrhythmia is the term applied to phasic variations in the underlying sinus rhythm P-P interval caused by the occurrence of ventricular contractions. Changes in the P-P interval may be due to the influence of the autonomic nervous system upon sinus discharge rate in response to changes in ventricular stroke volume. The most common example of ventriculophasic sinus arrhythmia occurs when complete AV block is present. In some cases of complete AV block, P-P cycles that contain a QRS complex may be shorter than P-P cycles without a QRS complex. The occurrence of a premature ventricular complex during normal sinus rhythm may be followed by a compensatory pause; lengthening of the subsequent P-P cycle is another example of a ventriculophasic sinus arrhythmia.

The general term sinus arrhythmia is applied to instances of phasic variation in sinus cycle length that are found frequently and are considered a normal event. In sinus arrhythmia, P wave morphology does not change and the P-R interval exceeds 120 m/sec and is also unchanged. Sinus arrhythmia appears in two basic forms: a respiratory form in which the P-P interval shortens during inspiration as a result of the reflex inhibition of vagal tone in a cyclic manner and a nonrespiratory form that is characterized by a phasic variation in P-P interval that cannot be related to the underlying respiratory events. Sinus arrhythmia commonly occurs in the young, especially in the respiratory form. The nonrespiratory form of sinus arrhythmia may be seen in instances of increased vagal tone, such as after digitalis therapy.[1]

Sinus arrest or sinus pause (see Braunwald, Fig. 22–3, p. 665) is characterized by a pause in the sinus rhythm for which the P-P interval limiting the pause does not equal a multiple of the basic underlying sinus P-P interval. The mechanism of this arrhythmia is believed to be a transient loss of spontaneous sinus-nodal automaticity and may be produced by excessive vagal tone, involvement of the sinus node during acute MI, degenerative fibrotic changes, and digitalis-induced effects. While brief episodes of sinus arrest may not require treatment, patients with chronic forms of sinus node disease with recurrent symptomatic sinus bradycardia or sinus arrest often require permanent pacing.

Sinoatrial (SA) exit block is also characterized by a pause during normal sinus rhythm, but in this arrhythmia the duration of the pause is a multiple of the basic P-P interval. The mechanism of SA exit block involves failure of a sinus impulse to emerge from the sinus node and depolarize the atria.[2] Two types of SA exit block, analogous to AV-nodal blocks, are recognized. Type I (Wenckebach) second-degree SA exit block is marked by the progressive shortening of sequential P-P intervals prior to the pause and by a pause duration that is less than 2 P-P cycles (see Braunwald, Fig. 22–4A, p. 666). Type II second-degree SA exit block is marked by a constant P-P interval, and a pause without P waves that is equal to approximately two, three, or even four times the normal P-P cycle (see Braunwald, Fig. 22–4B, p. 666). While in theory both first-degree and third-degree SA exit block may occur, their diagnosis with routine surface electrocardiography is not possible.

A variant of sinus arrhythmia known as wandering pacemaker occurs when the dominant pacemaker focus shifts from the sinus node to a latent pacemaker with a degree of automaticity close to but slightly less than that of the sinus node. The shift from the sinus focus to the ectopic focus occurs gradually over the duration of several beats, and is characterized by a gradual shortening of the P-R interval and a change in the P wave contour as the focus shifts (see Braunwald, Fig. 22–5, p. 666). Wandering pacemaker is considered to be a normal occurrence secondary to augmented vagal tone and may be seen particularly in young individuals and athletes.

REFERENCES

1. Hrushesky, W.J., Fader, D., Schmitt, O., and Gilbertson, V.: The respiratory sinus arrhythmia: The measure of cardiac age. Science *224*:1001, 1984.

2. Asseman, P., Berzin, B., Desry, D., Vilarem, D., Durand, P., Delmotte, C., Sarkis, E.H., Lekieffre, J., and Thery, C.: Persistent sinus nodal electrograms during abnormally prolonged post pacing atrial pauses in sick sinus syndrome in humans: Sinoatrial block versus overdrive suppression. Circulation 68:33, 1983.

187-B, 188-E, 189-C, 190-E   (Braunwald, pp. 868–878)

The development of drugs to inhibit the renin-angiotensin system has resulted in several new antihypertensive agents that have significant advantages over previously available drugs. The juxtaglomerular cells of the kidney sense blood Na^+ concentration and in response secrete the enzyme renin. This secretion can be inhibited by adrenoceptor blockers such as methyldopa because stimulation of renal nerves releases renin as well. Renin acts on renin substrate produced by the liver to form angiotensin I, which is then converted to the active octapeptide angiotensin II by converting enzyme in the lungs. Captopril is a specific inhibitor of this enzyme and thus prevents formation of angiotensin II. Enalapril differs from captopril in lacking a sulfhydryl group; also it is a "prodrug" that is hydrolyzed after ingestion to form enalaprilat, the active inhibitor. This makes enalapril slower in onset but longer in duration of action than captopril.

Angiotensin II is a potent vasoconstrictor that also acts on the adrenal cortex to increase aldosterone secretion, thereby causing sodium retention. These direct effects can be blocked by the competitive antagonist saralasin.

Ketanserin[1] is a serotonin antagonist that may be useful in some forms of hypertension.

The converting-enzyme inhibitors are a double-edged sword with regard to renovascular hypertension. On the one hand, they are effective in lowering BP.[2] However, by decreasing angiotensin II levels, which maintain efferent renal arteriolar resistance and renal perfusion pressure, they may lower renal perfusion leading to renal failure in patients with renal artery stenosis.[3] Hydralazine and minoxidil, which act primarily as arteriolar vasodilators, maintain cardiac output and renal perfusion pressure by virtue of their ability to activate the arterial baroreceptor reflex; therefore, they are much less likely to precipitate renal failure.

REFERENCES

1. Houston, S.D., and Vanoutte, P.M.: Serotonin and the vascular system. Role in health and disease, and implications for therapy. Drugs 31:149, 1986.
2. Reams, G.P., Bauer, J.H., and Gaddy, P.: Use of the converting enzyme inhibitor enalapril in renovascular hypertension. Hypertension 8:290, 1986.
3. Wenting, G.J., Tan-Tjiong, H.L., Derkx, F.H.M., deBruyn, J.H.B., Man in't Veld, A.J., and Schalekamp, M.A.D.H.: Split renal function after captopril in unilateral renal artery stenosis. Br. Med. J. 288:886, 1984.

191-B, 192-B, 193-B, 194-C   (Braunwald, pp. 698–700)

Torsades de pointes ("turning of the points") was originally described in the setting of bradycardia due to complete heart block. The term is presently used to describe a syndrome characterized by the appearance of a typical varying appearance of ventricular tachycardia as the QRS complexes "twist" around the isoelectric baseline, changing amplitude and contour (see Braunwald, Fig. 22–36A, p. 699). Q-T interval prolongation occurs as part of the syndrome. Although a U wave may be seen prominently, its role in the syndrome itself is unclear. Ventricular tachycardia that is morphologically similar to torsades but that occurs in patients with normal Q-T intervals is termed polymorphic ventricular tachycardia.

The most common predisposing factors for the development of torsades are severe bradycardia, drugs capable of inducing Q-T prolongation (such as quinidine, procainamide, disopyramide, and phenothiazines), and potassium depletion. Therapy of torsades is aimed at correction of the underlying cause of Q-T prolongation, cessation of provocative drugs, and acceleration of the heart rate by temporary pacing or isoproterenol in an attempt to overdrive the ventricular tachycardia.

The long Q-T syndrome occurs in two main categories. In the first, primary or idiopathic, are the inherited disorders that may (Jervell and Lange-Nielsen syndrome) or may not (Romano-Ward syndrome) be associated with deafness. Also, an acquired long Q-T syndrome may be caused by a variety of drugs such as quinidine, disopyramide, phenothiazines, or tricyclic antidepressants, as well as metabolic abnormalities such as hypokalemia and starvation, and as a consequence of the liquid protein diet. This acquired form may or may not have associated episodes of torsades de pointes. The syndrome has also been identified in patients with central nervous system lesions, dysfunction of the autonomic nervous system, and ischemic heart disease.

For patients with idiopathic long Q-T syndromes without a family history of sudden cardiac death, complex ventricular arrhythmia, or any history of syncope, no specific therapy is currently recommended. Patients with a positive family history or those who have experienced syncope are at increased risk of sudden death and should undergo evaluation in the electrophysiology laboratory with attempts to suppress provokable ventricular arrhythmias. Interestingly, the Valsalva maneuver is sometimes useful diagnostically because it may cause a further prolongation of the Q-T interval and provoke ventricular tachycardia in some patients.[1] In asymptomatic patients with complex ventricular ectopy or a family history of sudden death, maximal beta blocker therapy is recommended. In symptomatic patients, beta blockers may be combined with phenytoin and/or phenobarbital. Patients who remain resistant to drug therapy may require sympathetic ganglionectomy to interrupt the left stellate ganglion.[2] Patients unable to respond to this intervention may ultimately require an implantable defibrillator.

REFERENCES

1. Mitsutake, A., Takeshita, A., Kuroiwa, A., and Nakamura, M.: Usefulness of the Valsalva maneuver in management of the long QT syndrome. Circulation 63:1029, 1981.
2. Moss, A.J., Schwartz, P.J., Crampton, R.S., Locati, E., and Carleen, E.: The long QT syndrome: A prospective international study. Circulation 71:17, 1985.

195-B, 196-C, 197-D, 198-E *(Braunwald, pp. 404–420)*

There are many physiological mechanisms that regulate the contractility of the myocardial cell. Increases in heart rate cause increases in the rate of force development and developed force and also shorten the time to peak tension with accelerated relaxation. This response is called the *force-frequency relationship*. The positive inotropic action presumably reflects an increase in intracellular calcium resulting from the increased number of depolarizations. There does not appear to be a shift of the ventricular function curve, i.e., the relation between ventricular end-diastolic pressure and stroke work with an increase in heart rate. Instead, there appears to be an increase in stroke power at any given level of filling pressure consistent with an increase in myocardial contractility. It is likely that, under normal conditions in the conscious state, venous return to the heart is reflexly and metabolically stabilized so that varying heart rate between 60 and 160 beats/min has little effect on cardiac output despite the force-frequency relationship.[1] However, if the diastolic volume of the heart is maintained by increasing venous return such as would occur during exercise, then there is an increase in cardiac output. Also, it is likely that tachycardia plays a major role in increasing cardiac output under conditions of exercise. In contrast, when the heart is paced at a very rapid rate by electrical stimulation of the atrium such as during a pacing test, there is much less inotropic effect because the reflexes that maintain an increase in venous return are absent and also the diastolic filling time permitted is much less. This effect obviously has important implications for ventricular pacing with implanted pacemakers and illustrates the importance of the development of rate-responsive ventricular pacemakers that can respond to appropriate physiological needs.[2]

Laplace's law states that the average circumferential wall stress (force per unit of cross-sectional area of wall) is related directly to the product of intraventricular pressure and internal radius and inversely to wall thickness. Thus, as the ventricle hypertrophies (wall thickness increases) there is a decrease in circumferential wall stress. As the heart dilates (increase in the radius), there is an increase in average circumferential wall stress. Therefore, concentric hypertrophy (such as with stenotic valvular disease) maintains normal wall stress while eccentric hypertrophy (such as with regurgitant valvular disease) increases wall stress. The normal right ventricle is more compliant than the left ventricle, not because of any intrinsic difference in muscle stiffness but because it has a smaller radius and hence less wall stress.

The *Anrep effect* is the name given to "homeometric autoregulation," by which is meant the fact that a positive inotropic effect follows an abrupt elevation of systolic aortic and left ventricular pressure. This effect occurs during the first minutes after aortic pressure is abruptly elevated and appears to be related to recovery from transient subendocardial ischemia.

The *Cushing reflex* is a common manifestation of cerebral ischemia and consists of an increase in peripheral vascular resistance, constriction of the capacitance vessels, and bradycardia. The Cushing effect is particularly common during stroke and intracerebral hemorrhage, during which the rise in blood pressure and bradycardia can be dramatic. These phenomena are to be differentiated from the other effects of the chemoreceptor responses. One of these is hyperventilation, which by itself causes reflex phenomena. It should be noted that the chemoreceptors in aortic arch and carotid bodies are stimulated by reductions in arterial PO_2 and pH, by elevations of arterial PCO_2, by hemorrhage, and by sympathetic efferents. Among the variety of effects mediated by the chemoreceptors are bradycardia, vasoconstriction, positive inotropy, and hyperventilation.[3]

An increase in heart rate following expansion of blood volume is called the *Bainbridge reflex*. With volume loading it has been shown that heart rate increases in proportion to cardiac output even though the elevation of arterial pressure would tend to oppose the increase by activation of the carotid sinus reflex. On the other hand, volume depletion causes tachycardia as well, presumably as a consequence of reflex activation, with reduced stimulation of arterial blood pressure receptors.[4]

REFERENCES

1. Mitchell, J.H., Wallace, A.C., and Skinner, N.S., Jr.: Intrinsic effects of heart rate on left ventricular performance. Am. J. Physiol. 205:41, 1963.
2. Narahara, K.A., and Blettel, M.L.: Effect of rate on left ventricular volumes and ejection fraction during chronic ventricular pacing. Circulation 67:323, 1983.
3. Fujii, I., and Vatner, S.F.: Sympathetic mechanisms regulating myocardial contractility in conscious animals. *In* Fozzard, H.A., et al. (eds.): The Heart and Cardiovascular System. New York, Raven Press, 1986, pp. 1119–1132.
4. Vatner, S.F., and Boettcher, D.H.: Regulation of cardiac output by stroke volume and heart rate in conscious dogs. Circ. Res. 42:557, 1978.

199-C, 200-E, 201-A, 202-B *(Braunwald, pp. 783–790)*

Each of the conditions listed is associated with sustained increases in cardiac output that may precipitate heart failure in the appropriate clinical setting. Hyperthyroidism leads to an increase in cardiac output by a variety of mechanisms, including (1) vasodilation due to augmented metabolic rate; (2) increased heat production (both of these contribute to the decreased systemic vascular resistance in this condition); (3) increases in blood volume and mean circulatory filling pressure; (4) direct effects of thyroid hormone on myocardial contractility; and (5) effects of the sympathoadrenal system on a variety of cardiovascular functions. Clinical findings in hyperthyroidism include constitutional changes such as nervousness, diaphoresis, heat intolerance, and fatigue as well as cardiovascular manifestations such as palpitations, atrial fibrillation with a relatively rapid ventricular response, and sinus tachycardia with a hyperkinetic heart action. Examination of the heart may therefore reveal tachycardia, widened pulse pressure, brisk arterial pulsations, and a variety of findings associated with the hyperkinetic state. These may include a prominent S_1, the presence of an S_3 and/or S_4, and a midsystolic murmur along the left sternal border secondary to increased flow. When a particularly hyperdynamic cardiac effect is seen, this murmur may have an unusual scratching component known as the *Means-Lerman scratch*. This is thought to be caused by the rubbing together of normal pleural and pericardial surfaces. The ECG in thyrotoxicosis often reveals widespread, nonspecific ST and T wave abnormalities with terminal T-wave inversion and shortening of the Q-T interval in approximately 25 per cent of patients.[1] Treatment of hyperthyroidism is directed at the specific endocrine abnormality. However, control of the cardiac manifestations of the disorder may be achieved by use of antiadrenergic agents[2] in an adjunctive manner, although these are capable of controlling symptomatology only and do not reduce the elevated metabolic rate. Furthermore, the use of beta-adrenoreceptor blockade may be difficult and even contraindicated in patients with thyrotoxic heart disease and heart failure.

Systemic arteriovenous fistulas may be acquired as a result of trauma or they may be congenital. The increase in cardiac output that such lesions create is related to the size of the communication and the resultant reduction in the systemic vascular resistance that it promotes. In general, systemic AV fistulas lead to a widened pulse pressure, brisk arterial pulsations, and mild tachycardia. *Branham's sign*, defined as the slowing of heart rate after manual compression of the fistula,[3] is commonly present. The maneuver may also raise arterial and lower venous pressure. Congenital AV fistulas most frequently involve vessels of the lower extremities and on physical examination may reveal varices, swelling, increases in limb length, and warmth. Treatment is difficult in part because surgical excision is often not feasible technically. Acquired AV fistulas occur most often due to traumatic injuries such as stab or gunshot wounds or as a consequence of surgical procedures such as nephrectomy, laminectomy, cholecystectomy, and percutaneous vascular catheterizations. In addition, high-output congestive heart failure may be precipitated by the AV shunts that are intentionally placed to provide access for chronic hemodialysis. In general, surgical repair of AV fistulas is the recommended treatment.

Osler-Weber-Rendu disease or hereditary hemorrhagic telangiectasia is a specific inherited condition that may be associated with AV fistulas, especially in the liver and the lungs. The disease may produce a hyperkinetic circulation with abdominal bruits and hepatomegaly due to intrahepatic arteriovenous connections.[4] Because these connections may lead to the presence of oxygenated blood in the inferior vena cava and right atrium, Osler-Weber-Rendu disease may be a factor in the misdiagnosis of atrial septal defect in selected patients.[5]

Beriberi heart disease is a rare condition caused by severe thiamine deficiency that is found most frequently in the Far East. The absence of thiamine as a coenzyme for transketolase in the pentose phosphate pathway of glucose metabolism accounts for the basic pathophysiology in this condition. Elevation in cardiac output in beriberi heart disease is presumed to be due to a reduction in systemic vascular resistance and an augmentation of venous return. This occurs as a result of lesions created in the sympathetic nervous system nuclei by the absence of thiamine. Patients with beriberi may present with findings of the high-output state, severe generalized

malnutrition, and vitamin deficiency. Evidence is noted of peripheral neuropathy with paresthesias of the extremities, decreased or absent knee and ankle jerks, anemia, hyperkeratinized skin lesions, and painful glossitis. The presence of edema characterizes "wet beriberi" and differentiates this condition from the "dry" form. Beriberi heart disease is characterized by biventricular failure, an S_3 and an apical systolic murmur, and a hyperkinetic state with wide pulse pressure. The ECG demonstrates low voltage, Q-T interval prolongation, and inversion of T waves. It should be emphasized that, especially in Western society, alcoholic cardiomyopathy may contribute to or overlap with this clinical picture because of the tendency for alcoholics to become vitamin deficient from a low intake of vitamin B_1 and high carbohydrate ingestion. "Shoshin" beriberi is a fulminating form of the disease that may lead to severe illness or death within 48 hours.[6] Treatment of all forms of beriberi involves the administration of thiamine first intravenously and subsequently orally, as well as digitalis and diuretics to treat concomitant congestive heart failure.

The carcinoid syndrome is an uncommon disease which results from the release of serotonin and other vasoactive substances by carcinoid tumors. Physical findings may include cutaneous flushing, telangiectasia, diarrhea, and bronchial constriction due to release of humoral mediators. The syndrome may be accompanied by an elevation in cardiac output with a reduction in arterial–mixed venous oxygen difference.[7] This results from a reduction in systemic vascular resistance due either to mediator release and/or to shunting of blood to the carcinoid tumors themselves.

REFERENCES

1. Hoffman, I., and Lowrey, R.D.: The electrocardiogram in thyrotoxicosis. Am. J. Cardiol. 8:893, 1960.
2. Grossman, W., Robin, N.I., Johnson, L.W., Brooks, H.L., Selenkow, H.A., and Dexter, L.: Effects of beta blockade on the peripheral manifestations of thyrotoxicosis. Ann. Intern. Med. 74:875, 1971.
3. Branham, H.H.: Aneurysmal varix of the femoral artery and vein following a gunshot wound. Int. J. Surg. 3:250, 1890.
4. Baranda, M.M., Perez, M., DeAndres, J., De La Hoz, C., Merino, J., and Aguirre, C.: High-output congestive heart failure as first manifestation of Osler-Weber-Rendu disease. J. Vasc. Dis. 35:568, 1984.
5. Radtke, W.E., Smith, H.C., Fulton, R.E., and Adson, M.A.: Misdiagnosis of atrial septal defect in patients with hereditary telangiectasia (Osler-Weber-Rendu disease) and hepatic arteriovenous fistulas. Am. Heart J. 95:235, 1978.
6. Jeffrey, F.E., and Abelmann, W.H.: Recovery of proved Shoshin beriberi. Am. J. Med. 50:123, 1971.
7. Schwaber, J.R., and Lukas, D.S.: Hyperkinemia and cardiac failure in the carcinoid syndrome. Am. J. Med. 32:846, 1962.

203-B, 204-D, 205-C, 206-C *(Braunwald, pp. 454–455)*

Patient A has values typical of those in normal human subjects. Left ventricular mass increases in response to chronic pressure or volume overload or secondary to primary myocardial disease. With predominant pressure overload, as in aortic stenosis, there is an increase in mass with little change in chamber volume (concentric hypertrophy) (Patient B). In contrast, hypertrophy due to volume overload (as in aortic or mitral regurgitation), or due to primary myocardial disease, is caused by ventricular dilatation with only a small increase in wall thickness (eccentric hypertrophy). In regurgitant disease (Patient C) there is usually a nearly normal ejection fraction in the compensated state, while in cardiomyopathy there is impaired systolic function (Patient D). In mitral regurgitation there may be a paradoxically elevated ejection fraction caused by the decreased afterload afforded by the left atrium.

207-B, 208-A, 209-D, 210-B   (Braunwald, pp. 834–836)

The pathogenesis of essential hypertension is, by definition, still unknown but probably involves the effects of many regulatory hormones and the ionic consequences of their actions on target tissues. Among these hormones are the ouabain-like natriuretic factor, which, as postulated by deWardener and coworkers,[1] is increased in response to a rise in vascular volume and acts to inhibit the Na^+,K^+-ATPase. This results in increased renal sodium absorption and urinary intracellular Na^+. In turn this may increase intracellular Ca^{++} in smooth muscle leading to increased tone. Angiotensin II may play a pivotal role in the development of hypertension since it stimulates aldosterone production with secondary retention of sodium and also stimulates a rise in smooth muscle cell Ca^{++} and increase in vascular tone.[2] Atriopeptins are a family of 24–25 amino acid peptides synthesized in the atria. They are direct vasodilators by virtue of increasing vascular smooth muscle cell cyclic GMP; also, they induce a natriuresis without affecting Na^+,K^+-ATPase activity.[3] Renin is an important enzyme. It hydrolyzes angiotensin I to angiotensin II but has little direct effect on vascular smooth muscle tone. Oxytocin has powerful effects on uterine smooth muscle but not vascular smooth muscle.

REFERENCES

1. DeWardener, H.E., and Clarkson E.M.: Concept of natriuretic hormone. Physiol. Rev. 65:658, 1985.
2. Lebel, M., Brown, J.J., Kremer, D., Robertson, J.I.S., Schalekamp, M., Davies, D.L., Lever, A.F., Tree, M., Beevers, D.G., Frazier, R., Morton, J.J., and Wilson, A.: Sodium and the renin-angiotensin system in essential hypertension and mineralocorticoid excess. Lancet 2:308, 1974.
3. Needleman, P., and Greenwald, J.E.: Atriopeptin: A cardiac hormone intimately involved in fluid electrolyte and blood pressure homeostasis. N. Engl. J. Med. 314:528, 1986.

211-C, 212-A, 213-D, 214-E   (Braunwald, pp. 721–731)

Pacemaker functions are defined by a five-position code. The positions are:

1. Chamber paced: A, atrium; V, ventricle; D, both atrium and ventricle; S, either atrium or ventricle; O, neither.

2. Chamber sensed: same letters and indications as in 1.

3. Pacemaker response to sensed spontaneous electrical activity: O, no sensing; I, inhibited from delivery of stimulus for a certain time; T, a stimulus is discharged (triggered) in response; D, dual-chamber sensing—the detection of an atrial stimulus inhibits the ventricular discharge for a certain time, after which ventricular sensing takes precedence.

4. Pacemaker noninvasive programming capability: P, either rate and/or output alterable; M, more than two functions alterable; C, communicating function, e.g., telemetry; *, response to sensory input or hysteresis.

5. Tachycardic function: P, pacing; C, pacing and synchronous cardioversion; D, defibrillation; O, no capability.

The four general classes of pacemakers are:

1. Atrial and ventricular demand pacemakers (AAI, AAT, VVI, and VVT). VVI, a ventricular demand pacer, is the most commonly implanted pacer. It paces the ventricle (V), senses ventricular activity (V), and is inhibited (I) from discharging by sensed ventricular events.

2. Atrial synchronous ventricular pacemakers (VAT, VDD). These dual-chamber pacers preserve the atrial contribution to ventricular filling and maintain sinus control over ventricular rate. The VAT senses atrial activity and after a certain delay paces the ventricle. Its activity is limited by atrial rate; with bradycardia it becomes an asynchronous ventricular pacer (VOO) and with tachycardia it converts to 2:1 AV conduction. The VDD is more advanced in that it has a VVI mode during atrial bradycardia.

3. AV sequential pacemakers (DVI, DDI). These dual-chamber pacemakers preserve the atrial contribution to ventricular filling in the presence of both abnormal sinus node function and impaired AV conduction by pacing both atrium and ventricle. The DVI senses only ventricular activity but paces both atrium and ventricle.

4. Universal pacemaker (DDD). This dual-chamber pacemaker senses and paces both atrium and ventricle. It functions as an atrial demand pacer (AAI) during normally conducted sinus bradycardia, as an atrial synchronous pacer (VDD) during normal sinus rates that undergo AV conduction delay, and as an AV sequential pacer (DVI) during sinus bradycardia with AV block.

215-E, 216-A, 217-C, 218-B   (Braunwald, pp. 585–595)

The cardiac transmembrane potential consists of five distinct phases: Phase 0, upstroke or rapid depolarization; Phase 1, early rapid repolarization; Phase 2, plateau; Phase 3, final rapid repolarization; and Phase 4, the resting membrane potential in diastolic depolarization. Each phase results from the movement of ions down electrochemical gradients that are established and maintained by active ion pumps and exchange mechanisms.

When a stimulus arrives at excitable tissue, an action potential is generated once the membrane potential is reduced to a threshold value. As this occurs, Phase 0 or rapid depolarization is initiated in a "all-or-none" manner. Following Phase 0, the membrane repolarizes rapidly due to inactivation of sodium currents and inward movement of chloride down its concentration gradient. This reduces the newly reached positive membrane voltage back toward zero. Phase 1, early rapid repolarization, is particularly well-defined and separated from Phase 2 in the cardiac Purkinje fibers. Phase 2 of the action potential, or the plateau phase, may last several hundred milliseconds; during this time membrane conductance to all ions falls to relatively low values. Phase 3 of the action potential is final rapid repolarization, which leads directly into Phase 4, the resting membrane potential and diastolic depolarization phase.

Under normal conditions, the membrane potential of atrial and ventricular muscle cells remains steady throughout diastole. Potassium is the major ion determining this resting potential primarily because during diastole the cell membrane remains permeable to potassium and relatively impermeable to sodium. A knowledge of the action potential and its phases is important for the understanding of both mechanisms of arrhythmogenesis and the mode of action of antiarrhythmic therapeutic agents.

219-B, 220-D, 221-A, 222-C   (Braunwald, pp. 868–877)

Because there are many classes of antihypertensive agents, these drugs display a diversity of side effects. Thus, amiloride as well as the other potassium-sparing diuretics triamterene and spironolactone can cause hyperkalemia in patients with high potassium intake or sudden decreases in renal function. Methyldopa is unique in that it causes significant autoimmune side effects, including a positive antinuclear antibody test in 10 per cent of patients and red cell autoantibodies in about 20 per cent. However, hemolytic anemia is rare.[1]

Hydrochlorothiazide, like all thiazide diuretics, can cause hypokalemia, which is associated with leg cramps and muscle weakness. Many diuretics also cause hypomagnesemia, a condition that may contribute to these symptoms. Hypokalemia from diuretics may also be associated with increased ventricular ectopic activity and a rise in plasma lipids.[2] Clonidine is a central adrenergic agonist like methyldopa, but it does not cause autoimmune or inflammatory side effects. As an alpha-adrenoreceptor agonist, clonidine also acts on presynaptic alpha receptors and lowers norepinephrine release. Thus, upon discontinuation, catecholamine levels rise within 12 to 18 hours and may overshoot, causing tachycardia, restlessness, sweating and hypertension. This withdrawal reaction may be a problem especially in postoperative patients who are predisposed to increased adrenoceptor side effects.[3]

REFERENCES

1. Kelton, J.C.: Impaired reticuloendothelial function in patients treated with methyldopa. N. Engl. J. Med. 313:596, 1985.
2. Kaplan, N.M., Carnegie, A., Raskin, P., Heller, J.A., and Simmons, M.: Potassium supplementation in hypertensive patients with diuretic-induced hypokalemia. N. Engl. J. Med. 312:746, 1985.
3. Houston, M.C.: Abrupt cessation of treatment in hypertension: Consideration of clinical features, mechanisms, prevention, and management of the discontinuation syndrome. Am. Heart J. 102:415, 1981.

223-D, 224-A, 225-C, 226-D   (Braunwald, pp. 871–878)

Many antiadrenergic drugs are available which can be categorized on the basis of their site of action (central and peripheral) and their adrenoreceptor specificity (alpha and beta). Guanethidine, reserpine, and related compounds are peripheral neuronal inhibitors that deplete or prevent the release of norepinephrine from peripheral adrenergic neurons. Guanethidine inhibits release of norepinephrine from adrenergic neurons; because of its low lipid solubility it does not enter the brain so that sedation and depression are less common than with reserpine. Because of the significant postural hypotension, it is not frequently prescribed.

Prazosin is a selective postsynaptic alpha₁ receptor antagonist.[1] The mode of action of prazosin can be understood by considering the role of the presynaptic nerve in the mechanism of action of adrenoreceptor-blocking drugs. When the presynaptic nerve is stimulated, norepinephrine is released and binds to postsynaptic alpha₁- and beta-adrenoreceptors. In vascular smooth muscle, alpha₁ stimulation causes constriction and beta stimulation causes relaxation. The released norepinephrine can also bind to alpha₂ and beta receptors on the presynaptic nerve terminal to inhibit or stimulate further release of norepinephrine. Since the presynaptic alpha receptor (alpha₂) is not blocked by prazosin, the feedback loop for inhibition of norepinephrine release by circulating norepinephrine is intact. Thus, prazosin blocks peripheral vasoconstriction but preserves reflex feedback, resulting in an antihypertensive effect with no tachycardia, tolerance, or activation of the renin-angiotensin system. Other advantages include maintenance of cardiac output, no increase in serum lipids, and no adverse effects in renal insufficiency.

Labetalol combines alpha and beta blockade in a ratio of approximately 1:5. The predominant effect on BP is secondary to a decrease in peripheral resistance with maintenance of cardiac output.[2] Postural hypotension is the most common side effect. Because of its dual receptor blockade labetalol is useful in hypertensive crises, as in pheochromocytoma.

Clonidine, like methyldopa, is a central alpha-adrenoreceptor *agonist* reducing the sympathetic outflow from the central nervous system. Blood pressure decreases as a result of a fall in peripheral resistance with little change in cardiac output. Advantages include preservation of renal blood flow, little postural hypotension, and availability in a transdermal preparation that provides therapy for as long as one week.[3] Side effects include fluid retention, sedation, dry mouth, impotence, and rebound hypertension after discontinuation of therapy.

REFERENCES

1. Beretta-Piccoli, C., Ferrier, C., and Weidmann, P.: Alpha₁-adrenergic blockade and cardiovascular pressor responses in essential hypertension. Hypertension 8:407, 1986.
2. Lund-Johansen, P.: Pharmacology of combined alpha–beta blockade. II. Haemodynamic effects of labetalol. Drugs 28(Suppl. 2):35, 1984.
3. Weber, M.A., Drayer, J.I.M., McMahon, F.G., Hamburger, R., Shah, A.R., and Kirk, L.N.: Transdermal administration of clonidine for treatment of high blood pressure. Arch. Intern. Med. 144:1211, 1984.

227-B, 228-D, 229-A, 230-C, 231-C   (Braunwald, pp. 802–813)

Distinguishing between causes of pulmonary hypertension may be difficult on both clinical and pathologic grounds. The term "Eisenmenger syndrome" was popularized by Dr. Paul Wood in reference to patients with congenital cardiac lesions and severe pulmonary hypertension in whom reversal of a left-to-right shunt had occurred across an existing pulmonary-systemic communication. In the patients described originally by Eisenmenger, a ventricular septal defect was present. However, any right-to-left shunt that undergoes reversal due to increasing pulmonary pressures is referred to as *Eisenmenger syndrome*. In this syndrome, the progressive pathophysiological process that leads to obliterative changes in the pulmonary vasculature involves a variety of anatomical changes. These begin with hypertrophy of small muscular pulmonary arteries, progress through dilation and so-called "plexiform lesions" of the muscular pulmonary arteries and arterioles, and end in complex lesions with accompanying necrotizing arteritis. These changes have been carefully classified by Heath and Edwards.[1] Once the pulmonary vascular resistance increases to equal or exceed systemic resistance, resulting in a predominantly right-to-left shunt and end-stage changes of the pulmonary vessels, surgical closure of the intracardiac communication is contraindicated. This is because of the sudden increase in the load on the already overburdened RV which may be precipitated by such an intervention and which may lead to a more rapid death.

Primary pulmonary hypertension is by definition idiopathic, or unexplained. While controversy exists regarding the precise pathophysiology of this syndrome, most patients considered to have primary pulmonary hypertension have no evidence of an associated tendency toward thromboembolism, congenital or immunologic abnormalities, collagen vascular disease, or drug ingestion. Patients with primary pulmonary hypertension do appear to have increased pulmonary vascular reactivity and a more marked vasospastic or constrictive tendency.[2] There are several common pathological findings in primary pulmonary hypertension, including intimal thickening of smaller pulmonary arteries and arterioles with accompanying fibrosis, which is referred to as "onion skinning." In addition, plexiform lesions similar to those seen in patients with Eisenmenger syndrome may develop. Dilated, thin-walled branches of muscular pulmonary arteries may lead to the lesions that are responsible for the phrase "plexogenic pulmonary arteriopathy," which is frequently used to characterize the pathological changes in primary pulmonary hypertension. The finding of such lesions on lung biopsy mandates exclusion of any intracardiac shunts as an explanation for their presence.

The differential diagnosis for elevated pulmonary pressures includes silent mitral stenosis for both of the lesions noted. In some instances, the characteristic diastolic murmur of mitral stenosis is not appreciated, and echocardiographic visualization of the mitral valve with exclusion of the presence of any transvalvular pressure gradient may be necessary to exclude this disorder. Other conditions to be considered in the differential diagnosis include cor triatriatum, which must be recognized by appropriate hemodynamic studies and angiographic visualization of the left atrial membrane; pulmonary embolism; and pulmonary venous obstruction. Other diagnoses to be excluded include pulmonary parenchymal disease, collagen vascular disease, and pulmonary veno-occlusive disease.

REFERENCES

1. Heath, D., and Edwards, J.E.: The pathology of hypertensive pulmonary vascular disease. A description of 6 grades of structural changes in the pulmonary arteries with special reference to congenital cardiac septal defects. Circulation *18*:533, 1958.
2. Haworth, S.G.: Primary pulmonary hypertension. Br. Heart J. *49*:517, 1983.

232-A, 233-B, 234-B, 235-A *(Braunwald, pp. 633–636 and Table 21–1, pp. 622–623)*

Propranolol is a nonselective beta-adrenoreceptor blocking agent that has found application as an antiarrhythmic agent primarily in the treatment of supraventricular tachyarrhythmias. Bretylium tosylate, an agent originally introduced as an antihypertensive drug, has been shown to be useful in the treatment of life-threatening recurrent ventricular tachyarrhythmias that have not responded to first-line agents. Bretylium is selectively concentrated in sympathetic ganglia and postganglionic adrenergic nerve terminals, where it initially causes release of norepinephrine and subsequently prevents release of norepinephrine from sympathetic nerve terminals. Therefore, chronic administration may lengthen the duration of the action potential and increase refractoriness of cardiac Purkinje fibers. The aforementioned initial release of catecholamines may aggravate some arrhythmias such as those due to digitalis excess or myocardial infarction.[1] In contrast, propranolol has proven useful in the treatment of digitalis-induced arrhythmias such as nonparoxysmal junctional tachycardia, premature ventricular complexes, and ventricular tachycardia, in part because of the central nervous system effects of the drug. In addition, propranolol may be useful in the treatment of ventricular arrhythmias associated with the prolonged Q-T syndrome.[2]

For patients with ischemic heart disease, however, propranolol in general has not prevented episodes of chronic recurrent ventricular tachycardia that may occur during times when ischemia is not active. Bretylium is currently recommended for use in patients with life-threatening recurrent ventricular tachyarrhythmias that have not responded to a first-line agent such as lidocaine, quinidine, or procainamide[3] and has proven quite useful in treating victims of out-of-hospital ventricular fibrillatory arrest. Propranolol may be given in either oral or intravenous forms and is primarily metabolized through a hepatic mechanism in which the effects of first-pass hepatic metabolism reduce the bioavailability of oral propranolol to about 30 per cent. In contrast, bretylium is eliminated almost exclusively by a renal mechanism and is approved only for intravenous administration because of the erratic gastrointestinal absorption of the oral form.

Both drugs are capable of causing hypotension. In the case of bretylium, this side effect appears to occur by blockade of the efferent limb of the baroreceptor reflex due to the prevention of norepinephrine release. The hypotension caused by bretylium is more evident with orthostasis and can be prevented by tricyclic drugs such as protriptyline.

Of note, the worsening of arrhythmias due to digitalis excess, as well as sinus tachycardia and transient hypertension, may accompany the early phase of bretylium administration. The worsening may be due to the initial release of catecholamines stimulated by the drug. Propranolol may also cause bradycardia as a result of sinus bradycardia or AV block and may worsen preexisting congestive heart failure by exerting negative inotropic effects on cardiac contractility. Sudden withdrawal of propranolol may occasionally precipitate worsening of angina, cardiac arrhythmias, and myocardial ischemia, possibly because of a heightened sensitivity to beta agonists caused by the previous beta blockade.[4] It is therefore prudent to withdraw propranolol in a stepwise fashion. Other side effects of propranolol include exacerbation of underlying bronchospastic pulmonary disease, depression, fatigability, dream disturbances, elevation of serum lipid levels, impaired sexual function, and worsening of peripheral vascular disease or Raynaud's phenomenon. The last two side effects mentioned may arise as a result of the peripheral vasoconstriction caused by blockade of beta$_2$ receptors in the blood vessels.

REFERENCES

1. Duff, H.J., Roden, D.M., Yacobi, A., Robertson, D., Wang, T., Maffucci, R.J., Oates, J.A., and Woosley, R.L.: Bretylium: Relations between plasma concentrations and pharmacologic actions in high-frequency ventricular arrhythmias. Am. J. Cardiol. 55:395, 1985.
2. Schwartz, P.J.: Idiopathic long Q-T syndrome: progress and questions. Am. Heart J. 109:399, 1985.
3. Stang, J.M., Washington, S.E., Barnes, S.A., Dutko, J.H., Cheney, B.D., Easter, C.R., O'Hara, J.T., Kessler, J.H., Schaal, S.F., and Lewis, R.P.: Treatment of prehospital refractory ventricular fibrillation with bretylium tosylate. Ann. Emerg. Med. 13:234, 1984.
4. Nattel, S., Rango, R.E., and Vanloon, G.: Mechanism of propranolol withdrawal phenomenon. Circulation 59:1158, 1979.

236-D, 237-D, 238-C, 239-B   *(Braunwald, pp. 871–876)*

The wide variety of beta blockers available reflects their popularity, which is in part due to their relative effectiveness with few serious side effects. They can be classified on the basis of cardioselectivity, intrinsic sympathomimetic activity (ISA), and lipid solubility, although all are equally effective at lowering BP.

Acebutolol, atenolol, and metoprolol are relatively more selective for cardiac beta$_1$ receptors than beta$_2$ adrenoreceptors present in bronchi, vascular smooth muscle, and other areas. However, it should be noted that at the doses usually prescribed, cardioselective effects are often lost.

Pindolol, acebutolol, alprenolol, and oxprenolol have ISA, which means that they possess partial agonist activity but still block the effects of endogenous catecholamines on adrenoceptors. Thus, these drugs cause relatively smaller decreases in heart rate and cardiac output and smaller increases or no changes in serum lipids.[1, 2] These drugs may be useful in patients with bradycardia and/or peripheral vascular disease.

The relative lipid solubility of the beta blockers is reflected in the relative degree of clearance by hepatic uptake (high lipid solubility) and renal excretion (low lipid solubility). The least lipid-soluble drugs—atenolol and nadolol—share two theoretical advantages: longer serum half-lives due to decreased hepatic metabolism and fewer central nervous side effects due to lower brain concentrations.

REFERENCES

1. Choong, C.Y.P., Roubin, G.S., Harris, P.J., Tokuyasu, Y., Shen, W.F., Bautovich, G.J., and Kelly, D.T.: A comparison of the effects of beta blockers with and without intrinsic sympathomimetic activity on hemodynamics and left ventricular function at rest and during exercise in patients with coronary artery disease. J. Cardiovasc. Pharmacol. 8:441, 1986.
2. Johnson, B.F., Weiner, B., Marwaha, R., and Johnson, J.: The influence of pindolol and hydrochlorothiazide on blood pressure, and plasma renin and plasma lipid levels. J. Clin. Pharmacol. 26:258, 1986.

PART III: DISEASES OF THE HEART, PERICARDIUM, AORTA, AND PULMONARY VASCULAR BED

CHAPTERS 30 THROUGH 48

DIRECTIONS: Each question below contains five suggested responses. Select the ONE BEST response to each question.

240. In the presence of a coronary artery obstruction, the effective pressure perfusing the subendocardium is best described as:

A. the gradient between aortic pressure in systole and diastole
B. the gradient between peak LV end-systolic pressure and aortic diastolic pressure
C. the gradient between aortic diastolic pressure and LV end-diastolic pressure
D. the gradient between diastolic coronary pressure distal to the obstruction and LV end-diastolic pressure
E. none of the above

241. A 45-year-old man comes to the office because of recurrent chest discomfort and shortness of breath. He rides his bicycle daily to and from work and this past winter noticed occasional episodes of chest discomfort during bicycling. An exercise tolerance test (ETT) was performed for 12 minutes with a standard Bruce protocol without the development of significant symptoms or ECG findings. He was placed on a beta blocker, but his symptoms have persisted. You perform a repeat ETT, which again is negative, except for upsloping ST segment depressions present at 85 per cent of maximal predicted heart rate. You would recommend next:

A. switching medications to nifedipine
B. no further workup
C. echocardiography
D. stress thallium-201 scintigraphy
E. coronary arteriography

242. A 44-year-old farmer develops fever, chills, and a cough. He is treated by his local physician with tetracycline for 1 week and feels improved. However, a week later he again develops a low-grade fever associated with myalgias. Over the next few days he has several episodes of palpitation and chest tightness which are worse with exertion. He is referred to you for further evaluation. On examination he has a temperature of 99.5°F, pulse 90/min, respirations 16/min, BP 130/85. His lungs are clear. There is no jugular venous distention and the carotid upstrokes are normal. The LV impulse is not displaced; S_1 and S_2 are normal. There is a grade II/VI midsystolic murmur that increases with handgrip. A midsystolic click is also present. The rest of the examination is unremarkable. His chest x-ray and ECG are normal. Laboratory findings include Hgb 14.2 mg/dl; WBC 15,000/mm³ with 80 per cent polys, 3 per cent bands, 17 per cent lymphs; Na 140 mEq/liter, Cl 100, K 5.0, HCO₃ 25; urinalysis: clear, pH 6.6, 1+ protein, no WBC, 2 to 3 RBC/hpf. What would you order now?

A. Exercise testing
B. Exercise thallium testing
C. Ambulatory Holter monitor
D. Blood cultures
E. 1-week course of erythromycin

243. True statments about the clinical history in patients with acute myocardial infarction (AMI) include all of the following EXCEPT:

A. Approximately one-third of these patients may present with symptoms of unstable angina that have been present for longer than 24 hours
B. The duration of analgesic requirement after hospital admission is positively correlated with the likelihood of AMI being confirmed
C. The pain associated with AMI probably represents pain caused by infarcted myocardial tissue
D. Nausea and vomiting occur in more than half of patients with transmural MI
E. Between 20 and 60 per cent of nonfatal myocardial infarctions are unrecognized by the patient and are discovered on routine electrocardiographic examination

244. True statements about effusive-constrictive pericarditis include all of the following EXCEPT:

A. In effusive-constrictive pericarditis, removal of pericardial fluid by aspiration does not lead to a normal right atrial pressure
B. Idiopathic or presumed viral pericarditis is a common cause of effusive-constrictive pericarditis
C. Physical findings in effusive-constrictive pericarditis resemble chronic constrictive pericarditis more than cardiac tamponade
D. The diagnosis of effusive-constrictive pericarditis is made by careful hemodynamic monitoring before and after pericardiocentesis
E. Treatment of effusive-constrictive pericarditis consists of total parietal and visceral pericardiectomy

245. Each of the following is a potential cause of constrictive pericarditis EXCEPT:

A. myxedema
B. tuberculosis
C. rheumatoid arthritis
D. mediastinal irradiation
E. viral infection

246. True statements about the electrocardiogram in congenital heart disease include all of the following EXCEPT:

A. T-wave inversions may be seen in normal neonatal electrocardiograms
B. By the time the infant is 72 hours of age the T-waves should be inverted in V_1 to V_3
C. The presence of right ventricular hypertrophy suggests single ventricle or inversion of the ventricles
D. An electrocardiographic pattern of myocardial infarction may indicate an anomalous origin of a coronary artery
E. T-wave inversion in the lateral precordial leads may be observed in subendocardial ischemia

247. All of the statements about surgical therapy of tetralogy of Fallot are correct EXCEPT:

A. The most common palliative procedure that has been used for tetralogy of Fallot is the Blalock-Taussig shunt
B. Adult patients with tetralogy of Fallot and a palliative shunt that is functioning appropriately need not undergo total surgical repair
C. Total correction of tetralogy of Fallot is ordinarily best performed during the first 4 years of life
D. Common postsurgical anatomical problems in tetralogy of Fallot include persistent obstruction to right ventricular outflow and/or pulmonary regurgitation
E. Ventricular ectopy and more serious ventricular tachyarrhythmias may be late consequences of operative repair of tetralogy of Fallot

248. Each of the following statements about ventricular septal defect (VSD) is true EXCEPT:

A. A significant number of VSDs undergo spontaneous closure
B. Membranous VSD is the most common form of this anomaly
C. In the absence of aortic regurgitation or infective endocarditis, congestive heart failure is generally not associated with VSD after infancy
D. With a small VSD, the most common electrocardiographic finding is right axis deviation
E. In the adult patient with a small VSD, the chest x-ray is usually normal

249. Each of the following statements about coarctation of the aorta is true EXCEPT:

A. Coarctation of the aorta usually occurs just proximal to the left subclavian artery
B. Coarctation is frequently associated with a bicuspid aortic valve
C. The most common symptoms of coarctation are headaches, intermittent claudication, and leg fatigue
D. Simultaneous palpation of the upper and lower extremity pulses may reveal the diagnosis
E. A suprasternal thrill is common in this condition

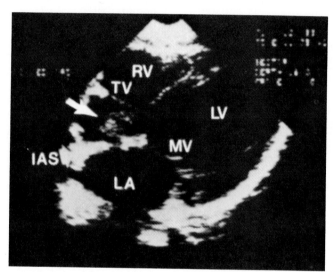

RV = right ventricle, TV = tricuspid valve, LV = left ventricle, MV = mitral valve, LA = left atrium. (From Panadis, I.P., et al.: Am. Heart J. *107*:745, 1984.)

250. The two-dimensional echocardiogram illustrated most likely demonstrates the presence of:

A. a right atrial myxoma
B. a left atrial myxoma
C. a rhabdomyoma
D. a lymphosarcoma
E. a pericardial cyst

251. True statements about coronary thrombolysis in acute myocardial infarction (AMI) include all of the following EXCEPT:

A. The GISSI trial of intravenous streptokinase in AMI demonstrated a significant reduction in mortality in patients treated within the early hours after onset of MI
B. The sum of clinical trial data available suggests that the use of fibrinolytic therapy in AMI leads to a highly significant reduction in mortality
C. Uncontrolled hypertension is a relative contrain-

dication to the use of intravenous fibrinolytic therapy in the setting of AMI

D. Tissue plasminogen activator has been shown to be a more effective lytic agent in the restoration of coronary patency than streptokinase

E. Patients with AMI who are treated with thrombolytic agents appear to experience more in-hospital reinfarctions than patients who do not receive this therapy

---

252. True statements about atrial infarction include all of the following EXCEPT:

A. Atrial infarction occurs in less than 20 per cent of autopsy-proven cases of MI

B. Atrial infarction is seen more commonly in the right atrium

C. Atrial infarction may lead to rupture of the atrial wall

D. Atrial arrhythmias are relatively uncommon in atrial infarction

E. Atrial infarction may often be seen in conjunction with left ventricular infarction

---

253. True statements about the percutaneous treatment of valvular stenosis include all of the following EXCEPT:

A. Balloon valvuloplasty has essentially replaced surgical repair for valvular pulmonic stenosis

B. In general, rheumatic mitral stenosis does not allow for successful balloon valvuloplasty repair

C. The development of moderate or severe mitral regurgitation following balloon mitral valvuloplasty for mitral stenosis is rare

D. In patients without left atrial thrombus, there appears to be no evidence of systemic embolization due to mitral valvuloplasty

E. In general, application of balloon valvuloplasty to aortic stenosis leads to a smaller improvement in orifice area than that obtained with valve replacement

---

254. Potential benefits arising from rehabilitation of patients with coronary artery disease include all of the following EXCEPT:

A. a decrease in reinfarction rates
B. favorable physiological adaptations
C. relief of symptoms
D. a sense of well-being
E. preservation of the patient's family role

---

255. Common signs and symptoms of left atrial myxomas include all the following EXCEPT:

A. fever
B. anemia
C. clubbing

D. mitral valve diastolic murmur
E. mitral valve systolic murmur

---

256. A 3-month-old infant is referred to you because of failure to thrive and cardiomegaly. Gestation and delivery were normal. The physical examination shows evidence of congestive heart failure and poor skeletal muscle tone. Chest x-ray shows cardiomegaly and mild pulmonary edema. ECG reveals tall broad QRS complexes consistent with left ventricular hypertrophy and a P-R interval of 0.08 sec. The most likely diagnosis is:

A. endocardial fibroelastosis
B. coarctation of the aorta
C. Shone syndrome
D. Type II glycogen storage disease (Pompe's)
E. Friedreich's ataxia

---

257. Which of the following factors has *not* been shown to be associated with increased cardiovascular mortality from atherosclerosis?

A. Consumption of more than 2 oz alcohol/day
B. Vasectomy
C. Heavy coffee consumption ($\geq$ 9 cups/day)
D. Cardiac transplantation
E. Elevated blood fibrinogen levels

---

258. All of the following are true statements about the pathophysiology of cardiac tamponade EXCEPT:

A. Cardiac tamponade occurs when the intrapericardial pressure is equal to the RA and RV diastolic pressures

B. In the presence of hypovolemia, the rise of the RA and intrapericardial pressures is less obvious; therefore, cardiac tamponade may be more difficult to detect

C. Equalization of intrapericardial and ventricular filling pressures may lead initially to a small increase in stroke volume

D. Sinus bradycardia may occur during severe cardiac tamponade

E. Hemodynamic deterioration during tamponade is dependent upon atrial compression during diastole

---

259. A 67-year-old woman, a Russian immigrant, comes to your office complaining of rapid heartbeat, fatigue, weight loss, and swelling of her ankles. She also complains of a sensation of fullness in her neck. She has been in apparent good health for all of her life until the last 6 months. She is taking no medications except furosemide. Examination discloses clear lungs, an irregular pulse, prominent jugular veins, a nearly pansystolic murmur that exhibits respiratory variation in intensity, and marked peripheral edema. There are no cardiac heaves or lifts. She also tells you that she has had several episodes

of flushing and diarrhea. The most likely cause of her illness is:

A. subacute bacterial endocarditis
B. carcinoid syndrome
C. Ebstein's anomaly
D. chronic pulmonary emboli disease
E. Marfan's syndrome

260. True statements about rupture of the free wall of the ventricle in acute myocardial infarction (AMI) include all of the following EXCEPT:

A. Rupture of the free wall occurs more commonly in women
B. Rupture of the free wall occurs more commonly in hypertensive patients
C. Rupture of the free wall usually involves the distribution of the left anterior descending coronary artery
D. Rupture of the free wall occurs most commonly 7 to 10 days following the infarct
E. Rupture of the free wall usually occurs near the junction of the infarct and normal myocardial tissue

261. True statements about neoplastic pericarditis include all of the following EXCEPT:

A. A large majority of pericardial effusions associated with Hodgkin's disease are of malignant origin
B. Lung and breast cancer are among the most common tumors associated with malignant pericarditis
C. Neoplastic pericarditis is the most common *specific* etiology of acute pericarditis in developed countries
D. Dyspnea is the most common symptom in patients with malignant pericarditis
E. A normal chest x-ray in patients with neoplastic pericarditis is uncommon

262. All of the following clinical findings would be possible in a patient with a 95 per cent stenosis of the left anterior descending artery during an ischemic episode EXCEPT:

A. paradoxical splitting of the second heart sound
B. a presystolic filling wave and sustained cardiac impulse
C. fixed splitting of the second heart sound
D. a diastolic murmur
E. a late systolic murmur

263. True statements about the clinical findings in patients with atrial septal defect (ASD) include all of the following EXCEPT:

A. A midsystolic ejection murmur and a diastolic rumbling murmur at the lower left sternal border may both be features of the cardiac examination in ASD

B. Patients with ostium primum defects usually show RV hypertrophy, a small rSR' pattern in the right precordial leads, and normal axis on the ECG
C. P-R interval prolongation may be seen with any of the types of ASD
D. Echocardiographic features of ASD include RV and pulmonary arterial dilatation as well as paradoxical septal motion
E. In children with a large left-to-right shunt, catheterization often reveals normal right-sided pressures

264. True statements about the appearance of bradyarrhythmias in acute myocardial infarction (AMI) include all of the following EXCEPT:

A. Sinus bradycardia is the most common early arrhythmia in AMI
B. Isolated sinus bradycardia that is uncomplicated by hypotension or ventricular ectopy may be initially observed rather than treated
C. If symptomatic sinus bradycardia requires treatment, atropine is the initial drug of choice
D. When administered to patients with AMI and sinus bradycardia, atropine not uncommonly aggravates ischemia by increasing heart rate and myocardial oxygen consumption
E. Sinus bradycardia occurring after the first 6 hours of AMI is often caused by a mechanism other than vagal hyperactivity

265. True statements about right ventricular infarction (RVI) include all of the following EXCEPT:

A. RVI may be accompanied by Kussmaul's sign
B. ST segment elevation in lead V_4 is commonly present in RVI
C. Echocardiography may help distinguish RVI from pericardial effusion and tamponade
D. Marked hypotensive responses to small doses of nitroglycerin may suggest the possibility of RVI
E. Sequential atrioventricular pacing may be of benefit in selected patients with RVI

266. Of the following bacteria, the one *most* likely to cause symptomatic myocarditis is:

A. *Mycobacterium tuberculosis*
B. *Salmonella typhimurium*
C. Diphtheria bacillus
D. Eikenella
E. Acinetobacter

267. True statements about the surgical management of abdominal aortic aneurysm (AAA) include all of the following EXCEPT:

A. All such aneurysms greater than 6 cm in diameter should be treated by elective surgical repair
B. The usual surgical repair consists of resection of

the aneurysm with insertion of a synthetic prosthesis

C. Marked hypotension following release of the aortic crossclamp continues to be a cause of perioperative morbidity

D. Approximately half of the perioperative deaths following AAA repair are due to myocardial infarction

E. The operative risk in the lowest-risk patients who undergo elective AAA repair is approximately 2 to 5 per cent

---

268. All of the following features suggest acute as opposed to chronic mitral regurgitation (MR) EXCEPT:

A. no cardiomegaly on chest x-ray
B. a normal ECG
C. a systolic murmur that radiates to the neck
D. a systolic murmur that clearly ends before S_2
E. normal jugular venous pressure

---

269. True statements about the clinical manifestations of cardiac tamponade include all of the following EXCEPT:

A. Patients in whom cardiac tamponade develops slowly usually complain of dyspnea
B. Patients with rapid development of severe cardiac tamponade due to intrapericardial hemorrhage most commonly demonstrate pulsus paradoxus
C. Jugular venous distention is a common physical finding in patients with cardiac tamponade
D. Massive pulmonary embolism may be difficult to distinguish from cardiac tamponade
E. Tamponade may be present in a patient in whom the physical examination is normal except for a moderate elevation of jugular venous pressure

---

270. True statements about precipitating factors in acute myocardial infarction (AMI) include all of the following EXCEPT:

A. In most patients, no precipitating factor can be identified
B. Surgical blood loss is correlated with an increased frequency of AMI
C. Emotional stresses may precipitate AMI
D. Trauma does not cause true AMI
E. Neurological disturbances may precipitate AMI

---

271. The M-mode echocardiogram illustrated *in the right column* would most likely be observed in a patient with which disease?

A. Hypertrophic obstructive cardiomyopathy
B. Marfan syndrome
C. Mitral stenosis

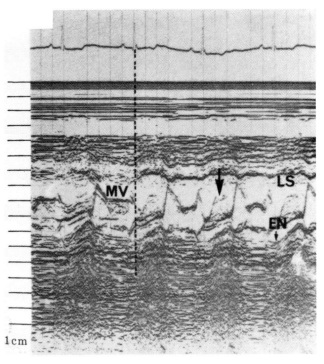

From Feigenbaum, H.: Echocardiography, 4th ed. Philadelphia, Lea & Febiger, 1986, p. 526.

D. Ruptured papillary muscle
E. Aortic regurgitation

---

272. Each of the following statements about congenital valvular aortic stenosis (AS) is true EXCEPT:

A. This anomaly occurs more frequently in males than in females
B. Most children with congenital AS grow and develop normally and are asymptomatic
C. The presence of left ventricular hypertrophy with "strain" on the ECG in childhood usually indicates severe AS
D. Any child with clinical evidence of AS should undergo cardiac catheterization
E. Antibiotic prophylaxis for endocarditis is indicated in all patients with this disorder, regardless of the severity of obstruction

---

273. True statements about congenital heart disease in infancy and childhood include all of the following EXCEPT:

A. Children with congenital heart disease are more commonly male
B. Patent ductus arteriosus is found more commonly in females
C. Approximately one-third of infants with both cardiac and extracardiac congenital anomalies have an established syndrome
D. The rubella syndrome may be accompanied by patent ductus arteriosus or pulmonic valvular stenosis

E. Maternal systemic lupus erythematosus may lead to congenital cardiac defects including ventricular septal defect and pulmonic stenosis

274. All of the following statements about the physical examination in the patient with acute pericarditis are true EXCEPT:

A. The pericardial friction rub is pathognomonic of acute pericarditis
B. The presystolic component of the pericardial friction rub is often loudest and most easily heard
C. A single-component rub is more likely to occur in patients with atrial fibrillation
D. A single-component pericardial friction rub may be mistaken for a systolic murmur of mitral regurgitation
E. Exercise may help establish the presence of a classic three-component rub

275. A 60-year-old man comes to the coronary care unit with severe chest pain. His ECG reveals 2 mm ST-segment elevations in leads II, III, and aV_F. The initial cardiac examination is unremarkable. On the second day a faint late systolic murmur is heard, and by the third day this murmur has increased to Grade III/VI. The patient has mild dyspnea, and a chest x-ray shows pulmonary vascular redistribution. The *most* likely explanation for the murmur is:

A. ruptured posterior papillary muscle
B. ruptured anterior papillary muscle
C. infarcted posterior papillary muscle
D. infarcted anterior papillary muscle
E. ruptured chordae tendineae

276. True statements about abdominal aortic aneurysms (AAA) include all of the following EXCEPT:

A. The majority of AAA are asymptomatic
B. Aneurysms may be sensitive and even tender to palpation
C. Careful physical examination is among the most accurate of noninvasive methods for evaluating AAA
D. Half of all aneurysms greater than 6 cm in diameter rupture within 1 year
E. Recent studies suggest that aneurysms expand by approximately 0.4 to 0.5 cm in diameter each year

277. A 36-year-old white woman complains of a heavy substernal chest discomfort. She consistently develops this discomfort each morning while eating breakfast and watching the morning news. She has no chest pain with exertion. There is no family history of heart disease, and the cholesterol level is normal as is the physical examination. Clinical features, which suggest that her symptoms may be due

to Prinzmetal's angina, would include all of the following EXCEPT:

A. clustering of symptoms after meals
B. cigarette smoking
C. a history of migraine headaches and Raynaud's phenomenon
D. relatively younger age than patients with classic angina
E. association between episodes of chest pain and emotional distress

278. True statements concerning the diastolic murmur of mitral stenosis (MS) include all of the following EXCEPT:

A. The intensity of the murmur is closely related to the severity of stenosis
B. In severe stenosis the murmur is holodiastolic
C. A myxoma in the left atrium may sound identical to MS
D. The duration of the murmur is a rough guide to the severity of stenosis
E. The murmur is reduced during inspiration and during the strain of the Valsalva maneuver

279. True statements about acute pericarditis include all of the following EXCEPT:

A. Acute pericarditis may not be apparent clinically
B. Viral and uremic pericarditis are common forms of the disorder
C. Few pathological changes are noted in acute pericarditis
D. The chief complaint in pericarditis often is chest pain
E. Acute pericarditis may be associated with dyspnea

280. True statements about laboratory tests in the diagnosis of acute myocardial infarction (AMI) include all of the following EXCEPT:

A. Determination of total lactic dehydrogenase (LDH) levels is a sensitive but not specific test for the diagnosis of MI
B. The heart contains principally LDH isozyme type 1
C. Peak total creatinine phosphokinase (CPK) activity usually occurs approximately 12 hours after the onset of symptoms of infarction
D. CPK values in women are normally approximately two-thirds of those in men
E. Elevations in CPK-MB levels may occur in the setting of a normal total CPK value

281. True statements about bacterial pericarditis include all of the following EXCEPT:

A. Uremic pericarditis with a preexisting pericardial effusion may predispose to the development of purulent bacterial pericarditis

B. Direct extension into the pericardium of bacterial pneumonia accounts for the majority of cases of purulent pericarditis

C. Bacterial pericarditis is most often an acute fulminant illness that develops over a few days

D. Long-term survival after purulent bacterial pericarditis remains poor despite the availability of antibacterial therapy

E. High concentrations of antibiotics may be achieved in pericardial fluid

282. A 16-year-old boy requests a physical examination before competing in high school athletics. His mother states that a cousin died suddenly during a basketball game and she recalls that there was something wrong with his heart. The boy has no symptoms. His vital signs are heart rate 64/min, respirations 12/min, and blood pressure 120/75. His cardiac examination is remarkable for a Grade II/VI systolic ejection murmur along the left sternal border, which decreases with squatting and increases with sudden standing. An ECG shows evidence of left ventricular hypertrophy and a chest x-ray shows an increased cardiothoracic ratio. You would recommend:

A. no competitive sports

B. noncontact competitive sports

C. noncontact competitive sports with beta-blocker therapy

D. high-intensity competitive sports

E. high-intensity competitive sports with beta-blocker therapy

283. True statements about atrial septal defect (ASD) include all of the following EXCEPT:

A. Sinus venosus type ASD is frequently associated with anomalous pulmonary venous connections

B. An incomplete seal of the foramen ovale occurs in approximately 25 per cent of adults

C. Approximately 10 to 20 per cent of patients with ostium secundum ASD have associated mitral valve prolapse

D. Children with ASD often experience easy fatigability and exertional dyspnea

E. Atrial arrhythmias are uncommon in children with ASD

284. Changes in left ventricular function and hemodynamics in isolated moderately severe aortic stenosis (AS) include all of the following EXCEPT:

A. normal cardiac output at rest

B. elevated left ventricular end-diastolic pressure

C. elevated left ventricular end-diastolic volume

D. increased *a* waves in the left atrial pressure pulse

E. normal left ventricular stroke volume

285. True statements about the use of noninvasive imaging in acute myocardial infarction (AMI) include all of the following EXCEPT:

A. Cardiomegaly on the chest x-ray is usually associated with left ventricular dysfunction

B. M-mode echocardiography is most useful in imaging the anterior left ventricular wall

C. Wall motion abnormalities are observed by two-dimensional echocardiography in more than two-thirds of patients with AMI

D. Most mechanical complications of AMI are well diagnosed by two-dimensional echocardiography

E. The severity of mitral or tricuspid regurgitation following AMI may be defined by Doppler echocardiography

286. All of the following are absolute indications for surgical intervention in prosthetic valve endocarditis EXCEPT:

A. fungal etiology

B. congestive heart failure

C. vegetations observed on echocardiography

D. new heart block in aortic valve endocarditis

E. positive blood cultures despite 2 weeks of appropriate antibiotic therapy

287. True statements with regard to differences among the calcium channel antagonists include all the following EXCEPT:

A. Verapamil is the most likely to cause constipation and gastrointestinal symptoms

B. Nifedipine is the least likely to cause left ventricular dysfunction

C. Verapamil is the most likely to cause flushing and headache

D. Nifedipine is the least likely to cause decreased heart rate and/or AV block in patients with conduction system disease

E. None of the calcium channel antagonists cause significant bronchoconstriction

288. True statements about tuberculous pericarditis include all of the following EXCEPT:

A. Tuberculous pericarditis usually develops by retrograde spread from adjacent lymph nodes or by early hematogenous spread from the primary infection

B. The tuberculous pericardial effusion usually develops slowly

C. Acute pericardial chest pain is not commonly found in tuberculous pericarditis

D. It is often difficult to establish a definitive bacteriological diagnosis of tuberculous pericarditis

E. Initial therapy for tuberculous pericarditis should include a standard three-drug regimen as well as corticosteroids to reduce pericardial inflammation

289. A 32-year-old woman complains of dizzy spells and one syncopal episode. She had been asymptomatic until the previous summer when she developed mild arthritis and a knee effusion. Her orthopedist found no evidence of infection and thought that she might have injured herself while on vacation in Nantucket, Massachusetts.

On examination, she appeared healthy and no abnormalities were found except for a resting pulse of 48/min. ECG was normal except for a P-R interval of 0.24 sec. A 24-hour ambulatory Holter ECG showed many episodes of Mobitz type II second-degree AV block. Although her erythrocyte sedimentation rate was elevated to 77 mm/hr, the antinuclear antibody titer was negative. The most likely diagnosis is:

A. subacute rheumatic fever
B. Lyme disease
C. systemic lupus erythematosus
D. *Trichinella spiralis* infection
E. hemochromatosis

290. All of the following are commonly associated with myocardial contusion EXCEPT:

A. congestive heart failure
B. ECG findings of pericarditis
C. elevated CPK-MB isoenzyme
D. positive uptake of technetium pyrophosphate
E. sinus node dysfunction

291. Correct statements with regard to "early" prosthetic valve endocarditis (PVE) include all of the following EXCEPT:

A. Initial antibiotic therapy should be oxacillin and an aminoglycoside
B. The most common class of organisms isolated is staphylococci
C. Fungal infection is more common in early than in late PVE
D. By definition, early PVE occurs within 60 days after operation
E. Early PVE has a five- to tenfold higher case fatality rate than late PVE

292. True statements about conduction disturbances in acute myocardial infarction (AMI) include all of the following EXCEPT:
A. Most patients with first-degree AV block and AMI have an intranodal conduction disturbance
B. Digitalis toxicity may be the cause of first-degree AV block in AMI
C. Of patients with AMI and second-degree AV block, the majority have Mobitz type I or Wenckebach second-degree AV block

D. Mobitz type II second-degree AV block in AMI is almost always found with anterior infarction
E. In patients with anterior infarction who develop third-degree AV block, the conduction disturbance usually occurs without prior intraventricular conduction abnormalities

293. True statements about the natural history of untreated ventricular septal defect (VSD) include all of the following EXCEPT:

A. The natural history of VSD may differ depending on the size of the defect and the magnitude of the pulmonary vascular resistance
B. Regardless of size, the presence of a VSD confers an increased risk for endocarditis
C. Progressive pulmonary vascular disease with reversal of shunting (Eisenmenger complex) usually occurs during the 5th decade of life in those patients with VSD who will develop this complication
D. Infundibular pulmonic stenosis may develop gradually in occasional adult patients with isolated VSD
E. Women with VSDs that lead to ratios of pulmonary to systemic flow less than 2:1 generally tolerate pregnancy well

294. A 21-year-old intravenous drug abuser came to the hospital with fever and malaise of 3 weeks' duration. His chest x-ray showed right-sided pneumonia and bilateral pleural effusions. The initial examination was remarkable for inspiratory wheezes and dullness at the right base. There were prominent *c-v* waves in his jugular venous pulse and a hyperdynamic precordium was noted. A Grade III/VI systolic murmur was audible most prominently along the left sternal border. Five of six blood cultures were positive for *Pseudomonas aeruginosa* and he was started on tobramycin and ticarcillin. However, after 2 weeks he had persistent fever to 100°F and 1+ pedal edema, and blood cultures were again positive for *Pseudomonas*. Appropriate therapy at this time would be:

A. an additional 4 weeks of treatment with higher doses of tobramycin and ticarcillin
B. antibiotics changed to tobramycin and piperacillin and given for an additional 4 weeks
C. tricuspid valvulectomy (with replacement by a prosthetic valve) followed by antibiotic treatment for 4 weeks
D. tricuspid valvulectomy with replacement by a Hancock porcine prosthesis and antibiotics for 4 weeks
E. tricuspid valvulectomy with replacement by a St. Jude mechanical prosthesis and continued antibiotics for 4 weeks

295. A 57-year-old white woman comes to the office complaining of dyspnea. She has no history of chest pain, denies smoking, and has never been hypertensive. She has a complicated medical history, including a long history of arthritis and adult-onset diabetes mellitus now requiring insulin. Her only current medication is NPH insulin. On examination she is a well-tanned woman with heart rate 90/min, respirations 16/min, blood pressure 140/85. Lungs: inspiratory crackles at the bases. Heart: elevated jugular venous pressure at 10 cm; normal carotid upstrokes and volume; normal cardiac impulse; S_1 and S_2 normal, loud S_3; holosystolic murmurs at left sternal border and apex, the former increasing with inspiration and the latter with handgrip. The liver is firm and palpable 2 cm below the right costal margin. There is 2+ pitting edema of both legs. ECG is unremarkable. The most likely cause for her dyspnea is:

    A. hemochromatosis
    B. sarcoidosis
    C. amyloidosis
    D. Fabry's disease
    E. ischemic cardiomyopathy

296. Each of the following statements about tetralogy of Fallot is correct EXCEPT:

    A. Classic tetralogy of Fallot is composed of a large ventricular septal defect (VSD), infundibular and/or valvular pulmonic stenosis, right ventricular hypertrophy, and overriding aorta
    B. In some cases, the VSD communicates with the right ventricle in an area just distal to the outflow tract obstruction
    C. Survival of patients with tetralogy of Fallot into adult life usually reflects mild to at most moderate obstruction of right ventricular outflow
    D. Pseudotruncus arteriosus is a variant of tetralogy of Fallot in which complete ventricular outflow tract obstruction occurs
    E. Congestive heart failure is unusual in patients with tetralogy of Fallot

297. True statements about atheromatous emboli include all of the following EXCEPT:

    A. The most common cause of atheromatous emboli is surgical manipulation of an atherosclerotic aorta
    B. Cardiac catheterization may lead to embolism of atheromatous material
    C. Hepatitis is an important complication of atheromatous embolism
    D. Cholesterol emboli may be visible on direct inspection of the retinal arteries
    E. Livido reticularis is one manifestation of atheromatous emboli

298. True statements about acute myocardial infarction (AMI) include all of the following EXCEPT:

    A. Approximately one-fourth of all deaths in the United States are due to AMI
    B. The majority of deaths caused by AMI occur during hours 2 to 4 after the beginning of the event
    C. A decline by 25 per cent or more in the incidence of AMI has occurred in recent years in the United States
    D. Most deaths among patients hospitalized with AMI are attributable to left ventricular failure and shock
    E. Careful monitoring of cardiac rhythm and treatment of primary arrhythmias have reduced the incidence of in-hospital death from AMI

299. All of the following characteristics of a chest pain would be unusual for coronary artery ischemia-induced angina EXCEPT:

    A. a pain that begins gradually and reaches maximum intensity over a period of minutes
    B. a pain aggravated or precipitated by one deep breath
    C. a pain relieved within seconds of lying horizontally
    D. a pain localized to an area the size of the tip of a finger
    E. a pain relieved within a few seconds by one or two sips of water

300. True statements about supravalvular aortic stenosis (AS) include all of the following EXCEPT:

    A. The clinical picture of supravalvular obstruction is indistinguishable from that of other forms of AS
    B. Williams' syndrome is a distinctive clinical picture produced by coexistence of supravalvular AS and a multiple-system disorder
    C. Accentuation of the aortic valve closure sound is a feature characteristic of supravalvular AS
    D. A continuous murmur may be heard on physical examination of some patients with known or suspected supravalvular AS
    E. Echocardiography is the most valuable technique for localization of the site of obstruction in supravalvular AS

301. A 65-year-old woman with an aortic valve replacement has a 2-week history of malaise and fever. After developing severe right flank pain, she seeks medical attention. On examination, she has a temperature of 100°F, heart rate 100/min, and respirations 16/min. Her lungs are clear. The cardiac examination is remarkable for a Grade III/VI systolic ejection murmur and a soft diastolic blowing murmur. Laboratory results include Hgb 10 gm/dl, WBC 14,000/mm³ with 80 per cent neutrophils, 5 per cent bands, and 15 per cent lymphocytes;

urinalysis reveals 3+heme; microscopic examination reveals 15 rbc/high-power field. The most likely diagnosis is:

A. focal glomerulonephritis
B. renal infarction
C. diffuse glomerulonephritis
D. cortical necrosis
E. renal abscess

302. All of the following statements with regard to *primary* endocardial fibroelastosis (EFE) are correct EXCEPT:

A. The condition is often familial
B. The mitral and aortic valve leaflets are usually thickened and distorted
C. The murmur of mitral stenosis is the most common murmur heard
D. Symptoms of primary EFE usually develop between 2 and 12 months of age
E. Echocardiographic features include a reduced ejection fraction and increased LA and LV dimensions

303. A 26-year-old construction worker comes to the emergency room on Monday morning, January 2, in atrial fibrillation. He states that for the last few months he has had occasional episodes of palpitation, almost always on Mondays. His vital signs include heart rate 140/min, respirations 16/min, and blood pressure 160/95. His physical examination is unremarkable except for a soft systolic murmur, and while being observed in the hospital, he spontaneously reverts to normal sinus rhythm. The most likely precipitating drug or condition is:

A. caffeine
B. "uppers"
C. alcohol
D. hypertension
E. mitral valve prolapse

304. True statements about the diagnosis of pulmonary embolism include all of the following EXCEPT:

A. Clinical symptoms and signs often are not helpful in discriminating between patients with evidence of pulmonary embolism on a pulmonary arteriogram and those without such evidence
B. Dyspnea and pleuritic chest pain are common symptoms in pulmonary embolism
C. A majority of patients with pulmonary embolism have a normal respiratory rate
D. The differential diagnosis in suspected pulmonary embolism includes asthma
E. The differential diagnosis in outpatients with suspected pulmonary embolism includes rib fracture

305. A 48-year-old man is seen in the office because of episodes of cardiac palpitation. His other symptoms include paroxysmal nocturnal dyspnea, nocturnal

enuresis, and mild angina. His wife adds that he snores loudly. There is a history of several recent auto accidents. On examination, his blood pressure is elevated at 190/100 and he is mildly overweight. Laboratory examination reveals a hematocrit of 58 mm Hg. The most likely cardiac finding would be:

A. mitral valve stenosis
B. aortic valve stenosis
C. right ventricular hypertrophy
D. pulmonary valve stenosis
E. atrial septal defect

306. True statements about the coronary and pathological anatomy of acute myocardial infarction (AMI) include all of the following EXCEPT:

A. One-third to two-thirds of patients who die from AMI have critical obstruction of a single coronary artery at necropsy
B. In series of patients studied at necropsy, a small number of patients with MI are found to have normal coronary vessels
C. Angiography is relatively safe even during the acute phase of MI
D. During the early hours of transmural MI, 90 per cent of infarct-related vessels are totally occluded
E. Spontaneous thrombolysis may decrease the incidence of totally occluded vessels found in the period following MI

307. True statements about pulmonic stenosis (PS) with intact ventricular septum include all of the following EXCEPT:

A. Valvular PS is the most common form of isolated right ventricular obstruction
B. The most common symptoms from PS during infancy are acidemia and hypoxemia
C. Normal heart size and primarily left ventricular forces on electrocardiography are characteristic of PS with intact ventricular septum
D. Percutaneous transluminal balloon valvuloplasty is the initial procedure of choice in patients with typical valvular PS and moderate to severe degrees of obstruction
E. The severity of obstruction due to PS is often suggested by findings on physical examination

308. All of the following are HACEK organisms which cause endocarditis EXCEPT:

A. Hemophilus
B. Actinobacillus
C. Cardiobacterium
D. *Escherichia coli*
E. Kingella

309. A 1-year-old child presents with evidence of pericarditis. Three weeks earlier he had a fever that lasted for 10 days despite penicillin therapy. Asso-

ciated findings at that time included congestion of the ocular conjunctivae and erythema of the palms and feet, a nonerupting rash, and dry, erythematous, and fissured lips. One week ago there was membranous desquamation of the fingertips. Present findings include ECG evidence of pericarditis and echocardiographic documentation of decreased LV function. The most likely diagnosis is:

A. acute rubella myocarditis
B. Coxsackie B myocarditis
C. *Hemophilus influenzae* myocarditis
D. Kawasaki's disease
E. Stevens-Johnson syndrome

310. True statements about the physical examination in acute myocardial infarction (AMI) include all of the following EXCEPT:

A. The majority of patients with uncomplicated AMI have mild systolic hypertension
B. The majority of patients with AMI have tachycardia
C. The majority of patients with AMI develop a mild fever
D. The majority of patients with AMI demonstrate a muffled S_1
E. S_4 is audible in the majority of patients with AMI

311. True statements with regard to the HMG CoA reductase inhibitors include all of the following EXCEPT:

A. These agents competitively inhibit 3-hydroxy-3-methyl glutaryl coenzyme A reductase
B. Their primary mechanism of action is to decrease cholesterol synthesis
C. About 2 per cent of patients taking these agents will have a sustained rise in serum transaminase levels to 3 times the upper limit of normal
D. These agents usually cause a significant decrease in hepatic LDL receptors
E. Their main indication is to treat elevated LDL cholesterol

312. Increases in the following parameters directly increase cardiac $M\dot{V}O_2$ EXCEPT:

A. external mechanical work
B. left ventricular systolic pressure
C. left ventricular wall tension
D. left ventricular end-diastolic volume
E. none of the above

313. True statements about peripheral pulmonary artery stenoses include all of the following EXCEPT:

A. Pulmonary artery stenoses may occur anywhere from the main pulmonary trunk to the smallest peripheral arterial branches

B. Most often peripheral pulmonary artery stenoses are isolated findings, but occasionally they may be seen in conjunction with other cardiovascular defects
C. Intrauterine rubella infection is an important cuase of pulmonary artery stenoses
D. Most children with peripheral pulmonary artery stenoses are asymptomatic
E. Percutaneous transcatheter balloon angioplasty may be used in the treatment of this disorder

314. A 59-year-old business executive complains of chest pain that is midsternal and that radiates primarily retrosternally. It is an aching, burning pain, occurring most frequently at night, occasionally awakening the patient shortly after he has fallen asleep. His internist prescribed nitroglycerin, which he has taken infrequently. However, it does relieve his pain, usually within 10 to 30 minutes. The previous day during a luncheon meeting, he had a severe episode while presenting a new financial plan; the pain seemed to lessen when he sat down and finished lunch. The most likely explanation for his chest pain is:

A. Prinzmetal's angina
B. esophageal reflux spasm
C. "fixed-threshold" angina
D. "variable-threshold" angina
E. biliary colic

315. Features common to Type II hyperlipoproteinemia include all of the following EXCEPT:

A. increased low-density lipoprotein (LDL) levels
B. xanthomas of the extensor tendons
C. corneal arcus
D. premature atherosclerosis
E. recurrent pancreatitis

316. True statements about congestive heart failure in neonates and infants include all of the following EXCEPT:

A. Scalp edema, ascites, pericardial effusion, and decreased fetal movements are all findings in fetal heart failure
B. In the preterm infant, the most common cause of cardiac decompensation is a persistently patent ductus arteriosus
C. Tachycardia and pulmonary rales are uncommon manifestations of heart failure in the infant
D. Pleural and pericardial effusions are rare in infants with cardiac decompensation
E. Hepatomegaly is a common finding in infants with heart failure

317. A 62-year-old black man comes to the hospital in congestive heart failure. His symptoms include a 2-month history of progressive dyspnea and orthopnea

and worsening pedal edema. The week prior to admission he had paroxysmal nocturnal dyspnea almost every night. He denies chest pain, fevers, or chills. His past history is remarkable for mild hypertension currently untreated with medication. He developed anemia 2 years ago, when a diagnosis of multiple myeloma was made. He has been stable since then on chlorambucil (Leukeran) 10 mg daily, and requiring transfusion of 1 unit of blood monthly.

On examination the heart rate was 100/min, respirations 22/min, and BP 100/60. The chest showed inspiratory crackles halfway up the lung fields. His jugular venous pulse was 10 cm above the clavicle. The cardiac impulse was displaced laterally. S_1 and S_2 were normal; a loud S_3 was present. A Grade II/VI holosystolic murmur radiated to the axilla. There was mild hepatosplenomegaly and 2+ pedal edema. Chest x-ray showed cardiomegaly, bilateral pleural effusions, and pulmonary vascular redistribution. ECG was normal except for low voltage. The most likely cause for his congestive heart failure is:

A. sarcoid heart disease
B. cardiac amyloidosis
C. Leukeran cardiotoxicity
D. alcoholic cardiomyopathy
E. hemochromatosis

318. The most important intrinsic vasodilator present in states of diminished coronary perfusion is:

A. adenosine triphosphate (ATP)
B. calcium
C. hypoxanthine
D. adenosine
E. cyclic adenosine monophosphate (cAMP)

319. Based on survival data for medically treated patients in the Coronary Artery Surgery Study (CASS) Registry, the patient group with the lowest survival at 4 years would most likely be:

A. 1 diseased vessel, LV ejection fraction (EF) 35 to 50 per cent
B. 1 diseased vessel, LV EF <35 per cent
C. 2 diseased vessels, LV EF 35 to 50 per cent
D. 2 diseased vessels, LV EF <35 per cent
E. 3 diseased vessels, LV EF 35 to 50 per cent

DIRECTIONS: Each question below contains five suggested answers. For EACH of the FIVE alternatives listed you are to respond either YES (Y) or NO (N). In a given item ALL, SOME, OR NONE OF THE ALTERNATIVES MAY BE CORRECT.

320. Acute myocardial infarction (AMI) may occasionally result from nonatherosclerotic causes. Examples of nonatherosclerotic causes of AMI include which of the following?
A. Endocarditis
B. Kawasaki's disease
C. Systemic lupus erythematosis
D. Amyloidosis
E. Cocaine abuse

321. Noninvasive studies may be useful in the evaluation of patients with tetralogy of Fallot. True statements about such studies include which of the following?

A. The electrocardiogram in tetralogy of Fallot is characterized by right ventricular hypertrophy
B. The boot-shaped heart (coeur en sabot) is characteristic of the chest x-ray in infants and children
C. The chest x-ray in tetralogy of Fallot is less typical in adults
D. An abnormal relationship between the aortic annulus and the interventricular septum is rarely visible on M-mode echocardiography
E. Magnetic resonance imaging may be helpful in assessment of tetralogy of Fallot

322. True statements with respect to the diagnosis of Prinzmetal's or variant angina include:

A. Usually there is elevation of ST segments with pain
B. Exercise testing of patients with variant angina is most likely to yield ST segment elevation at low work thresholds
C. Approximately two-thirds of patients have severe coronary artery stenosis at the site of the spasm
D. Patients with normal coronary arteries and Prinzmetal's angina have a higher incidence of right coronary artery spasm and a more benign course
E. Ergonovine testing with intravenous administration of 1 to 10 mg is sensitive and specific for provoking coronary artery spasm

323. With reference to the ostium primum atrial septal defect (ASD), true statements include which of the following?

A. Ostium primum ASDs often displace and disfigure both the anterior and posterior leaflets of the mitral valve

B. The clinical features of ostium primum ASDs are quite similar to those of ostium secundum variety

C. Chest roentgenography usually reveals both RA and RV enlargement

D. The presence of an ostium primum ASD along with a ventricular septal defect in the postero-basal portion of the ventricular septum comprises the entity known as complete atrioventricular canal defect

E. Streaming of contrast material through the ostium primum ASD into the right heart during left ventriculography creates the characteristic "gooseneck" deformity.

---

324. The use of permanent pacing in patients who survive acute myocardial infarction (AMI) is still somewhat controversial. True statements about the use of permanent pacing in this population include which of the following?

A. Transient type II second-degree AV block or complete third-degree AV block in the presence of inferior infarction does not appear to require permanent pacing

B. The occurrence of transient high-grade AV block in the presence of bundle branch block heralds a greater risk of *recurrent* high-degree AV block

C. Most patients with AMI and bundle branch block with transient high-degree AV block who die do so because of recurrent high-degree block

D. Late in-hospital ventricular fibrillation in coronary care unit survivors is increased in patients with anteroseptal AMI complicated by either right or left bundle branch block

E. Persistent Mobitz type II second-degree AV block is an absolute indication for permanent pacing following AMI

---

325. Correct statements regarding diphtheritic myocarditis in children include:

A. Cardiac involvement is secondary to direct endocardial and myocardial invasion by the bacillus

B. Cardiac dysfunction is secondary to depletion of myocardial carnitine

C. Cardiac involvement is clinically evident in about 10 per cent of patients with diphtheria

D. Development of right or left bundle branch block and complete AV block is associated with mortality rates in excess of 50 per cent

E. Following recovery from an acute episode of diphtheritic cardiomyopathy, the prognosis is poor for about 50 per cent of children

---

326. True statements about the clinical manifestations of aortic dissection include which of the following?

A. Men are more frequently affected than women

B. Severe pain is the most common presenting symptom

C. Patients with aortic dissection usually present with hypotension

D. Aortic regurgitation is seen in the majority of patients with distal aortic dissection

E. Pulse deficits are more common in proximal than in distal aortic dissection

---

327. Surgical *repair* of the mitral valve (e.g., annuloplasty and/or suture repair of the valve with repair of the chordae tendineae as necessary) might be prudent and likely to be successful in which of the following patients?

A. A 33-year-old man with Marfan syndrome and myxomatous degeneration

B. A 62-year-old man with severe MR due to annular dilatation following MI

C. A 40-year-old woman with MR due to a ruptured chordae tendineae with active infective endocarditis

D. A 70-year-old woman with rheumatic heart disease, combined MS and MR with calcified mitral valve, and deformed leaflets

E. A 23-year-old man with a congenitally cleft mitral valve

---

328. With reference to management of ventricular septal defect (VSD), true statements include which of the following?

A. In the absence of evidence of pulmonary hypertension, elective hemodynamic evaluation of VSD should occur between the ages of 3 and 6 years

B. Surgical treatment for children with normal pulmonary arterial pressures and shunts greater than 1.2:1.0 should be carried out before the beginning of school

C. Right bundle branch block is the most significant surgically induced conduction system abnormality in the repair of VSD

D. The presence of right bundle branch block with left anterior hemiblock and transient complete heart block in the postoperative period is an indication for permanent pacemaker therapy

E. In patients who have repair of VSD, a normal resting pulmonary arterial pressure makes the presence of normal pulmonary pressures during exercise likely

---

329. Intraventricular conduction disturbance may complicate acute myocardial infarction (AMI). Which of the following are true statements concerning intraventricular block in the setting of AMI?

A. The presence of isolated left anterior fascicular block is associated with increased risk of death in patients with AMI

B. In general, a larger infarct is required to create

left posterior fascicular block than left anterior fascicular block

C. New onset of right bundle branch block in the setting of AMI often is associated with the development of AV block
D. Left bundle branch block in the setting of AMI leads to complete AV block more frequently than does right bundle branch block
E. Preexisting bundle branch block or divisional block is less likely to progress to complete heart block in patients with AMI than are conduction defects acquired during the course of the infarct itself

330. A 62-year-old woman returns to the office for evaluation of mitral valve disease. Fifteen years earlier she had undergone a closed mitral commissurotomy with excellent results. Five years ago she developed atrial fibrillation that persisted despite several attempts at cardioversion. Three years ago she was placed on warfarin because she suffered a small stroke. Her symptoms now include progressive dyspnea on exertion, rapid heart beat, and left-sided chest pain on exertion. Her clinical examination is consistent with moderate to severe mitral stenosis (MS). An echocardiogram reveals normal LV function, a markedly dilated left atrium, a heavily calcified poorly mobile aortic valve, and some mitral regurgitation. The other valves appear normal. You would advise the following:

A. cardiac catheterization
B. open commissurotomy and mitral valve repair
C. balloon mitral valvuloplasty
D. mitral valve replacement with a mechanical prosthetic valve
E. no further treatment

331. With regard to the management of tetralogy of Fallot, true statements include which of the following?

A. Early definitive repair is indicated
B. The size of the pulmonary arteries is the single most important determinant in assessing candidacy for primary repair of tetralogy of Fallot
C. If early corrective operation is not possible, a palliative procedure that leads to increased pulmonary blood flow is usually recommended
D. Postoperative increase in pulmonary venous return may lead to mild to moderate RV decompensation
E. Bleeding problems are a common complication in the postoperative period following repair of tetralogy of Fallot

332. Correct statements concerning the M-mode echocardiogram displayed *at right* include:

A. The mitral valve leaflets are thickened
B. The *a* wave is exaggerated
C. During diastole leaflet separation is decreased

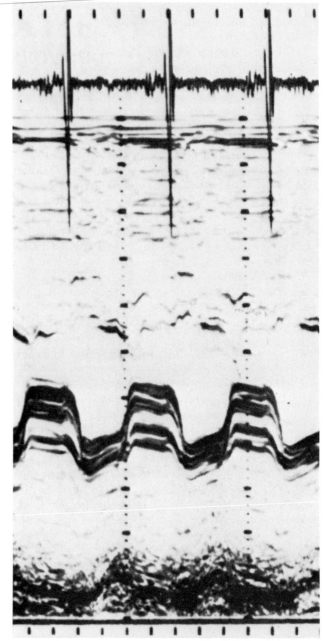

From Bloomfield, P., O'Boyle, J.E., and Parisi, A.F.: Non-invasive Investigations for the Diagnosis of Mitral Valve Disease. *In* Ionescu, M.I., and Cohn, L.H. (eds.): Mitral Valve Disease: Diagnosis and Treatment. London, Butterworths, 1985, p. 58.

D. The mitral valve area is probably normal
E. During diastole the posterior mitral valve leaflet moves posteriorly

333. Left ventricular aneurysm may develop as a consequence of acute myocardial infarction (AMI). True statements about left ventricular aneurysm include which of the following?

A. Left ventricular aneurysm complicating AMI is usually due to total occlusion of the left anterior descending artery
B. Aneurysms usually range in size from 1 to 8 cm in diameter

C. Inferoposterior anerysms are slightly more common than apical aneurysms

D. When mortality in patients with left ventricular aneurysm is compared with that in patients without aneurysm but with similar ejection fractions, no substantial difference is evident

E. Persistent ST-segment elevation in an electrocardiographic area of infarction indicates a large infarct but does not necessarily indicate an aneurysm

---

334. Which of the following are true statements about the pathophysiology of constrictive pericarditis?

A. Constriction leads to equalization of diastolic pressures in all four cardiac chambers

B. Diastolic filling is unimpeded in early diastole in constrictive pericarditis

C. Most ventricular filling occurs within the initial portion of diastole in constrictive pericarditis

D. In general, the x descent is steeper than the y descent in constrictive pericarditis

E. In constrictive pericarditis, the greatest acceleration of venous blood flow returning to the heart occurs during systole

---

335. Features typical of patients with familial myxoma include:

A. transmission in an autosomal recessive fashion

B. presence of multiple myxomas

C. earlier age of initial presentation than for patients with sporadic myxoma

D. increased incidence of pigmented nevi and lentigines

E. increased incidence of myxomas outside the left atrium

---

336. Postinfarction angina may complicate acute myocardial infarction (AMI). True statements about postinfarction angina include which of the following?

A. Both short- and long-term mortality are higher in patients with postinfarction angina

B. Most patients who develop spontaneous angina in the early days following AMI should undergo cardiac catheterization

C. No absolute increase in mortality is noted in patients who have true infarct extension

D. Infarct extension occurs in less than 1 per cent of patients with AMI during the first 10 days after infarction

---

337. Which of the following are true statements about the management of constrictive pericarditis?

A. The therapy of choice for constrictive pericarditis is resection of the pericardial tissue from the anterior and inferior surfaces of the RV

B. The operative mortality for pericardiectomy is approximately 10 to 15 per cent

C. Most patients develop a low-output syndrome immediately following pericardiectomy for constrictive pericarditis

D. Symptomatic improvement is reported in approximately 90 per cent of survivors of pericardiectomy

E. In general, pericardiectomy should be performed early in the course of constrictive pericarditis in symptomatic patients

---

338. Myocarditis is not uncommon in association with which of the following viruses?

A. Coxsackie

B. Mumps

C. Variola and vaccinia

D. Echovirus

E. Influenza

---

339. Perfusion lung scanning is a key diagnostic test used in screening for pulmonary embolism. True statements about perfusion lung scanning in the diagnosis of pulmonary embolism include which of the following?

A. A completely normal perfusion lung scan essentially rules out all but the smallest pulmonary emboli

B. The four designations *low, moderate, high,* and *indeterminate probability* for pulmonary embolism on perfusion lung scanning have been standardized by the American Society of Radiology

C. In general, patients with perfusion defects that are segmental or greater in size and with normal ventilation on scintigraphy in the same areas as the perfusion defects have an increased likelihood of pulmonary embolism

D. The presence of a chest x-ray abnormality in the area of a perfusion defect leads to the designation "indeterminate scan"

E. Subsegmental and nonsegmental perfusion defects that match ventilation defects may be present in patients with normal pulmonary angiography

---

340. On the basis of the National Institutes of Health Cholesterol Consensus Conference recommendations, which of the following patients should receive treatment for elevated cholesterol level (diet and/or drugs)?

A. 19-year-old male, cholesterol 200

B. 30-year-old male, cholesterol 200

C. 45-year-old male, cholesterol 260

D. 60-year-old female, cholesterol 260

E. 30-year-old female, cholesterol 215

---

341. With respect to the assessment of prognosis in the period following myocardial infarction (MI), true statements include which of the following?

A. A predischarge submaximal exercise test is useful for early screening and detection of ischemia

B. A maximal exercise test 4 to 6 weeks following discharge will identify a number of patients with residual myocardial ischemia not identified on a predischarge submaximal exercise test

C. Decreased left ventricular ejection fraction and ventricular ectopy are independent risk factors for post-MI mortality

D. Ambulatory electrocardiographic monitoring should be carried out in all patients who have recently had MI

E. A fall in left ventricular ejection fraction during exercise determined by radionuclide ventriculography is usually an indication for cardiac catheterization in the post-MI patient

---

342. True statements with regard to the presentation of the patient with the illustrated valve *shown below* include:

A. The abnormality was most likely congenital

B. A systolic ejection murmur would be likely

C. Endocarditis frequently leads to this lesion

D. Diabetes mellitus and hypercholesterolemia are risk factors for development of this lesion

E. A loud diastolic blowing murmur would be likely

---

343. While few absolute contraindications to physical activity exist for healthy people, there are cardiovascular contraindications to an exercise program. Which of the following are absolute contraindications to such a program?

A. Resting blood pressure greater than 200/110 mm Hg

B. Unpaced third-degree heart block

C. Diabetes

D. Cardiomyopathy

E. Ischemia

---

344. Which of the following are true statements about the use of percutaneous transluminal coronary angioplasty (PTCA)?

A. The risk of occlusion of the side branch of a coronary artery in PTCA involving coronary bifurcations is less than 5 per cent

B. The primary success rate in dilatation of a coronary artery which has been totally occluded for less than 3 months is approximately 60 per cent

C. In patients with multivessel disease who undergo PTCA of a single vessel, recurrent angina is more likely to occur than in patients in whom no residual stenoses exist

D. Controlled comparison of multivessel PTCA

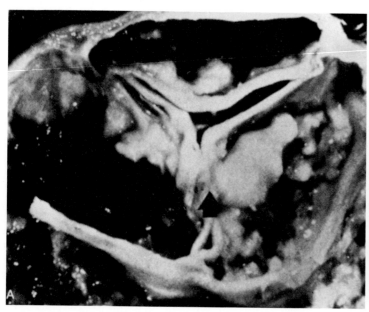

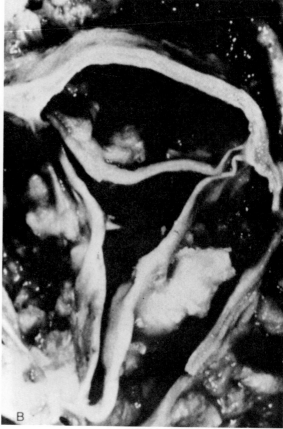

From Salem, D.N., and Isner, J.M.: Chest 92:326, 1987.

with bypass surgery reveals no significant difference in 1-year mortality in patients with three-vessel disease and normal ventricular function
  E. A significant number of patients with unstable angina have lesions that are amenable to PTCA

345. Which of the following are appropriate steps in the *initial* management of acute pericarditis?

  A. Bed rest
  B. Hospitalization
  C. Corticosteroid therapy
  D. Low-dose oral anticoagulants
  E. Antibiotics

346. Clinical features typical of mitral stenosis (MS) include:

  A. greater incidence in women than men
  B. a loud first heart sound (S_1)
  C. presence of a third heart sound (S_3)
  D. hyperdynamic, enlarged LV
  E. presence of a presystolic murmur

347. True statements about pericardiocentesis include which of the following?

  A. Hydration prior to pericardiocentesis may prove useful
  B. A major risk of percutaneous pericardiocentesis is laceration of the heart, coronary arteries, or lung
  C. The size of the effusion is not well correlated with the probability of successfully obtaining pericardial fluid
  D. Cardiac tamponade associated with malignant pericardial effusion can often be managed by pericardiocentesis
  E. Pericardiocentesis is especially useful in situations in which a loculated effusion is present

348. Correct statements with regard to graft patency rate and prognosis in coronary artery bypass surgery include:

  A. The patency rate of internal mammary artery (IMA) grafts at 1 year is about 95 per cent
  B. After 7 to 10 years the patency rate of IMA grafts is about 50 per cent
  C. Although the diameter of a saphenous vein graft is closer to that of the recipient coronary artery than that of an IMA, the increased tendency for intimal hyperplasia results in decreased vein graft patency
  D. Total blood flow through an IMA is less than through a saphenous vein graft
  E. Blood flow through vein grafts greater than 45 ml/min is predictive of increased graft patency

349. True statements about the typical evolution of the ECG in acute pericarditis include which of the following?

  A. In general, the serial appearance of four stages of abnormalities of the ST segments and T waves characterizes the electrocardiographic evolution of acute pericarditis
  B. Stage I changes, or ST-segment elevation, are not often of great diagnostic value
  C. The ST-segment elevation in stage I of acute pericarditis is usually most prominent in inferior leads
  D. In acute pericarditis, the ST segment usually returns to baseline before the appearance of T-wave inversion
  E. Stage IV electrocardiographic change is the reversion of T-wave changes to normal which may occur weeks or months following the acute episode of chest pain

350. True statements with regard to the clinical history of aortic stenosis (AS) include:

  A. Average survival from the onset of syncope is approximately 3 years
  B. Average survival from the onset of congestive heart failure is approximately 2 years
  C. Average survival from the onset of angina pectoris is approximately 1 year
  D. Sudden death in patients with AS usually occurs in previously symptomatic individuals
  E. Development of atrial fibrillation is usually well tolerated in patients with moderately severe AS

351. Correct statements with regard to the coronary artery morphology observed at cardiac catheterization in patients with unstable compared with stable angina include:

  A. Lesions with a narrow neck, irregular borders, or both are more common in patients with unstable angina
  B. Rapid progression of an insignificant to a significant lesion is more common in unstable angina
  C. The right coronary artery is the most commonly affected vessel in patients with unstable angina
  D. Intracoronary filling defects are more common in patients with unstable angina
  E. The majority of patients with unstable angina have obstructive three-vessel disease

352. Which of the following are features of the post-myocardial infarction syndrome (Dressler syndrome)?

  A. Usual occurrence 2 to 3 weeks following infarction
  B. Antimyocardial antibodies identified as the principal cause

C. Specific histological appearance of the pericardium

D. Mild, atypical chest pain in approximately 50 per cent of patients

E. Need for hospitalization for observation

353. Asymmetric or disproportionate septal hypertrophy may sometimes be documented by echocardiography in which of the following patients or illnesses?

A. 6-month-old infant
B. Pulmonic stenosis
C. Beriberi
D. Hyperthyroidism
E. Following an anterior myocardial infarction

354. True statements with regard to penetrating chest wounds include:

A. Post-traumatic pericarditis is a common complication
B. Injuries to the atria are associated with a higher survival than are injuries to the ventricles
C. Rupture of the interventricular septum is often a late complication
D. The right coronary artery is the most commonly lacerated coronary artery

355. Correct statements with regard to the mechanisms of action of nitrates in ischemic heart disease include:

A. Nitrates directly relax vascular smooth muscle
B. The vasodilator effects of nitrates predominate in the arterial circulation
C. Coronary arteries containing significant atherosclerotic plaque (>70 per cent stenosis) often dilate in response to nitrates
D. Nitrates increase myocardial contractility directly
E. An intact endothelium is required for nitrate-induced vasodilation

356. A 60-year-old woman with a history of progressive symptoms secondary to calcific aortic stenosis undergoes porcine aortic valve replacement. Post-operatively she does well except for a persistent fever to 99.5°F. On the seventh postoperative day a new diastolic murmur is appreciated. That evening cardiac telemetry reveals a gradually increasing P-R interval. True statements regarding her condition include:

A. Blood cultures would likely grow *Staphylococcus aureus*
B. The risk of her developing complete heart block is small
C. Surgical treatment is likely to be required
D. Initial antibiotic management should include vancomycin and an aminoglycoside

E. Appearance of right bundle branch block suggests endocarditis involving the mitral valve

357. Patients at high risk for infective endocarditis and who should therefore receive prophylactic antibiotics include those with which of the following?

A. Isolated ostium secundum ASD
B. Post-coronary artery bypass
C. Hypertrophic obstructive cardiomyopathy
D. One year following repair of an ostium secundum ASD without a patch
E. Ventriculoatrial shunt for hydrocephalus

358. Which of the following clinical findings would be *unusual* in a patient with hypertrophic obstructive cardiomyopathy?

A. A prominent *a* wave in the jugular pulse
B. A slowing of the carotid upstroke
C. The murmur of aortic regurgitation
D. The murmur of mitral regurgitation
E. An S_3

359. Correct statements with regard to the oxygen-derived free radical system in myocardial ischemia include:

A. The superoxide anion is denoted as $\cdot O_2-$
B. The superoxide anion can give rise to either hydrogen peroxide (H_2O_2) or the hydroxyl radical ($\cdot OH$)
C. Superoxide dismutase enzymes produce superoxide from hydrogen peroxide
D. Xanthine oxidase in the presence of xanthine may produce oxygen radicals
E. Free radicals are normally involved in cellular reactions such as oxidative phosphorylation

360. Features typical of patients with variable-threshold angina as compared with fixed-threshold angina include:

A. precipitation of angina by sudden exposure to cold temperatures
B. presence of an underlying significant coronary artery stenosis
C. a higher incidence of nonfatal MI
D. an episodic pain syndrome with "good days" when substantial physical activity is possible and "bad days" when angina may occur at rest
E. a higher likelihood of two- and three-vessel coronary artery disease

361. Significant involvement of the heart causing hemodynamic compromise is typical in amyloidosis associated with which of the following diseases or conditions?

A. Rheumatoid arthritis
B. Multiple myeloma
C. Tuberculosis
D. Advanced age
E. B cell lymphoma

362. On the basis of the findings of the Coronary Artery Surgery Study (CASS) and of the Veterans Administration Cooperative Study, which of the patients with chronic stable angina listed below are candidates for coronary artery bypass surgery?

A. Angina pectoris that results in a New York Heart Association Class III or IV
B. A left main coronary artery stenosis of 30 per cent
C. Three-vessel disease (>70 per cent stenoses) with normal resting LV ejection fraction (EF)
D. Three-vessel disease (>70 per cent stenoses) with impaired resting LV function (EF <50 per cent)
E. Two-vessel disease (>70 per cent stenoses) with poor exercise tolerance (unable to complete Bruce Stage II) associated with 2 mm ST-segment depression after 4 minutes

DIRECTIONS: Each question below contains four suggested responses of which ONE OR MORE ARE CORRECT. Select

A   if 1, 2, and 3 are correct
B   if 1 and 3 are correct
C   if 2 and 4 are correct
D   if 4 is correct
E   if 1, 2, 3, and 4 are correct

363. Correct statements with regard to pathophysiological events associated with myocardial reperfusion following prolonged ischemia include:

1. Severely ischemic myocytes may demonstrate accelerated necrosis
2. Infarcts are more likely to be hemorrhagic with reperfusion
3. The reintroduction of oxygen causes marked damage to the sarcolemma and may lead to Ca^{++} overload in ischemic myocytes
4. The "no-reflow" phenomenon refers to the fact that mildly ischemic myocardium maintains sufficient vascular tone to prevent reperfusion

364. The Doppler echocardiogram illustrated *on the following page* was obtained during evaluation of the mitral valve. Correct statements include:

1. Mitral stenosis is present
2. Early diastolic flow is abnormal at 2.5 meters/sec
3. Mitral regurgitation is present
4. The "atrial kick" is absent

365. True statements with regard to the demonstration of vegetations in endocarditis by echocardiography include:

1. Patients with one or more vegetations that are seen on echocardiography are at a higher risk for developing complications than those patients with no vegetations
2. Fungal endocarditis is more likely than bacterial endocarditis to reveal vegetations

3. *Streptococcus viridans* endocarditis rarely has demonstrable vegetations
4. A persistent vegetation usually indicates treatment failure

366. Associations of Ebstein's anomaly of the tricuspid valve include:

1. pulmonic stenosis
2. paroxysmal supraventricular tachycardia
3. Wolff-Parkinson-White syndrome
4. delay in tricuspid valve closure relative to mitral closure on M-mode echocardiography

367. A 48-year-old man has a 2-week history of postprandial indigestion and nausea. On the evening of admission, after an argument with his wife, he developed abdominal pain in addition to his usual symptoms and sought medical attention. In the emergency room he had an unremarkable physical examination but his ECG showed 2 mm ST-segment elevation in leads II, III, and aV_F. While preparations were being made for transfer to the CCU he stated that his pain suddenly disappeared; but within the next 30 seconds his heart rate decreased to 30/min and his systolic pressure fell to 68 mm Hg. The most likely explanation(s) is (are):

1. the Anrep effect
2. the Bezold-Jarisch reflex
3. rupture of an abdominal viscus
4. reperfusion of a thrombosed coronary artery

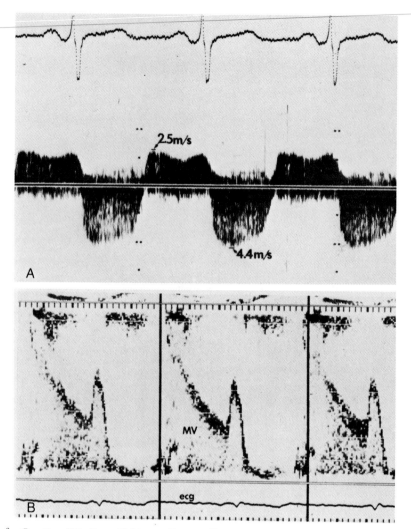

Illustration for Question 364. From Nishimura, R.A., Miller, F.A., Callahan, M.J., Benassi, R.C., Seward, J.B., and Tajik, A.J.: Doppler Echocardiography: Theory, Instrumentation, Technique, and Application. Mayo Clin. Proc. 60:326, 1985.

368. A 42-year-old man presents with Löffler's endocarditis. Typical findings include:

1. eosinophilia
2. ejection fraction ≤30 per cent
3. right ventricular pressure tracing showing a "square root" sign
4. asthma and nasal polyposis

369. A 55-year-old woman seeks medical attention because of progressive exertional dyspnea and rapid heart action. At age 12 she had rheumatic fever and has had a heart murmur since then. She has been in atrial fibrillation for 2 years with good rate control on digoxin 0.25 mg qid. Her vital signs are heart rate 80/min, BP 130/80, and respirations 16/min. She has inspiratory rales at the lung bases. Her cardiac impulse is displaced laterally and is prominent. There are a loud S_1, single S_2, an opening snap, a holodiastolic rumbling murmur at the apex, and a soft diastolic blowing murmur along the left sternal border. Isometric handgrip augments the diastolic murmur while administration of amyl nitrite diminishes the murmur. She has 1+ peripheral edema. Her ECG is illustrated *on the following page.* The most likely diagnosis(es) is (are):

1. tricuspid stenosis
2. aortic regurgitation
3. mitral regurgitation
4. mitral stenosis

370. Characteristics of the opening snap (OS) in mitral stenosis (MS) include:

1. The A_2-OS interval varies directly with left atrial pressure
2. A short A_2-OS interval (<0.08 sec) is a reliable indicator of significant MS
3. Sudden standing narrows the A_2-OS interval
4. During exercise the A_2-OS interval narrows

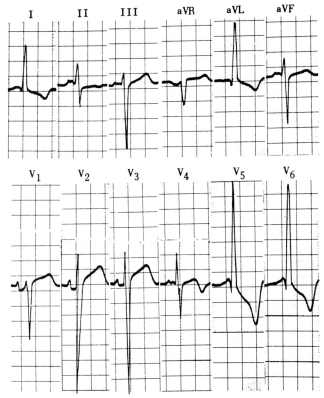

Illustration for Question 369. From Massie, E., and Walsh, T.J.: Clinical Vectorcardiography and Electrocardiography. Chicago, Year Book Medical Publishers, 1960, p. 136.

371. Descriptions of the hemodynamic measurements characteristically obtained at cardiac catheterization in patients with cardiac tamponade include:

1. prominent *y* descent
2. an elevated right ventricular diastolic pressure
3. an intrapericardial–right atrial pressure difference of 2 to 5 mm Hg
4. the absence of a dip-and-plateau configuration in the right ventricular pressure tracing

372. Correct statements with regard to Chagas' disease include:

1. The causative organism is *Brucella cruzi*
2. The classic echocardiographic findings are those of a dilated cardiomyopathy with an apical aneurysm
3. The most common ECG abnormality in chronic Chagas' disease is left bundle branch block
4. The disease is transmitted to humans by the reduviid bug

373. Mechanisms that have been identified for cardiac dysfunction associated with excessive alcohol consumption include:

1. direct toxic effect of alcohol and/or its metabolites
2. beriberi heart disease
3. toxic effects due to additives in the beverage (e.g., cobalt)
4. hyperkalemia-induced contractile dysfunction

374. Which of the following statements about the rhythm displayed *below* are true in the setting of acute myocardial infarction (AMI)?

1. This rhythm is present in between 10 and 15 per cent of patients with AMI
2. This rhythm is a consequence of left atrial ischemia in most cases
3. This rhythm in association with hemodynamic compromise should be treated by electrical cardioversion
4. This rhythm is the least common of atrial arrhythmias associated with AMI

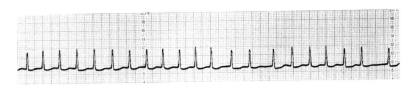

375. The Coronary Primary Prevention Trial (CPPT) involved 3806 men who at entry were free of clinical manifestations of coronary artery disease, were between the ages of 35 and 59, and had Type II hyperlipoproteinemia with serum cholesterol values greater than 265 mg/dl. All participants were placed on a diet that lowered cholesterol by an average of 4 per cent. The control group received placebo and the treatment group cholestyramine. Correct statements with regard to the results of this trial include:

1. Cholesterol levels in the treated group decreased on average by 30 per cent
2. A 1 per cent reduction in cholesterol reduced the risk of developing coronary disease by 2 per cent
3. Overall mortality from all causes in the treated group was significantly lower than in the control group
4. The reduction in cardiovascular deaths was paralleled by decreases in the development of angina pectoris, positive exercise tests, and number of patients requiring bypass surgery

376. Patent ductus arteriosus (PDA) in premature infants is characterized by:

1. significant deterioration in approximately one-third of infants
2. a normal cardiac silhouette on chest radiography
3. pharmacological responsiveness to indomethacin that leads to constriction and frequently to closure of the PDA
4. an absence of clinical findings on the cardiovascular examination

377. Correct statements regarding hemodynamic findings in patients with hypertrophic obstructive cardiomyopathy with disproportionate septal hypertrophy include:

1. Systolic function is usually impaired to a greater extent than diastolic function
2. The majority of ventricular emptying is more rapid than usual
3. Left ventricular end-diastolic pressure is usually normal
4. Ejection fraction is usually normal

378. Dynamic maneuvers to produce changes in the timing and intensity of the systolic click and murmur in the mitral valve prolapse (MVP) syndrome are helpful diagnostically. Correct statements include:

1. Sudden standing causes the click and murmur to occur earlier in systole
2. Administration of propranolol causes the click and murmur to increase in intensity and to occur earlier
3. Handgrip causes a delay in onset of the click and murmur

4. During the straining phase of the Valsalva maneuver the click and murmur occur later in systole

379. True statements with regard to electrocardiographic changes observed during ambulatory monitoring associated with myocardial ischemia include:

1. The most common finding is pseudonormalization of previously inverted or flat T waves
2. ST-segment depression occurs in a high percentage of patients with ischemic chest pain
3. Ischemic chest pain usually occurs 60 to 120 seconds *after* the onset of ST–T-wave changes
4. Ischemic chest pain invariably is associated with either ST-segment elevation or depression

380. In patients with combined aortic regurgitation (AR) and aortic stenosis (AS), the cardiac output used in the Gorlin formula to calculate valve area should be the:

1. Fick output
2. dye indicator output
3. pulmonary artery saturation output
4. angiographic LV output

381. Which of the following are characteristics of aortic injuries due to blunt trauma?

1. Evidence of other thoracic trauma
2. An abnormal chest x-ray
3. An absence of specific symptoms
4. Survival for the majority of patients who reach the hospital alive

382. Persistent patent ductus arteriosus is characterized by:

1. exercise intolerance
2. wide arterial pulse pressure
3. normal sinus rhythm
4. diagnostic M-mode echocardiogram

383. True statements regarding hypertension in infants and children include:

1. Secondary causes of hypertension are more common than essential hypertension
2. Blood pressure cuff sizes should be appropriate, since a cuff that is too small will produce spuriously low readings
3. The most common cause of secondary hypertension is renal disease
4. There is no familial tendency for susceptibility to hypertension

384. Treatment of myocardial contusion would normally include which of the following?

  1. Bed rest with gradual ambulation over 7 to 10 days
  2. Analgesia with nonsteroidal anti-inflammatory agents for chest pain
  3. Cardiac monitoring for 3 to 5 days
  4. Anticoagulation to prevent systemic embolization

385. Appropriate steps in the management of patients with acute aortic dissection include:

  1. combined sodium nitroprusside and beta-blocker therapy
  2. administration of a loop diuretic
  3. surgical repair for cases of proximal dissection
  4. surgical repair for cases of distal dissection

386. Characteristics of abrupt coronary artery closure immediately following percutaneous transluminal coronary angioplasty (PTCA) include:

  1. occurrence in approximately 12 per cent of patients
  2. successful reopening upon repeat dilatation approximately half the time
  3. an absence of myocardial damage, even in patients undergoing emergency surgical revascularization
  4. improved management due to the availability of special perfusion or "shunt" catheters

387. The following may be considered primary hypercoagulable states:

  1. anti-thrombin III deficiency
  2. presence of lupus anticoagulant
  3. protein C deficiency
  4. oral contraceptive use

388. Correct statements about the arrhythmia illustrated *below* when seen in the setting of acute myocardial infarction (AMI), include:

  1. This rhythm may be seen in up to 20 per cent of patients with AMI

  2. This rhythm confers a small but significant increase in morbidity and mortality
  3. This rhythm commonly occurs due to slowing of the sinus rhythm
  4. This rhythm is initiated almost exclusively by the occurrence of a premature beat

389. Which of the following events will increase the gradient and systolic murmur of hypertrophic obstructive cardiomyopathy?

  1. sudden standing from a squatting position
  2. a spontaneous premature contraction
  3. administration of amyl nitrite
  4. the Müller maneuver

390. The intensity of exercise in patients with coronary artery disease is an important determinant in achieving desired training effects. True statements about exercise intensity include:

  1. Cardiac patients should train at about 50 to 75 per cent of maximal oxygen uptake
  2. Most persons maintain an exact target heart rate
  3. A heart rate of 70 to 85 per cent of maximal capacity corresponds to 50 to 75 per cent levels of maximal oxygen uptake required for training
  4. Maximal heart rate values obtained from a previous exercise test should *not* be used to compute subsequent target heart rate zones in cardiac patients

391. Which of the following drugs is (are) relatively contraindicated in the therapy of patients with hypertrophic obstructive cardiomyopathy?

  1. digitalis
  2. disopyramide
  3. furosemide
  4. verapamil

392. A 52-year-old man suffered a large anterior myocardial infarction (MI) (CPK maximum, 4000 given intravenously) 2 months ago. Since then he has had symptoms of persistent mild congestive heart failure despite taking 80 mg furosemide qid. His ECG shows ST-segment elevations in V_2–V_4. An enlarged

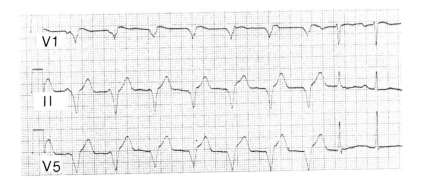

cardiac silhouette is present on chest x-ray. Correct statements with regard to diagnosis and management include:

1. Anticoagulation for 4 to 6 months is prudent
2. Biplane left ventriculography is more likely to define his problem than two-dimensional echocardiography
3. He is likely to have multivessel coronary artery disease
4. Surgical intervention should be planned within the next 1 to 2 weeks

393. A 55-year-old businessman presents to the office complaining of increasing fatigue and shortness of breath. He has also noticed that he is more comfortable sleeping on three pillows. He denies any change in his usual habits and also denies chest pain or pleuritic pain. His only medications are hydrochlorthiazide and a beta blocker for hypertension of 10 years' duration. His past medical history is remarkable for an appendectomy. He smokes one-half to 1 pack of cigarettes per day. He drinks whiskey socially and admits to one or two martinis at lunch. There is no family history of heart disease.

On examination the heart rate is 104/min, respirations 20/min, BP 150/90. There are grade II hypertensive changes in the fundi. His lungs reveal bibasilar rales over the lower third of the lung fields; the carotid upstrokes are normal. The apical impulse is laterally displaced and sustained. S_1 and S_2 are normal with an increased A_2. There is a loud S_4 and a moderately loud S_3. There is a Grade II/VI holosystolic murmur that radiates to the axilla. The remainder of the examination is normal except for a trace of pedal edema. The chest x-ray and ECG show left ventricular hypertrophy. The most likely cause(s) for this man's congestive heart failure is (are):

1. hypertension
2. alcohol
3. coronary atherosclerosis
4. idiopathic hypertrophic subaortic stenosis

394. True statements with regard to blood flow in the subendocardium as compared with the subepicardium include:

1. Systolic flow is less in the subendocardium
2. Total subendocardial flow under normal conditions is equal to or greater than subepicardial flow
3. An elevation of ventricular end-diastolic pressure will reduce subendocardial flow to a greater extent than subepicardial flow
4. The reserve for vasodilatation in the subendocardium is greater than in the subepicardium

395. Tissue plasminogen activator (tPA) may play a role in the thrombolytic treatment of acute pulmonary embolism. True statements about tPA in this setting include:

1. tPA causes more fibrin-specific thrombolysis and less hemorrhage than either urokinase or streptokinase in animal models
2. The majority of patients who receive tPA demonstrate significant clot lysis within 6 hours
3. In clinical trials to date, there is approximately a 5 per cent incidence of major bleeding with tPA
4. For large or massive pulmonary embolism, tPA is the current therapy of choice

396. True statements regarding sarcoid heart disease include:

1. Less than 10 per cent of patients with pulmonary sarcoidosis have clinical manifestations of sarcoid heart disease
2. Conduction disturbances are the most frequent clinical indication of sarcoid heart disease
3. Endomyocardial biopsy may reveal noncaseating granulomas and fibrosis
4. Sarcoid involvement of the cardiac valves may lead to mitral and/or aortic stenosis

397. Characteristics of radiation pericarditis include:

1. an association with mantle field radiation therapy of Hodgkin's disease
2. a variable time course for the onset of pericardial injury
3. an association with constrictive pericarditis in patients who undergo drainage by a pericardial window
4. an association with constrictive pericarditis in children

398. Aortic valve replacement is indicated in which of the following?

1. A patient with infective endocarditis, aortic regurgitation (AR), and heart failure
2. A patient with severe chronic AR and minimal symptoms who shows serial decreases in ejection fraction during exercise measured by radionuclide angiography
3. A patient with severe, chronic AR who is symptomatic with an echocardiographic end-systolic left ventricular dimension of 6 cm
4. A 60-year-old man with severe chronic AR who is symptom-free with an ejection fraction of 65 per cent

399. True statements regarding primary tumors of the heart include:

1. Benign tumors are more common than malignant tumors
2. The most common malignant cardiac tumors are angiosarcomas and rhabdomyosarcomas
3. The presence of a hemorrhagic pericardial effusion is indicative of a malignant tumor

4. Malignant tumors are more likely to occur on the left side of the interatrial septum

---

400. True statements with respect to chylomicrons include:

1. They are composed mainly of triglycerides
2. Chylomicrons are frequently present in fasting plasma
3. Chylomicronemia per se is not thought to contribute to premature coronary artery disease
4. Chylomicrons are cleared from the blood in the liver by action of the enzyme acyl cholesterol acyl transferase (ACAT)

---

401. Which of the following is (are) commonly associated with viral pericarditis?

1. Coxsackie virus group B
2. peak incidence in the spring and fall
3. frequent prodromal syndrome
4. short-term recurrence rate of between 15 and 40 per cent

---

402. Correct statements with respect to low-density lipoproteins (LDLs) include:

1. LDLs are the major cholesterol-carrying components of plasma
2. The major lipid components of LDL are triglyceride and esterified cholesterol
3. LDL is mainly formed from VLDL breakdown
4. Apo E is the dominant protein present in LDL

---

403. A 66-year-old woman with chronic stable angina returns to her home from a Florida vacation. After carrying her suitcases up two flights of stairs, she develops her usual anginal pain. She cannot locate her nitroglycerin pills in her purse, so she uses some pills on the window sill in her kitchen. Despite taking three tablets, she obtains no relief. Finally, she locates her other nitroglycerin and obtains relief in 5 minutes. Her other medications include propranolol 40 mg qid and isosorbide dinitrate 40 mg qid. The most likely explanation(s) for the failure of the initial three pills to relieve her angina is (are):

1. poor absorption due to dry mouth
2. development of an anxiety state
3. loss of potency
4. nitrate tolerance

---

404. Which of the following are physical examination features of constrictive pericarditis?

1. pulsus paradoxus
2. systolic retraction of the apical impulse
3. midsystolic pericardial knock
4. hepatomegaly

---

405. Passive collapse of a stenotic coronary artery when myocardial flow increases is due to which of the following hemodynamic principles?

1. As flow increases, there is an exponential rise in the pressure gradient across the stenosis
2. As flow increases, turbulence causes a rise in intraluminal pressure
3. A rise in the transstenotic pressure gradient causes a fall in intraluminal pressure
4. As flow increases intramyocardial pressure rises, which causes increased extrinsic compression of blood vessels

---

406. Criteria that necessitate prophylaxis for deep venous thrombosis (DVT) and pulmonary embolism in general surgical patients include:

1. obesity
2. age equal to or greater than 40 years
3. a surgical procedure greater than 1 hour in duration
4. known cancer

---

407. Of the following drugs that typically are used for treatment of chronic stable (exercise-induced) angina, which one(s) may cause detrimental effects in patients with Prinzmetal's angina?

1. Ca^{++} channel antagonists
2. aspirin
3. nitrates
4. beta blockers

---

408. True statements with regard to the Coronary Artery Surgery Study (CASS) findings for the treatment of patients with mild angina include:

1. There was no statistically significant difference in survival among patients with one- or two-vessel disease who were assigned to medical or surgical treatment
2. A significant advantage was observed for surgical treatment of patients with three-vessel disease and LV ejection fraction of between 35 and 50 per cent
3. In patients with severe angina and three-vessel disease, surgery improved survival regardless of LV ejection fraction
4. In patients with LV ejection fraction below 26 per cent, survival with surgical therapy was not different from that of patients with medical therapy

---

409. True statements with regard to acquired aortic stenosis (AS) due to rheumatic disease as compared with degenerative (senile) calcific disease include:

1. AS secondary to rheumatic disease is more likely to have associated aortic regurgitation (AR)

2. Commissural fusion is the hallmark of the rheumatic aortic valve

3. There is an increased incidence of degenerative AS in patients with hypercholesterolemia or diabetes mellitus

4. In degenerative AS, calcific deposits at the tips of the valve leaflets narrow the opening to blood flow

410. Correct statements with regard to the severity of obstruction in pure mitral stenosis (MS) include:

1. Atrial contraction increases the presystolic transmitral valvular gradient by approximately 30 per cent

2. When the mitral valve area is ≤ 2.0 cm², little additional flow can be achieved regardless of the transvalvular pressure gradient

3. At any given valve area the transvalvular pressure gradient is a function of the square of the transvalvular flow rate

4. At any given valve area the transvalvular pressure gradient is directly proportional to the transvalvular flow rate

411. Secondary causes of Type IV hyperlipoproteinemia (primary increased VLDL) include which of the following diseases?

1. diabetes mellitus
2. hypothyroidism
3. nephrotic syndrome
4. neurofibromatosis

412. True statements concerning the relationship between clinical manifestations of angina and underlying coronary artery pathology include:

1. When infarction without angina is the first manifestation of ischemic heart disease, it is often associated with single-vessel disease

2. When angina occurs before infarction, two- or three-vessel disease is usually present

3. The incidence of coronary artery disease is about 90 per cent in patients with typical exercise-induced angina

4. Myocardial infarction is the most frequent clinical presentation of coronary artery disease in women

DIRECTIONS: The group of questions below consists of lettered headings followed by a set of numbered items. For each numbered item select the ONE lettered heading with which it is MOST closely associated. Each lettered heading may be used ONCE, MORE THAN ONCE, OR NOT AT ALL.

For each statement, match the appropriate substance.

A. Elevate(s) HDL cholesterol
B. Elevate(s) LDL cholesterol
C. Have (has) no significant effect on lipoproteins
D. Lower(s) cholesterol
E. Lower(s) VLDL cholesterol

413. Thiazide diuretics

414. Propranolol

415. Estrogens

416. Calcium channel antagonists

For each congenital cardiac abnormality listed, match the appropriate descriptive phrase.

A. Persistent truncus arteriosus
B. Coronary arteriovenous fistula
C. Anomalous pulmonary origin of the coronary artery
D. Ruptured aortic sinus aneurysm
E. Aortic arch obstruction

417. This defect is always accompanied by ventricular septal defect (VSD)

418. Myocardial infarction is the most common clinical presentation

419. This malformation usually involves the right coronary artery

420. This anomaly is frequently characterized by a history of chest pain of recent onset

Match the cell types potentially involved in atherogenesis listed below with the appropriate descriptive phrase.

A. Endothelial cell
B. Smooth muscle cells
C. Macrophage
D. Platelet

421. Demonstrate(s) proliferation in the intima in atherosclerosis

422. Is (are) the principal cell(s) of the fatty streak

423. Secrete(s) prostacyclin

424. Is (are) capable of little or no protein synthesis

For each disease, match the appropriate statement.

    A. Viral myocarditis
    B. Diphtheritic cardiomyopathy
    C. Trypanosomal myocarditis
    D. None of the above

425. Cardiac symptomatology may occur after a symptom-free interval of many years

426. The majority of children who develop this condition recover with few or no sequelae

427. Papillary muscle involvement may lead to a characteristic murmur of mitral regurgitation

428. The typical electrocardiographic presentation includes left ventricular hypertrophy and inverted T waves in the left precordial leads

429. Electrocardiographic changes range from ST-segment and T-wave changes to arrhythmias and conduction disturbances

---

For each aortic outflow tract disease, match the appropriate finding.

    A. Acquired nonrheumatic aortic stenosis
    B. Hypertrophic obstructive cardiomyopathy
    C. Congenital subvalvular stenosis
    D. Congenital supravalvular stenosis
    E. Congenital valvular stenosis

430. Normal carotid pulse on the right but slow rise on the left

431. Mitral regurgitation is frequently present

432. Aortic ejection sound is commonly present

433. Murmur of mitral regurgitation due to Gallavardin phenomenon is suggested

---

For each statement, match the appropriate eponym.

    A. Osler nodes
    B. Janeway lesions
    C. Roth spots
    D. Subungual hemorrhages
    E. Bracht-Wächter bodies

434. Small (1 to 4 mm diameter), irregular, erythematous nontender macules present on the thenar and hypothenar eminences of the hands

435. Small, raised red (or purple) tender lesions present

in the pulp spaces of the terminal phalanges of the fingers

436. Collections of lymphocytes in the nerve layer of the retina

437. Collections of lymphocytes and mononuclear cells in the myocardium

---

For each drug, match the appropriate statement.

    A. Nicotinic acid
    B. Neomycin sulfate
    C. Cholestyramine
    D. Probucol
    E. Gemfibrozil

438. May decrease prothrombin time in patients taking warfarin

439. May increase prothrombin time in patients taking warfarin

440. Most likely to cause impaired glucose tolerance and hyperuricemia

441. Most likely to lower HDL

For each drug(s) listed, match its (their) effect on concomitant use of beta-blocking agents.

    A. Cimetidine
    B. Aluminum hydroxide gel
    C. Barbiturates
    D. Lidocaine
    E. Calcium carbonate antacids

442. Enhance(s) metabolism of beta blockers and reduces plasma levels

443. Reduce(s) hepatic metabolism of beta blockers and increases plasma levels

444. Reduce(s) gastrointestinal absorption of beta blockers and reduces plasma levels

---

For each prosthetic device, match the appropriate statement.

    A. Starr Edwards valve
    B. Bjork-Shiley valve
    C. St. Jude valve
    D. Hancock valve
    E. Lillehei-Kaster valve

445. Certain models have been associated with sudden thrombosis or strut fracture

446. Lowest profile mechanical valve

447. Least thrombogenic valve

448. Valve most commonly associated with increased serum lactate dehydrogenase

For each organism listed, match the appropriate antibiotic regimen for treatment of native valve endocarditis

  A. Vancomycin (500 mg IV every 6 hr)
  B. Oxacillin (2 gm IV, every 4 hrs)
  C. Ampicillin (3 gm IV, every 6 hrs)
  D. Tobramycin (1.7 mg/kg IV, every 8 hrs) plus ticarcillin (3 gm IV, every 4 hrs)
  E. Nafcillin (1 gm IV, every 6 hrs)

449. *Staphylococcus epidermidis*, methicillin resistant

450. *Staphylococcus aureus* in a hospitalized patient, antibiotic sensitivity not available

451. *Pseudomonas aeruginosa*

452. *Escherichia coli*, community acquired

For each, match the most appropriate statement.

  A. Constrictive pericarditis
  B. Restrictive cardiomyopathy
  C. Both
  D. Neither

453. Atrial fibrillation, diffuse low QRS voltage

454. RV systolic pressure greater than 60 mm Hg

455. Normal motion of the crista supraventricularis present on angiography

456. 80 per cent of LV filling occurs in the first half of diastole

For each disease listed, match the most appropriate therapy.

  A. A fat-restricted diet and medium-chain triglyceride therapy
  B. HMG-CoA reductase therapy
  C. Dietary management alone may suffice
  D. Clofibrate therapy

457. Dysbetalipoproteinemia (Type III hyperlipoproteinemia)

458. Polygenic hypercholesterolemia (Type II hyperlipoproteinemia)

459. Heterozygous familial hypercholesterolemia (Type II hyperlipoproteinemia)

460. Lipoprotein lipase deficiency (Type I hyperlipoproteinemia)

461. Type IV hyperlipoproteinemia

Listed below are four sets of hemodynamic data and clinical information describing patients with acute myocardial infarction (AMI). Match each set of data with the most appropriate description that follows.

  A. Cardiac index (CI) 3.2 liters/minute/square meter, pulmonary capillary wedge pressure (PCW) 9 mm Hg
  B. CI 2.5, PCW 24
  C. CI 2.4, PCW 9, arterial pressure 88/60 mm Hg
  D. CI 1.6, PCW 30

462. Most compatible with a patient with hypovolemic hypotension

463. The patient for whom beta blockade may be appropriate therapy

464. Patient in the group whose mortality is approximately 10 per cent

465. The patient in whom acute mitral regurgitation or ventricular septal defect must be initially excluded

DIRECTIONS: The group of questions below consists of four lettered headings followed by a set of numbered items. For each numbered item select

A if the item is associated with (A) *only*
B if the item is associated with (B) *only*
C if the item is associated with *both* (A) and (B)
D if the item is associated with *neither* (A) nor (B)

Each lettered heading may be used ONCE, MORE THAN ONCE, OR NOT AT ALL.

A. Marfan syndrome
B. Ankylosing spondylitis
C. Both
D. Neither

466. Aortic stenosis is the most common valvular presentation

467. Conduction disturbances are common

468. Degeneration of the aortic wall media is frequently present

469. Aortic aneurysms are common

___

A. Supravalvular aortic stenosis
B. Discrete subaortic stenosis
C. Both
D. Neither

470. Mental retardation is commonly associated

471. Associated with idiopathic infantile hypercalcemia

472. Commonly accompanied by tricuspid stenosis

473. Mild degrees of aortic regurgitation are commonly observed

474. Dilatation of the ascending aorta is common

___

A. Heparin
B. Streptokinase–urokinase
C. Both
D. Neither

475. In the majority of studies, continuous intravenous infusion leads to a lower frequency of major hemorrhage than intermittent infusion

476. The most important adverse effect clinically is hemorrhage

477. Dissolution of recently formed thrombus is a major action

478. Randomized trials have demonstrated a decrease in mortality from pulmonary embolism after administration

479. In general, should be used along with an antiplatelet agent

___

A. Type II glycogen storage disease
B. Mucocutaneous lymph node syndrome (Kawasaki's disease)
C. Both
D. Neither

480. Inherited as an autosomal dominant disorder

481. Congestive heart failure may be an important complication

482. Intravenous gamma globulin may be a useful therapy

483. The etiology of the disorder remains unknown

484. The electrocardiogram may demonstrate a short P-R interval

___

A. Fatty streak
B. Fibrous plaque
C. Both
D. Neither

485. Earliest lesion of atherosclerosis

486. Lipid-filled smooth muscle cells are present

487. Is composed primarily of macrophages

488. Is commonly found within the length of the renal arteries

489. Is grossly white in appearance

___

A. Tricuspid stenosis
B. Pulmonic stenosis
C. Both
D. Neither

490. Usually rheumatic in origin

491. May be associated with carcinoid heart disease

492. Most adults are asymptomatic

493. Ascites is common on physical examination

494. Balloon valvuloplasty is the treatment of choice

    A. Emphysema
    B. Chronic bronchitis
    C. Both
    D. Neither

495. Cardiomegaly on chest x-ray

496. Pulmonary hypertension at rest

497. Markedly decreased oxygen-diffusing capacity

498. Repeated episodes of right heart failure

    A. ⎫
    B. ⎬ *See illustration below*
    C. Both
    D. Neither

499. The most common congenital cardiac anomaly

500. Patients having dental procedures require antibiotic prophylaxis

501. Often associated with ankylosing spondylitis

502. May be associated with aortic valve prolapse

503. May be associated with angina

    A. Acute ventricular septal rupture in the presence of acute myocardial infarction (AMI)
    B. Acute mitral regurgitation in the presence of AMI
    C. Both
    D. Neither

504. A murmur due to this lesion may decrease in intensity as arterial pressure falls

505. Pulmonary artery wedge pressure tracings may demonstrate large *v* waves

506. A characteristic diastolic murmur is usually present

507. Occurs primarily with large infarctions

    A. Chronic constrictive pericarditis
    B. Cardiac amyloidosis
    C. Both
    D. Neither

508. Right ventricular pressure tracing showing a deep and rapid early decline at the onset of diastole, with

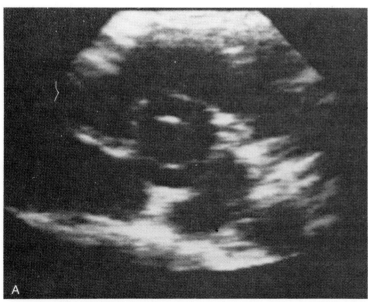

From Stewart, W.J., King, M.E., Gillam, L.D., Guyer, D.E., and Weyman, A.E.: Am. J. Cardiol. *54*:1277, 1984.

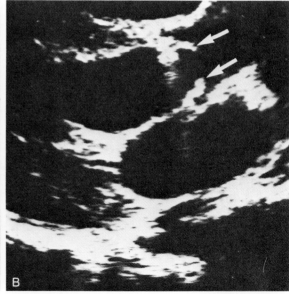

From Stewart, W.J.: *In* Miller, D.D., Burns, R.J., Gill, J.B., and Ruddy, T.D. (eds.): Clinical Cardiac Imaging. New York, McGraw-Hill, 1988, p. 466.

a rapid rise to a plateau in early diastole ("square root" sign)

509. Left ventricular end-diastolic pressure (LVEDP) 10 mm Hg greater than right ventricular end-diastolic pressure (RVEDP)

510. Peak RV systolic pressure = 35 mm Hg, RVEDP = 18 mm Hg

511. Pulmonary artery systolic pressure = 60 mm Hg, RVEDP = 15 mm Hg

---

A. Takayasu's arteritis
B. Giant cell arteritis
C. Both
D. Neither

512. Occurrence is predominantly in women

513. Onset is typically during teenage years

514. Jaw muscle claudication suggests the diagnosis

515. Fever is almost always present

516. Steroid therapy is a cornerstone of management

A. Mitral regurgitation (not due to prolapse)
B. Aortic stenosis
C. Both
D. Neither

517. Systolic murmur decreases in intensity during the strain of the Valsalva maneuver

518. Systolic murmur increases in intensity with handgrip

519. Systolic murmur becomes softer after administration of amyl nitrite

520. Systolic murmur intensity varies significantly from beat-to-beat in atrial fibrillation

---

A. Complete transposition of the great arteries
B. Total anomalous pulmonary venous connection
C. Both
D. Neither

521. An interatrial communication is frequently present

522. A majority of patients have symptoms during the first year of life

523. Cardiac murmurs are not a prominent clinical feature

524. The electrocardiogram most commonly shows right atrial enlargement and right ventricular hypertrophy

525. Balloon atrial septostomy may provide dramatic palliation

---

A. Amoxicillin 3 gm orally 1 hr before
B. Amoxicillin 1 gm IM or IV plus gentamicin 120 mg IM or IV; amoxicillin 0.5 gm orally or IM 6 hrs later
C. Both
D. Neither

526. Extraction of a wisdom tooth under local anesthetic in a patient with rheumatic mitral stenosis

527. Extraction of a wisdom tooth in a patient with a Hancock aortic valve prosthesis

528. Laminectomy under general anesthesia in a patient with hypertrophic obstructive cardiomyopathy

529. Surgical procedures for stress urinary incontinence associated with cystocele in a woman with a DDD pacemaker

---

A. Nifedipine
B. A beta blocker
C. Both
D. Neither

Decide which drug or drugs are most appropriate initially in patients who have chronic stable angina pectoris in conjunction with the following conditions:

530. Second-degree atrioventricular block

531. Moderate mitral stenosis

532. Aortic regurgitation

533. Raynaud's phenomenon

A. Patent ductus arteriosus
B. Complete atrioventricular canal defect
C. Both
D. Neither

534. A common AV orifice is frequently present

535. An association with rubella infection during the first trimester is noted

536. Heart failure in early infancy is common

537. A "gooseneck" deformity is seen during left ventricular angiography

538. A blowing, high-pitched decrescendo diastolic murmur is common at the left sternal border

   A. Cardiac myxoma
   B. Cardiac sarcoma
   C. Both
   D. Neither

539. May be accompanied by multiple blue nevi

540. The majority occur sporadically

541. Right atrial involvement is most common

542. The most common primary cardiac tumor

543. The most common morphology is sessile or polypoid

   A. Atenolol
   B. Propranolol
   C. Both
   D. Neither

544. Relatively lipid-soluble

545. Accumulates in renal failure

546. Has intrinsic sympathomimetic activity

547. Relatively selective for beta$_2$-adrenoceptors

PART III: DISEASES OF THE HEART, PERICARDIUM, AORTA, AND PULMONARY VASCULAR BED

———— CHAPTERS 30 THROUGH 48 ————

═══ ANSWERS ═══

240-D *(Braunwald, pp. 1201–1203)*

The development of subendocardial ischemia is directly related to changes in transmural blood flow. The delivery of oxygen to the subendocardium can be represented by the product of arterial oxygen content and the driving force for subendocardial blood flow, which depends on the integrated pressure difference between the aorta and the left ventricle during diastole, as formulated by Hoffman.[1] In the presence of a coronary artery obstruction, the effective pressure perfusing the subendocardial region is reduced to the gradient between the diastolic coronary pressure distal to the obstruction and the left ventricular end-diastolic pressure. Thus there is a dramatic reduction in the perfusion of the subendocardium distal to the obstruction. When left ventricular diastolic pressure is elevated, as occurs during ischemia, the endocardial-epicardial flow ratio declines. This further reduces subendocardial blood flow and intensifies subendocardial ischemia, creating a vicious circle. It has been shown by analysis of fractional uptake of radioactively labeled microspheres that both nitroglycerin and beta blockers redistribute blood flow to the subendocardium.[2] This may explain in part their effectiveness in myocardial ischemia.

REFERENCES

1. Hoffman, J.I.E.: Determinants of prediction of transmural myocardial perfusion. Circulation 58:381, 1978.
2. Becker, L.C., Fortuin, N.J., and Pitt, B.: Effect of ischemia and antianginal drugs on the distribution of radioactive microspheres in the canine left ventricle. Circ. Res. 28:263, 1971.

241-D *(Braunwald, pp. 1321–1325)*

This patient presents a difficult problem. He has a history that is consistent with exercise-induced chest pain but has had two negative standard exercise tolerance tests (ETTs). However, the relatively low sensitivity of exercise testing (approximately 73 per cent sensitivity for all coronary artery disease) and the fact that this patient appears to have variable threshold angina as indicated by the relationship of the pain to cold weather makes the standard ETT an unsatisfactory test to rule out coronary artery disease. In fact, the standard ETT is particularly insensitive for patients with single-vessel disease. In a study by Goldschlager et al., patients with single-vessel disease had a significantly lower incidence of downsloping ST segments or ST depression of 2 mm than that noted for patients with two- or three-vessel disease.[1]

Thus in this patient, in whom your clinical suspicion for coronary artery disease is relatively high, a further workup is mandatory. Of the other tests available, a stress thallium-201 scintigram would be the one most likely to yield a positive result.[2] Echocardiography might reveal other causes for chest pain, such as mitral valve prolapse, but again would not rule out significant coronary artery disease. Changing medications to nifedipine probably would be a successful therapeutic intervention but should be done only after further diagnostic workup. Coronary arteriography might eventually be indicated if the stress thallium study showed a large perfusion defect or if the patient was not helped by medical treatment.

Another option would be to perform an exercise radionuclide ventriculogram. This test has also been shown to have a high sensitivity and specificity for coronary artery disease, with measurement of both ejection fraction and regional wall motion aiding in the diagnosis. The greater sensitivity of the two radionuclide techniques compared with the standard ETT is probably related to the fact that abnormalities of perfusion and of left ventricular contraction occur at a lower ischemic threshold than does exercise-induced ST-segment depression. The sensitivity and specificity of both radionuclide techniques have been found to be similar in several studies.[3]

REFERENCES

1. Goldschlager, N., Selzer, A., and Cohn, K.: Treadmill stress tests and indicators of presence and severity of coronary artery disease. Ann. Intern. Med. 85:277, 1976.
2. Port, S.C., Oshima, M., Ray, G., McNamee, P., and Schmidt, D.H.: Assessment of single-vessel coronary artery disease: Results of exercise electrocardiography, thallium-201 myocardial perfusion imaging, and radionuclide angiography. J. Am. Cardiol. 6:75, 1985.
3. Gibson, R.S., and Beller, G.A.: Should exercise electrocardiography testing be replaced by radioisotope methods? In Rahimtoola, S.H. (ed.): Controversies in Coronary Artery Disease. Philadelphia, F.A. Davis Co., 1983, pp. 1–31.

242-D *(Braunwald, pp. 1094–1103)*

This patient probably has subacute infective endocarditis. The exact incubation period of subacute endocarditis is difficult to define. Starkebaum et al.[1] suggested that the time from transient bacteremia to the development of symptoms was about a week, with symptoms appearing in 2 weeks in 84 per cent of the patients. In many cases the onset of subacute infective endocarditis is characterized by the general manifestations of infection without any signs or symptoms specific to diseases of the heart or any other organ. This patient's complaints of malaise, myalgias, chills, and fever are nonspecific. The classic findings, such as subungual (splinter) hemorrhages, Osler nodes, Janeway lesions, and Roth spots, were much more prominent in the preantibiotic era than in the current era because of the previous longer course of active disease. Nevertheless, the presence of microscopic hematuria is consistent with renal emboli, which are quite common in subacute endocarditis, with renal infarcts detected in as many as 60 per cent of patients studied at autopsy.[2]

Although it is possible that the patient's murmur may be a consequence of acute endocarditis, it is more likely that the patient has had longstanding mitral valve prolapse. This is further suggested by his complaints of palpitations and chest pain; these could be due either to the endocarditis or to underlying mitral valve prolapse. Because of the uncertainty in diagnosis of mitral valve prolapse, it is difficult to determine precisely the contributing risk of mitral valve prolapse to endocarditis. In a case-controlled study of patients with valvular endocarditis, Clemens et al.[3] found that 13 of 51 (25 per cent) patients had mitral valve prolapse, while only 11 of 153 (7 per cent) of patients hospitalized for other causes had mitral valve prolapse. This indicates a three- to four-fold higher risk of endocarditis in such patients. Others have found a much lower relative risk,[4] suggesting that although the risk of bacterial endocarditis is greater in patients with mitral valve prolapse than in the patients without this lesion, the absolute risk remains low. As a generalization, it is probable that patients who have only a mitral valve click without significant mitral regurgitation are at minimal risk. On the other hand, patients with large myxomatous valves with significant mitral regurgitation probably are at significantly increased risk and should receive prophylactic therapy for dental manipulations and other procedures that could cause bacteremia.

REFERENCES

1. Starkebaum, M., Durack, D., and Beeson, P.: The "incubation period" of subacute bacterial endocarditis. Yale J. Biol. Med. 50:59, 1977.
2. Kerr, A., Jr.: Bacterial endocarditis revisited. Mod. Con. Cardiovasc. Dis. 33:831, 1964.
3. Clemens, J.D., Horwitz, R.J., Jaffee, C.C., Feinstein, A.K., and Stanton, B.F.: A controlled evaluation of the risk of bacterial endocarditis in persons with mitral valve prolapse. N. Engl. J. Med. 307:776, 1982.
4. Retchin, S.M., Fletcher, R.H., and Waugh, R.A.: Endocarditis and mitral valve prolapse: What is "risk?" Int. J. Cardiol. 5:653, 1984.

243-C *(Braunwald, pp. 1235–1236)*

The clinical history remains an important part of the diagnosis of acute myocardial infarction. While a prodrome may be elicited in between 20 to 60 per cent of these patients, it may not be disturbing enough to cause them to seek immediate medical attention. In fact, only about 20 per cent of all patients with prodromal symptoms will seek medical help in the first 24 hours.[1] Approximately one-third of such patients will have had symptoms for 1 to 4 weeks before hospitalization, and in many cases these symptoms are of unstable angina, occurring at rest or with less activity than usual.

Morphine is usually capable of relieving the pain of AMI, although a dull pressure or ache may persist following analgesic treatment. Interestingly, the longer a patient suspected of having ischemic chest pain requires administration of analgesic therapy after hospital admission, the more likely that the diagnosis of AMI will be confirmed.[2] A variety of studies, including those in patients receiving thrombolytic therapy, have supported the notion that the ischemic zone of viable myocardium surrounding the necrotic central area of infarction gives rise to the pain sensation. This has important clinical ramifications for the care of patients in the periinfarction setting.

The majority of patients with transmural myocardial infarction and chest discomfort have nausea and vomiting,[3] which is thought to be due to activation of vagal reflexes. Attempts to quantify the number of infarctions that occur in a "silent" fashion through population studies have suggested that between 20 and 60 per cent of nonfatal infarctions are unrecognized by the patient and are discovered at the time of routine ECG.[4] However, further analysis reveals that approximately half of these patients will indeed have some recollection of an event characterized by symptoms compatible with AMI and that the infarction was not truly silent. Unrecognized or silent infarction occurs more commonly in patients without prior angina pectoris and in those with a history of hypertension or diabetes, although the association with diabetes is still controversial.

REFERENCES

1. Harper, R.W., Kennedy, G., DeSanctis, R.W., and Hutter, A.M., Jr.: The incidence and pattern of angina prior to acute myocardial infarction: A study of 577 cases. Am. Heart J. 97:178, 1979.
2. Baker, P.: Suspected myocardial infarction: Early diagnostic value of analgesic requirements. Br. Med. J. 290:27, 1985.
3. Ingram, D.A., Fulton, R.A., Portal, R.W., and Aber, C.P.: Vomiting as a diagnostic aid in acute ischemic cardiac pain. Br. Med. J. 281:636, 1980.
4. Margolis, J.R., Kannel, W.B., Feinleib, M., Dawber, T.R., and McNamara, P.M.: Clinical features of unrecognized myocardial infarction: Silent and symptomatic. Eighteen-year follow-up: The Framingham Study. Am. J. Cardiol. 32:1, 1973.

244-C *(Braunwald, pp. 1507–1508)*

Effusive-constrictive pericarditis, which may represent an intermediate stage in the development of chronic constrictive pericarditis, is defined as the simultaneous presence of a tense pericardial effusion and of visceral pericardial restriction.[1] This pathophysiology leads to the hemodynamic hallmark of the condition, which is continued elevation of right atrial pressure following aspiration of the pericardial fluid and the resultant return of intrapericardial pressures to zero. The etiologies for this entity are the same as those for chronic constrictive pericarditis. The most common include idiopathic or presumed viral pericarditis, as well as tuberculosis, neoplastic infiltration of the pericardium, and mediastinal irradiation. The physical findings seen most commonly in effusive-constrictive pericarditis include pulsus paradoxus, abnormal or diminished pulse pressure, and jugular venous distention with a predominant x descent. They therefore more closely resemble the physical findings of cardiac tamponade than they do those of chronic constrictive pericarditis.

The chest x-ray in this condition usually shows cardiac enlargement and the ECG may reveal diffuse low QRS voltage and/or ST- and T-wave abnormalities. Echocardiography may demonstrate both the pericardial effusion and a thickened pericardium. The diagnosis of effusive-constrictive pericarditis is ultimately made at cardiac catheterization, with careful hemodynamic monitoring of intrapericardial and right atrial pressures before and after pericardiocentesis. Although restoration of intrapericardial pressure to zero following pericardiocentesis may allow some improvement in hemodynamics, pressures do not return entirely to normal. Wave forms may convert to a pattern more consistent with constrictive pericarditis following pericardiocentesis, with a prominent y descent in the left atrial pressure tracing as well as a dip-and-plateau pattern in the right ventricular pressure tracing. As might be expected from the pathophysiology, pericardiocentesis provides only partial and transient relief, and definitive therapy for this condition consists of total parietal and visceral pericardiectomy.

REFERENCE

1. Hancock, E.W.: Subacute effusive constrictive pericarditis. Circulation 43:183, 1971.

245-A (Braunwald, pp. 1502–1503)

Prior to the development of antituberculosis therapy, tuberculosis was the leading cause of constrictive pericarditis in the United States. While this is still true in developing nations, tuberculosis is no longer the major cause of constrictive pericarditis in modern Western society. Most cases of constrictive pericarditis today are attributed to clinically inapparent viral pericarditis and are referred to as idiopathic.[1] Other specific causes of constrictive pericarditis include chronic renal failure (especially in patients undergoing hemodialysis), rheumatoid arthritis, systemic lupus erythematosus and other connective tissue disorders, and neoplastic infiltration of the pericardium. Neoplastic infiltration is most commonly seen in breast cancer, lung cancer, lymphoma, and Hodgkin's disease. It should be noted that constrictive pericarditis may occur years following mediastinal irradiation for therapy of either breast cancer or Hodgkin's disease.

Infectious processes that lead to the accumulation of products of inflammation and fibrin deposition may also lead to chronic constrictive pericarditis. The disorder has been seen as a consequence of incomplete drainage of purulent pericarditis, as well as following fungal infections and parasitic infections. It is also being increasingly recognized as a complication of cardiac surgery and procedures involving hemopericardium.[2] While myxedema may lead to an acute pericarditis and a pericardial effusion, it is not associated with chronic constrictive pericarditis (see Braunwald, pp. 1807–1808).

REFERENCES

1. Blake, S., Bonar, S., O'Neill, H., Hanly, P., Drury, I., Flanagan, M., and Garrett, J.: Aetiology of chronic constrictive pericarditis. Br. Heart J. 50:273, 1983.
2. Fowler, N.O.: Constrictive pericarditis: New aspects. Am. J. Cardiol. 50:1014, 1982.

246-C (Braunwald, pp. 912–913)

In general, the electrocardiogram is less helpful in the diagnosis of congenital heart disease in premature and newborn infants than it is in older children or adults. Right ventricular hypertrophy is a normal finding in the neonate, and the range of normal voltages is wide in this age group. Initial septal depolarization may be assessed from the ECG even in the neonate. While septal Q waves may not be clearly seen in the lateral precordial leads in the first 72 hours of life, a *leftward, posteriorly directed septal vector* giving rise to Q waves in the right precordial leads is abnormal and may suggest the presence of marked right ventricular hypertrophy, single ventricle, or inversion of the ventricles.

T-wave inversions may be a normal finding in the neonatal ECG, and by the age of 72 hours T waves should be inverted in right precordial leads and upright in the lateral precordium. The persistence of upright T waves in right precordial leads is a sign of significant, abnormal right ventricular hypertrophy. Flattening or inversion of lateral T waves may suggest subendocardial ischemia or obstruction to left ventricular outflow. In addition, these findings may be seen in electrolyte disturbance, acidosis, and hypoxemia.

The electrocardiographic findings of myocardial infarction in an infant suggest the diagnosis of anomalous origin of a coronary artery. Finally, heart block or supraventricular tachycardia as well as other arrhythmias may be detected by the ECG. Thus, while the ECG is not as useful in neonates and infants as it is in older age groups, it is capable of offering significant clues to the presence of underlying cardiovascular disease.

247-B (Braunwald, pp. 990–991)

Because corrective surgery can now be carried out at a low risk, palliative operations are much less commonly performed than previously. However, a number of patients are still alive who have undergone a palliative procedure. The most common palliative procedure is the

Blalock-Taussig shunt, which involves an end-to-side anastomosis of a subclavian artery to the pulmonary artery. This iatrogenic left-to-right shunt allows an increase in pulmonary arterial flow and reduces hypoxia. Patients who have undergone palliation have a lower survival rate than that for patients with complete correction and, as a general rule, adult patients with tetralogy of Fallot who have a palliative shunt should undergo total surgical repair.[1] The total surgical repair of tetralogy may be undertaken in adults with a mortality rate comparable to that reported in children.[2] However, whenever possible, the total correction of tetralogy of Fallot should occur early in life; when the operation is performed prior to the age of 4 years, the development of accompanying left ventricular dysfunction may be avoided.

Patients who have undergone total repair of tetralogy of Fallot do quite well. Persistent obstruction to right ventricular outflow and/or pulmonary regurgitation, as well as a residual ventricular septal defect, are the most common anatomical findings following total repair.[3] Pregnancy seems to be well tolerated after successful total correction of tetralogy of Fallot. There are several reports of ventricular ectopy and more serious arrhythmias occurring as a late complication of total repair. These may require aggressive antiarrhythmic therapy.[4]

REFERENCES

1. Mattila, S., Luosto, R., Ketonen, P., Nieminen, M., Merikallio, E., and Kyllonen, K.E.J.: Total correction of tetralogy of Fallot in adults. Scand. J. Thorac. Cardiovasc. Surg. 18:23, 1984.
2. Hu, D.C.K., Seward, J.B., Puga, F.J., Fuster, V., and Tajik, A.: Total correction of tetralogy of Fallot at age 40 years and older: Long-term follow-up. J. Am. Coll. Cardiol. 5:40, 1985.
3. Tamer, D., Wolff, G.S., Ferrer, P., Pickoff, A.S., Casta, A., Mehta, A.V., Garcia, O., and Gelband, H.: Hemodynamics and intracardiac conduction after operative repair of tetralogy of Fallot. Am. J. Cardiol. 51:552, 1983.
4. Garson, A., Randall, D.C., Gillette, P.C., Smith, R.T., Moak, J.P., McVey, P., and McNamara, D.G.: Prevention of sudden death after repair of tetralogy of Fallot: Treatment of ventricular arrhythmias. J. Am. Coll. Cardiol. 6:221, 1985.

248-D   (Braunwald, pp. 985–988)

Ventricular septal defect is the most common congenital cardiac malformation reported in infants and children. A significant number of VSDs close spontaneously during infancy or childhood, and some may even close during adolescence.[1] Of the four major anatomical types of VSD the most common is the membranous variety, accounting for approximately three-fourths of all cases. Membranous VSDs are located inferior to the crista supraventricularis in the region of the membranous septum and in proximity to the septal leaflet of the tricuspid valve. Approximately 10 per cent of VSDs are of the muscular type and another 10 per cent are caused by atrioventricular canal defects. The least common type of VSD is the supracristal, which constitutes about 5 per cent. Patients with moderate or large VSDs without pulmonary vascular disease have significant left-to-right shunts and volume overload of the left side of the heart. However, congestive heart failure

is generally not part of the clinical history in patients over 2 years of age unless aortic regurgitation or infective endocarditis appears.[2]

The ECG in the adult with small, uncomplicated VSDs is usually normal. When a larger defect is present, both left atrial enlargement and left ventricular hypertrophy may be present. The presence or development of right axis deviation in the frontal plane suggests right ventricular hypertrophy secondary either to acquired infundibular obstruction or the development of pulmonary vascular obstructive disease. The chest x-ray is usually normal in adults with a small VSD. Larger defects may be characterized by increased pulmonary vascular markings as well as by enlargement of pulmonary arteries, left atrium, and left ventricle.

REFERENCES

1. Weidman, W.H., DuShane, J.W., and Ellison, R.C.: Clinical course in adults with ventricular septal defect. Circulation 56:178, 1977.
2. Corone, P., Doyon, F., Gaudeau, S., Guerin, F., Vernant, P., Ducan, H., Rumeau-Rouquette, C., and Gaudeau, P.: Natural history of ventricular septal defect: A study involving 790 cases. Circulation 55:908, 1977.

249-A   (Braunwald, pp. 994–997)

In most cases, coarctation of the aorta consists of an eccentric narrowing of the thoracic aortic lumen just *distal* to the origin of the subclavian artery, which is frequently dilated.[1] Less commonly the coarctation may be proximal to or involve the origin of the left subclavian artery itself. Coarctation is frequently associated with other congenital cardiac malformations, the most common of which are bicuspid aortic valve, patent ductus arteriosus, ventricular septal defect, and mitral valve abnormalities.[2] Adult patients with coarctation of the aorta are usually asymptomatic, and suspicion is the key to the diagnosis of this condition. In adults with this condition, the most common complaints are headaches, leg fatigue, and intermittent claudication. Patients may also come to medical attention because of symptoms associated with left ventricular failure, infective endarteritis, or aortic rupture or dissection. Endocarditis may occur on an associated bicuspid valve as another presentation of this disorder.

While patients with coarctation usually appear normal, this is the most common anomaly associated with Turner's syndrome and should be specifically sought in patients with this condition. In most cases, simultaneous palpation of pulses in the upper and lower extremities reveals diminished and delayed femoral when compared with radial pulses. In questionable cases, exercise may exacerbate the difference and accentuate these physical findings. A suprasternal thrill is often present in coarctation of the aorta. In addition, auscultation usually demonstrates an ejection murmur that may be caused by the coarctation itself or by an associated bicuspid aortic valve. The presence of an ejection click should raise further the possibility of this aortic valve abnormality.

REFERENCES

1. Maron, B.J.: Aortic isthmic coarctations. *In* Roberts, W.C. (ed.): Adult Congenital Heart Disease. Philadelphia, F.A. Davis, 1987, pp. 443–454.
2. Serfas, D., and Borow, K.M.: Coarctation of the aorta: Anatomy, pathophysiology, and natural history. J. Cardiovasc. Med. 8:575, 1983.

250-A *(Braunwald, pp. 1472–1473; 1477–1478)*

The two-dimensional echocardiogram illustrated demonstrates a tumor in the right atrium attached to the intraatrial septum (IAS). Since the tumor appears to be pedunculated, it is much more likely that it is a myxoma rather than a rhabdomyoma or a lymphosarcoma, both of which tend to be adherent to the wall. Myxomas are the most common type of primary cardiac tumor, comprising 30 to 50 per cent of total tumors in most pathological series. Approximately 85 per cent of myxomas occur in the left atrium; the number in the right atrium is only about 15 per cent. In more than 90 per cent of cases myxomas are solitary. The most common site of attachment for myxomas is in the area of the fossa ovalis. Rhabdomyosarcomas are tumors of smooth muscle, which usually diffusely infiltrate the myocardium. Lymphosarcomas are quite rare in contrast to metastatic systemic lymphoma, which involves the heart in 25 per cent of cases. Lymphosarcomas can mimic hypertrophic cardiomyopathy due to the extensive myocardial infiltration. A pericardial cyst would be relatively easy to discern based on the appearance of a liquid-filled space.

251-C *(Braunwald, pp. 1253–1257)*

Over the past decade the use of thrombolytic agents to restore patency to thrombosed coronary vessels has received widespread attention due to the potential value of such an intervention in salvaging jeopardized myocardial tissue and limiting the extent of MI. While earlier investigations focused on the use of intracoronary thrombolysis in the early hours of AMI, the ease and relative low cost of intravenous thrombolytic therapy has directed current attention to this latter treatment modality. Careful analysis of existing clinical trials of the use of fibrinolytic therapy in AMI reveals a statistically significant improvement in mortality in patients receiving such therapy.[1]

The GISSI trial conducted in hospitals throughout Italy has provided an important confirmation of the usefulness of fibrinolytic therapy in AMI.[2] In this study a total of 11,806 patients were randomized to receive either conventional therapy or conventional therapy plus 1.5 million units of intravenous streptokinase as soon as possible after randomization. It should be noted that those patients were excluded who had an *absolute contraindication* to intravenous fibrinolytic therapy, such as those with a prior cerebral vascular accident, a recent surgical or invasive procedure or trauma, uncontrolled hypertension, recent bleeding problems, or other life-threatening conditions. A highly significant reduction in in-hospital mortality was achieved in the streptokinase-treated group, especially in patients receiving therapy in the early hours

following the onset of symptoms. In patients who received streptokinase within the first hour, a nearly 50 per cent reduction in mortality by streptokinase was noted. The therapy appeared to be extremely useful in patients who were younger than 65 years of age, patients with anterior infarction, patients without previous infarction, and patients without complicating heart failure or shock. Interestingly, those patients treated with streptokinase experienced twice as many in-hospital reinfarctions as control patients in this study. Recent and ongoing studies are examining the use of tissue plasminogen activator in the AMI setting. This has been shown to be a more effective lytic agent than streptokinase and may prove to have less pronounced systemic lytic effects,[3] although the relative clinical benefits of these two fibrinolytic agents are still not clear as of this writing (November 1988).

REFERENCES

1. Yusuf, S., Collins, R., Peto, R., Furberg, C., Stampfer, M.J., Goldhaber, S.Z., and Hennekens, C.H.: Intravenous and intracoronary fibrinolytic therapy in acute myocardial infarction: Overview of results on mortality, reinfarction, and side effects from 33 randomized trials. Eur. Heart J. 6:556, 1985.
2. Gruppo Italiano Per Lo Studio Della Streptochinasi Nell'Infarcto Miocardico (GISSI): Effectiveness of intravenous thrombolytic treatment in acute myocardial infarction. Lancet 1:397, 1986.
3. Verstraete, M., Bory, M., Collen, D., Erbel, R., Lennane, R.J., Mathey, D., Michels, H.R., Schartl, M., Uebis, R., Bernard, R., Brower, R.W., DeBono, D.P., Huhmann, W., Lursen, J., Meyer, J., Rutsch, W., Schmidt, W., and Von Essen, R.: Randomized trial of intravenous recombinant tissue-type plasminogen activator versus intravenous streptokinase in acute myocardial infarction. Lancet 1:842, 1985.

252-D *(Braunwald, pp. 191; 1224)*

Autopsy studies over the last 4 decades have revealed that true atrial infarction occurs in between 7 and 17 per cent of autopsy-proven cases of MI.[1] Atrial infarction is often seen in conjunction with left ventricular infarction and it more commonly involves the right atrium. This may be due to the presence of well-oxygenated blood in the left atrium which may be capable of nourishing the thin atrial wall despite the presence of obstructive coronary disease involving the coronary arterial system perfusing the left atrium. Atrial infarction may lead to rupture of the atrial wall and is more frequently noted in the atrial appendages than in the lateral or posterior aspects of the atrium itself. Because right atrial infarction, the most common variety of atrial infarction, is usually associated with obstructive disease of the sinus node artery, it is frequently accompanied by atrial arrhythmias.

REFERENCE

1. Gardin, J.M., and Singer, D.H.: Atrial infarction: Importance, diagnosis and localization. Arch. Intern. Med. 141:1345, 1981.

253-B *(Braunwald, pp. 1390–1391)*

In 1982, pediatric cardiologists began to use balloon dilatation catheters with inflated diameters of 1 to 2 cm to produce commissural splitting of stenotic pulmonary valves and were able to achieve reductions of pulmonic valve gradients to approximately one-third of their baseline value. In addition, this technique proved to have a very high success rate and has now essentially replaced open surgical repair for valvular pulmonic stenosis. Theoretical concerns existed regarding the efficacy of balloon valvuloplasty in the treatment of adult acquired rheumatic and/or calcific stenosis of either the mitral or aortic valves. In 1985, despite these concerns, successful balloon valvuloplasty using a transseptal approach was first reported in young adult patients with rheumatic mitral stenosis.[1] This technique is now being used successfully in a variety of centers and is capable of achieving physiologically adequate enlargement of the mitral orifice. Moderate or severe mitral regurgitation occurs rarely following balloon valvuloplasty, provided that patients are preselected for the absence of left atrial thrombus. One minor complication without significant hemodynamic consequence is that approximately one-third of patients show some evidence of a persistent, small left-to-right shunt at the site of atrial septal puncture at the time of transseptal left heart catheterization.

Aortic valvuloplasty using a retrograde approach has also proven successful; however, the magnitude of orifice improvement during aortic valvuloplasty appears to be less than that achieved by the mitral procedure and restenosis occurs commonly. Despite this, in the appropriately selected patient, aortic valvuloplasty has proven to be useful, capable of improving both left ventricular performance and overall clinical status in patients studied to date.[2] In general, the degree of improvement in aortic orifice area following balloon valvuloplasty is less than that achieved by valve replacement. The technique may ultimately prove most useful as a temporizing measure for patients who are poor surgical risks.

REFERENCES

1. Lock, J.E., Khalilullah, M., Shrivastava, S., Bahl, V., and Keane, J.F.: Percutaneous catheter commissurotomy in rheumatic mitral stenosis. N. Engl. J. Med. 313:1545, 1985.
2. McKay, R.G., Safian, R.D., Lock, J.E., Diver, D.J., Berman, A.D., Warren, S.E., Come, P.C., Baim, D.S., Mandel, V.E., Royal, H.D., and Grossman, W.: Assessment of left ventricular and aortic valve function after aortic balloon valvuloplasty in adult patients with critical aortic stenosis. Circulation 75:192, 1987.

254-A   *(Braunwald, pp. 1395–1401)*

A comprehensive program of rehabilitation for the patient with coronary artery disease involves physical fitness, secondary prevention, psychosocial adaptations, and vocational counseling. Rehabilitation programs may be especially useful in patients who have undergone therapeutic procedures such as coronary artery bypass grafting or heart valve replacement. Despite therapeutic advances, return-to-work rates have diminished since 1970 for patients with uncomplicated myocardial infarction, although in general up to 80 per cent of patients who are previously employed and are less than 55 years of age do ultimately resume employment. In addition to return-to-work, other potential benefits include the ca-

pability of attaining near-maximal performance, favorable physiological adaptations (in part through increasing maximal oxygen uptake), relief of symptoms, creation of a sense of well-being, and preservation of the patient's role in both family and society. While most studies over the last decade have shown a lower mortality among survivors of MI randomized to an exercise training group than that among patients in a control group, little effect on the incidence of reinfarction has been noted.[1] The improved mortality appears to be more marked if exercise rehabilitation is begun early following MI.

REFERENCE

1. May, G.S., Eberlain, K.A., Furberg, C.D., Passamani, E.R., and DeMets, D.L.: Secondary prevention after myocardial infarction: A view of long-term trials. Prog. Cardiovasc. Dis. 24:331, 1982.

255-C   *(Braunwald, pp. 1470–1473)*

Cardiac myxomas produce a wide variety of systemic findings, including fever, cachexia, malaise, arthralgias, Raynaud's phenomenon, rash, and systemic and pulmonary emboli. A variety of abnormal laboratory findings are common, including hypergammaglobulinemia, elevated erythrocyte sedimentation rate, thrombocytosis, thrombocytopenia, polycythemia, leukocytosis, and anemia.

Among the classic cardiac manifestations of myxomas are mitral valve abnormalities. Most commonly, left atrial tumors mimic symptoms of mitral stenosis, including dyspnea, orthopnea, pulmonary edema, cough, hemoptysis, chest pain, peripheral edema, and fatigue. Tumors in the right atrium (which are rare) frequently produce right heart failure, including fatigue, peripheral edema, ascites, hepatomegaly, and prominent *a* waves in the jugular venous pulse. Myxomas occur more commonly in the left atrium (85 per cent) than the right atrium, so that mitral valve findings predominate. In cases of right atrial myxomas, right atrial hypertension may cause right-to-left shunting through a patent foramen ovale, producing systemic hypoxia, cyanosis, clubbing, and polycythemia.

256-D   *(Braunwald, p. 1013)*

The patient described has the classic clinical signs and findings of *type II glycogen storage disease*. This disease is a consequence of the deficiency of alpha-1,4-glucosidase (acid maltase), a lysosomal enzyme that hydrolyzes glycogen into glucose. The condition commonly presents in the neonatal period. Characteristic symptoms include failure to thrive, progressive hypotonia, lethargy, and a weak cry. Of all the glycogen storage diseases, type II (or Pompe's disease) is the most likely to cause cardiac symptoms. The ECG shows extremely tall, broad QRS complexes with a short P-R interval (commonly less than 0.09 sec). A short P-R interval may be the result of enhanced AV conduction due to myocardial glycogen deposition. Chest x-ray frequently shows cardiomegaly with pulmonary vascular redistribution. Diagnosis is confirmed by demonstrating the enzymatic deficiency in lymphocytes, skeletal muscle, or liver.[1]

Cardiac glycogenosis may be confused with other entities that cause cardiac failure, particularly in association with cardiomegaly in the early months of life. *Endocardial fibroelastosis*, a disease of unknown etiology, differs from Pompe's disease in lacking the short P-R interval and the fact that symptoms are limited to the cardiac system, while in Pompe's disease skeletal muscle hypotonia is prominent. Furthermore, in endocardial fibroelastosis, mitral regurgitation and abnormalities of the cardiac valves, especially mitral and aortic, are frequent. *Coarctation of the aorta*, another common cause of congestive heart failure in infants, can readily be distinguished by the presence of pulse and blood pressure discrepancies between the upper and lower extremities. *Myocarditis*, another cause of congestive heart failure in children, is usually of abrupt onset and is not associated with hypotonia. *Anomalous pulmonary origin of the left coronary artery* can cause cardiomegaly but usually has a distinctive ECG pattern of anterolateral MI.

Shone syndrome is a developmental complex that consists of four obstructive anomalies: (1) a supravalvular ring of the left atrium; (2) a parachute mitral valve; (3) subaortic stenosis; and (4) coarctation of the aorta. It frequently presents with mitral stenosis, since flow from the left atrium must pass through the intrachordal spaces of the mitral valve causing functional mitral stenosis. Pulmonary venous hypertension is a common finding in this illness because of left ventricular inflow and outflow obstruction. However, Shone syndrome frequently presents in early childhood rather than infancy and lacks the skeletal muscle changes of Pompe's disease.

Friedreich's ataxia is a hereditary autosomal recessive disease that affects the individual during late childhood and presents with progressive ataxia. The limbs, in addition to being ataxic, generally show considerable weakness. About 50 per cent of patients with Friedreich's ataxia have cardiac involvement, which typically presents as a hypertrophic cardiomyopathy associated with arrhythmias. Coronary arteries may either be normal or show extensive intimal proliferation leading to obstruction while atherosclerosis and thrombosis are generally not present.

REFERENCE

1. Caddell, J.L.: Metabolic and nutritional diseases. In Adams, F.H., and Emmanouilides, G.C. (eds.): Moss' Heart Disease in Infants. Infants, Children and Adolescents. 3rd ed. Baltimore, Williams & Wilkins, 1983, pp. 596–626.

257-B   (*Braunwald, pp. 1183–1185*)

Many large case-controlled studies have been performed to identify risk factors that affect cardiovascular mortality in addition to the established major risk factors, i.e. cigarette smoking, hypertension, elevated serum cholesterol, and diabetes mellitus. Among these other risk factors are sedentary life style, obesity, fat distribution, diet, family history, social and behavioral factors, stress and occupation, glucose intolerance, estrogens, and male gender. The data for many of these are quite controversial, and it is likely that a multitude of factors play a role in the determination of cardiovascular risk.

Several minor factors have been shown to be associated with increased or decreased cardiovascular mortality. It has been demonstrated that consumption of small to moderate amounts of ethanol is associated with a decreased incidence of cardiovascular mortality.[1] It appears that the relative cardiovascular risk of people drinking the equivalent of two glasses of wine/day is approximately 0.7 compared with those drinking no alcohol. However, consumption of excessive amounts of alcohol is associated with elevated blood pressure and an increased cardiovascular mortality.

Vasectomy has been shown to cause an increase in atherosclerosis in rhesus monkeys. However, large studies carried out in vasectomized men have shown no increase in the incidence of nonfatal MI.[2] At this time vasectomy does not appear to cause a significantly increased risk of cardiac mortality.

Heavy coffee consumption has been associated with an increase in serum cholesterol and in cardiovascular mortality. Consumption of more than nine cups of coffee a day significantly raised cholesterol and was associated with a two- to threefold greater risk of coronary artery disease in these persons compared with noncoffee drinkers.[3]

Cardiac transplantation is associated with accelerated atherosclerosis. It is unclear whether or not this is due to a chronic immune injury or to hypertension or hypercholesterolemia commonly associated with the post-transplantation condition. Nonetheless, these patients frequently develop painless cardiac ischemia, and early deaths due to myocardial infarction occur in 10 to 20 per cent of patients who have undergone cardiac transplantation.

A strong association has also been noted between blood fibrinogen concentration and coronary artery disease.[4] Fibrinogen is positively correlated with concentrations of cholesterol and triglyceride and therefore is associated with hyperlipidemia. It is also correlated with smoking, obesity, and socioeconomic stress. Furthermore, since over 90 per cent of patients with MI exhibit coronary thrombosis one might expect high concentrations of fibrinogen to predispose to thrombotic events.

REFERENCES

1. St. Leger, A.S., Cochrane, A.L., and Moore, F.: Factors associated with cardiac mortality in developed countries with particular reference to the consumption of wine. Lancet 1:1017, 1979.
2. Walker, A.M., Jick, H., Hunter, J.R., Danford, A., Watkins, R.N., Alhedeff, L., and Rothman, K.J.: Vasectomy and nonfatal myocardial infarction. Lancet 1:13, 1981.
3. LaCroix, A.Z., Mead, L.A., Liang, K.Y., Thomas, C.B., and Pearson, T.A.: Coffee consumption and the incidence of coronary heart disease. N. Engl. J. Med. 315:977, 1986.
4. Meade, T.W., Mellows, S., Brozovic, M., Miller, G.J., Cakrabarti, R.R., and North, W.R.: Haemostatic function and ischemic heart disease: Principal results of the Northwick Park Heart Study. Lancet 2:533, 1986.

258-C   (*Braunwald, pp. 1492–1493*)

The accumulation of pericardial fluid to the point of cardiac compression is termed cardiac tamponade and is characterized by an increase in intracardiac pressures, progressive limitation of diastolic filling of the ventricles, and an ultimate reduction in stroke volume. Normal intrapericardial pressures are several mm Hg lower than right and left ventricular diastolic pressures and are very close to intrapleural pressures. As fluid is accumulated in the pericardial space, intrapericardial pressure rises to the level of the RA and RV diastolic pressures, and cardiac tamponade occurs. At this point, the transpericardial pressure distending the cardiac chambers declines to zero. While the rise of RA and intrapericardial pressures may be less dramatic in the presence of hypovolemia, cardiac tamponade can occur during this state and may be masked because the pressures in these two spaces equalize at a lower absolute value. As intrapericardial fluid continues to accumulate, pericardial and RV diastolic pressures rise together toward the level of LV diastolic pressure. Subsequently, all three pressures equalize and, as they continue to rise, lead to a marked decrease in transmural distending pressures, with a decrease in the diastolic volumes of the ventricles and a fall in stroke volume.[1] Cardiac output in this setting may initially be maintained by a reflex tachycardia. However, as the accumulation of pericardial fluid continues, compensatory mechanisms are no longer able to maintain systemic blood pressure and cardiac output begins to decline, with an accompanying impairment of the perfusion of vital organs.

In the most extreme examples of cardiac tamponade, transmural diastolic ventricular pressures may actually be negative. This implies that ventricular filling in this situation occurs by diastolic suction. Both the cardiac depressor branches of the vagus nerve and sinoatrial node ischemia are believed to contribute to the sinus bradycardia that may occur during severe cardiac tamponade.[2] Hemodynamic deterioration during tamponade has been noted to be markedly influenced by the presence of atrial compression during diastole and subsequent impairment of cardiac filling. Echocardiographic studies have demonstrated that right atrial diastolic collapse is consistently present in patients with tamponade, while left atrial and left ventricular diastolic collapse is a more variable finding.[3]

REFERENCES

1. Spodick, D.H.: The normal and diseased pericardium: Current concepts of pericardial physiology, diagnosis and treatment. J. Am. Coll. Cardiol. 1:240, 1983.
2. Kostreva, D.R., Castaner, A., Pedersen, D.H., and Kampine, J.P.: Nonvagally mediated bradycardia during cardiac tamponade or severe hemorrhage. Cardiology 68:65, 1981.
3. Kronton, I., Cohen, M.L., and Winer, H.E: Diastolic atrial compression: A sensitive echocardiographic sign of cardiac tamponade. J. Am. Coll. Cardiol. 2:770, 1983.

259-B   (Braunwald, pp. 1072–1075)

This 67-year-old woman presents with the classic physical findings and symptoms of tricuspid regurgitation (TR). By history, the course of her illness is relatively rapid and includes systemic symptoms such as fatigue, weight loss, and peculiar episodes of rapid heartbeat, flushing, and diarrhea. The most likely diagnosis is the carcinoid syndrome. Carcinoid is a slowly growing tumor that leads to focal or diffuse deposits of fibrous tissue in the endo-

cardium of the valvular cusps and cardiac chambers. The white fibrous carcinoid plaques are most extensive on the right side of the heart, usually because the tumor begins in the portal circulation and drains through the inferior vena cava into the right side of the heart. The plaques are deposited on the ventricular surfaces of the tricuspid valve and cause the cusps to adhere to the underlying right ventricle, producing TR.[1] Carcinoid syndrome is suggested by the coexistence of TR, flushing, and diarrhea due to the release of vasoactive amines (predominantly 5'-hydroxytryptamine) by the tumor cells. Less common causes of TR include cardiac tumors (particularly right atrial myxomas), endomyocardial fibrosis, methysergide-induced valvular disease, and systemic lupus erythematosus.

The causes of isolated TR may be divided into those involving an anatomically abnormal valve and those involving an anatomically normal valve. The latter, in which functional TR is present due to dilatation of the RV and tricuspid annulus, is actually more common. The most common cause of functional TR is RV hypertension, especially as a result of mitral valve disease, RV infarction, congenital heart disease, primary pulmonary hypertension, or cor pulmonale. This woman had no evidence for chronic elevations in her pulmonary pressures, nor did she have an RV lift. RV infarction may also cause TR in the absence of pulmonary hypertension, secondary to RV dilatation.

A variety of disease processes may affect the tricuspid valve, directly leading to regurgitation. Among these are: (1) Ebstein's anomaly, in which there is abnormal attachment and elongation of the tricuspid valve with ventricularization of the atrium; (2) common atrioventricular canal, in which the tricuspid valve is involved in the formation of an aneurysm of the ventricular septum; (3) rheumatic fever, which usually causes both regurgitation and stenosis as well as coexisting mitral valve disease; (4) infarction, rupture, or ischemia of the papillary muscles of the RV in coronary disease; (5) infective endocarditis; and (6) Marfan syndrome.

REFERENCE

1. Callahan, J.A., Wroblewski, E.M., Reeder, G.S., Edwards, W.D., Seward, J.B., and Tajik, A.J.: Echocardiographic features of carcinoid heart disease. Am. J. Cardiol. 50:762, 1982.

260-D   (Braunwald, pp. 1281–1283)

Rupture of the free wall of the infarcted ventricle may occur in up to 10 per cent of patients who die in the hospital with AMI. This serious complication occurs more frequently in women and in elderly patients, much more commonly affects the left than the right ventricle, and only rarely affects the atria. Rupture of the free wall is more common in hypertensive patients. It is usually associated with a transmural infarction that damages at least 20 per cent of the left ventricle, and usually involves the lateral or anterior walls of the ventricle in the terminal distribution of the left anterior descending artery. The complication usually results from a frank tear in the myocardial wall or a dissection of a hematoma that perforates a necrotic area of the myocardium, in the area of the junction of the infarct and normal myocardial tissue (see Braunwald, Fig. 38–37, p. 1282). Although free wall rupture usually occurs between 1 day and 3 weeks following infarction, it is most commonly seen between the third and sixth days following infarction.

Occasionally, rupture of the free wall will occur in the center of an infarct. However, when rupture occurs here, it more often happens during the second week following the infarct. Rupture of the free wall is rare in a hypertrophied ventricle or in an area that is well supplied by collateralization. In general, the prognosis of this complication is poor, with survival depending largely upon immediate hemodynamic stabilization and surgical repair.[1]

REFERENCE

1. Coma-Canella, I., Lopez-Sendon, J., Gonzalez, L.N., and Ferrufino, O.: Subacute left ventricular free wall rupture following acute myocardial infarction: Bedside hemodynamics, differential diagnosis, and treatment. Am. Heart J. *106*:278, 1983.

261-A (Braunwald, pp. 1515–1516)

Pericardial involvement occurs in between 5 and 10 per cent of patients with malignant neoplasms. Lung and breast cancer, as well as hematological malignancies, acount for approximately 80 per cent of all reported cases of malignant pericarditis. In children, neuroblastomas, sarcomas, and Wilms' tumor also may lead to malignant pericarditis. In general, primary malignancies of the pericardium are rare and are predominantly due to mesothelioma. It should be noted, however, that patients with mediastinal malignancies such as lymphoma and Hodgkin's disease quite commonly have asymptomatic *nonmalignant* pericardial effusions that are detected during staging procedures.[1]

If idiopathic instances of pericarditis are excluded, neoplastic pericarditis is the most common *specific* etiology of acute pericarditis in Western society. The most common symptom of neoplastic pericarditis is dyspnea—chest pain, cough, orthopnea, and hepatomegaly are also commonly seen. The classic pericardial friction rub seen in viral pericarditis is an uncommon finding in the malignant form of the disease. Diagnosis of this disorder usually occurs only when evidence of cardiac compression becomes manifested clinically. The chest x-ray in patients with malignant pericarditis, which is abnormal in greater than 90 per cent of patients, may show a pleural effusion, an enlarged cardiac silhouette, mediastinal widening, or even an irregular nodular contour of the cardiac silhouette.[2] The cornerstone of the diagnosis of malignant pericarditis is a high index of suspicion in appropriate patients. The clinical findings of elevated jugular venous pressure, peripheral edema, and hepatomegaly in cancer patients should bring to mind a differential diagnosis that includes neoplastic pericarditis with cardiac compression as well as underlying left ventricular dysfunction (due to cardiac disease or Adriamycin cardiac toxicity), superior vena caval obstruction syndrome, malignant hepatic in-volvement with portal hypertension, and pulmonary lymphangitic spread of tumor. Echocardiography may provide further information about the pericardial involvement of a malignant process, and pericardiocentesis may provide diagnostic confirmation of the pericardial involvement of a malignant process. When patients with a malignant process thought to involve the pericardium are brought to cardiac catheterization, the possibility of coexistent superior vena caval obstruction must also be considered. Cyanosis, hypoxemia, and increased pulmonary vascular resistance should be sought as well, because this constellation of findings is more consistent with lymphangitic spread of the tumor process.

REFERENCES

1. Markiewicz, W., Gladstein, E., London, E.J., and Popp, R.L.: Echocardiographic detection of pericardial effusion and pericardial thickening in malignant lymphoma. Radiology *123*:161, 1977.
2. Posner, M.R., Cohen, G.I., and Skarin, A.T.: Pericardial disease in patients with cancer. Am. J. Med. *71*:407, 1981.

262-C (Braunwald, pp. 1320–1321; 1353)

Clinical examination of the patient with presumed ischemic heart disease can be quite revealing. First, the presence of murmurs of hypertrophic obstructive cardiomyopathy or aortic valve disease may suggest that ischemic chest pain is caused by other conditions in addition to coronary artery disease. Second, findings such as third or fourth heart sounds in association with early diastolic or presystolic filling waves suggest that ischemia is indeed present. These findings can be increased in intensity by having the patient perform handgrip exercise. These sounds and pulsations are related to the functional state of the left ventricle, particularly the pressure and compliance during diastole.

Paradoxical splitting of the second heart sound, which may occur during an anginal attack, appears to be related to asynergy and prolongation of left ventricular contraction as would be anticipated in a patient with severe disease of the left anterior descending coronary artery. It would be unlikely for fixed splitting of the second heart sound to occur in this setting. Equalization of pressures between the right and left atrium would be required, as occurs most typically in an atrial septal defect.

Several murmurs are characteristic of coronary artery disease. Perhaps most typical are transient apical systolic murmurs. These are attributed to reversible papillary muscle dysfunction, particularly in patients who have had a previous subendocardial infarction. However, occasionally a diastolic murmur or continuous murmur may be heard. This has been attributed to turbulent flow across a proximal coronary artery stenosis.[1]

REFERENCE

1. Sangster, J.F., and Oakley, C.M.: Diastolic murmur of coronary artery stenosis. Br. Heart J. *35*:840, 1973.

263-B *(Braunwald, pp. 916–917)*

There are a variety of clinical findings in ASD that may provide evidence of the underlying condition. On physical examination, common findings include a prominent RV impulse, palpable pulmonary artery pulsations, accentuation of the tricuspid valve closure sound leading to splitting of the first heart sound, and a midsystolic pulmonary ejection murmur due to increased flow across the pulmonic valve. If the shunt is large, a mid-diastolic rumbling murmur may be audible at the lower left sternal border. This murmur results from increased blood flow across the tricuspid valve.

The ECG may be particularly helpful in the diagnostic evaluation of a patient with suspected ASD. The ECG in patients with an ostium secundum ASD usually shows right-axis deviation and an rSR' or rsR' pattern in the right precordial leads with a normal QRS duration. The presence of left-axis deviation of the P wave in the frontal plane in association with the aforementioned constellation suggests the presence of a sinus venosus defect. Left-axis deviation and superior orientation of the QRS complex in the frontal plane suggest the presence of either an ostium primum defect or, less commonly, a secundum atrial defect in association with mitral valve prolapse. Prolongation of the P-R interval may be seen with all types of ASDs. It is believed to result both from the increased size of the atrium in this condition and the increased distance for intranodal conduction produced by the defect itself.[1]

Chest x-ray may reveal enlargement of the RA and RV, pulmonary arterial dilatation, and increased pulmonary vascular markings. Echocardiographic evaluation of ASD may reveal pulmonary arterial and RV dilatation as well as anterior systolic (paradoxical) supraventricular septal motion, especially if significant RV volume overload is present.[2] The defect itself may be visualized by two-dimensional echocardiography, particularly utilizing a subcostal view of the interatrial septum. In many institutions, two-dimensional echocardiography along with Doppler flow analysis has become the primary confirmatory test for ASD.[3] Cardiac catheterization may be employed in clinical situations in which the diagnosis is in question or if significant pulmonary hypertension is suspected. In children with ASD, pressures on the right side of the heart are usually normal, even in the presence of a large left-to-right shunt. Pulmonary hypertension and resultant right ventricular failure are serious complications of ASD and most commonly begin in the third or fourth decades of life.

REFERENCES

1. Clark, E.B., and Kugler, J.D.: Preoperative secundum atrial septal defect with coexisting sinus node and atrioventricular node dysfunction. Circulation 65:976, 1982.
2. DiSessa, T.G., and Friedman, W.F.: Echocardiographic evaluation of cardiac performance. *In* Friedman, W.F., and Higgins, C.B. (eds.): Pediatric Cardiac Imaging. Philadelphia, W.B. Saunders Company, 1984, p. 219.
3. Freed, M.D., Nadas, A.S., Norwood, W.I., and Castaneda, A.R.: Is routine preoperative cardiac catheterization necessary before repair of secundum and sinus venosus atrial septal defects? J. Am. Coll. Cardiol. 4:333, 1984.

264-D *(Braunwald, pp. 1263–1264)*

Between 25 and 40 per cent of patients presenting with AMI have electrocardiographic evidence of sinus bradycardia within the first hour after the onset of symptoms. This is the most common arrhythmia noted during the early phases of AMI.[1] Sinus bradycardia in this early periinfarction period is believed to be due to two factors: vagotonia and stimulation of cardiac vagoafferent receptors. Sinus bradycardia is particularly frequent in patients with inferior and posterior infarctions. Its incidence declines over the ensuing 4 to 6 hours following the onset of the MI. Some debate exists regarding the clinical significance of sinus bradycardia in the early hours of AMI. Some evidence suggests that this arrhythmia during these early hours may be an important risk factor for development of repetitive ventricular arrhythmias in hypotension.[2] It has also been suggested that increased vagal tone and resultant sinus bradycardia may produce a protective effect on the heart by reducing myocardial oxygen demands. The acute mortality rate in patients with sinus bradycardia does appear to be lower than that of patients without this bradyarrhythmia (see Braunwald, Table 38–9, p. 1263).

Uncomplicated sinus bradycardia in the first 4 to 6 hours following infarction may be observed and does not require immediate treatment. If, however, hypotension or ventricular ectopy appears to be exacerbated because of the slowing of heart rate, atropine may be given in doses of 0.3 to 0.6 mg every 3 to 10 minutes to a total dosage up to 2 mg to bring the heart rate up to the 60 beat/min range. Interestingly, atropine often contributes to restoration of arterial pressure in coronary perfusion and may cause regression of ST-T segment elevation with favorable effects upon any ischemia that existed in the setting of the sinus bradycardia (see Braunwald, Fig. 38–30, p. 1264).

When sinus bradycardia occurs more than 6 hours after the onset of AMI it is often due to sinus node dysfunction or atrial ischemia rather than vagal hyperactivity. Rarely, it is accompanied by hypotension or the exacerbation of ventricular ectopy.

REFERENCES

1. Graner, L.E., Gershen, B.J., Orlando, M.M., and Epstein, S.E.: Bradycardia and its complications in the prehospital phase of acute myocardial infarction. Am. J. Cardiol. 32:607, 1973.
2. Zipes, D.P.: The clinical significance of bradycardiac rhythms in acute myocardial infarction. Am. J. Cardiol. 24:814, 1969.

265-B *(Braunwald, pp. 1280–1281)*

Patients with right ventricular infarction (RVI) may have a hemodynamic profile resembling that of patients with pericardial disease. For example, elevations in right atrial and ventricular filling pressures, as well as a rapid right atrial *x* descent and an early diastolic dip-and-plateau ("square root sign"), may be present. In addition, Kussmaul's sign may occur in patients with RVI and is highly predictive for right ventricular involvement in the setting of inferior wall infarction.[1] Patients who are admitted with inferior wall infarction should have an ECG with the precordial leads placed on the right chest in a mirror-image pattern to the usual placement on the left chest. Most patients with right ventricular infarction have ST-segment elevation of 1 millimeter or more in lead V_4R.[2] Echocardiography may establish the absence of pericardial fluid and the presence of abnormal right ventricular wall motion, as well as right ventricular dilatation and depression of right ventricular function. RVI must be distinguished from other causes of hypotension with acute myocardial infarction, including pericardial tamponade as already mentioned, constrictive pericarditis, and pulmonary embolus.

Treatment is aimed at increasing right atrial, right ventricular and thus left-sided filling pressures by increasing total intravascular volume through the administration of intravenous saline. A marked hypotensive response to small doses of nitroglycerin may be a clinical clue to the presence of RVI.[3] Because atrial transport may be very important in patients with RVI, patients who become pacemaker dependent may benefit from atrioventricular sequential pacing, which has been shown to improve hemodynamics in this condition.[3]

REFERENCES

1. Baigrie, R.S., Haq, A., Morgan, C.D., Rakowski, H., Drobac, M., and McLaughlin, P.: The spectrum of right ventricular involvement in inferior wall myocardial infarction: A clinical hemodynamic and noninvasive study. J. Am. Coll. Cardiol. 1:1396, 1983.
2. Croft, C.H., Nicod, P., Corbett, J.R., Lewis, S.E., Huxley, R., Mukharji, J., Willerson, J.T., and Rude, R.E.: Detection of acute right ventricular infarction by right precordial electrocardiography. Am. J. Cardiol. 50:421, 1982.
3. Haffajee, C.I., Love, J., Gore, J.M., and Alpert, J.S.: Reversibility of shock by atrial or atrioventricular sequential pacing in right ventricular infarction. Am. J. Cardiol. 49:1025, 1982.

266-C   (Braunwald, p. 1444)

Although many bacteria commonly cause endocarditis, it is rather unusual for bacterial infection to lead to myocarditis. When this does occur, it is usually because of release of a bacterial toxin. The diphtheria bacillus is the most common organism to cause a toxic myocarditis, and indeed myocardial involvement is the most common cause of death in this infection. Myocardial involvement occurs in at least 25 per cent of cases of diphtheria and typically produces signs of cardiac dysfunction at the end of the first week of the illness. Cardiomegaly and severe congestive heart failure are often present. Elevation of serum transaminase levels may be seen, as well as ST- and T-wave abnormalities on the ECG. To prevent the serious effects of the toxin on the myocardium, diphtheria antitoxin should be administered as rapidly as possible when cardiac involvement is seen. It has also been suggested that treatment with carnitine may reduce the incidence of heart failure and lower mortality.[1] Symptomatic myocardial involvement during Salmonella infection is rare, although electrocardiographic abnormalities are sometimes seen. Myocarditis with congestive heart failure may be seen in children who are severely ill with salmonellosis and is associated with a high mortality. Tuberculosis rarely causes involvement of the myocardium, especially in patients treated with ap-

propriate drugs. Eikenella and Acinetobacter are among the group of less common enterobacteria which cause endocarditis. They are included in the mnemonic HA-CEK, which stands for Hemophilus influenzae, Acinetobacter, Corynebacterium, Eikenella, and Kingella bacteria.

Other bacteria which may cause myocarditis include beta-hemolytic streptococci, the meningococci, and Clostridium perfringens.

REFERENCE

1. Ramos, H.C., Elias, P.R., Barrucand, L., and Da Silva, J.H.: The protective effect of carnitine in human diphtheritic myocarditis. Pediatr. Res. 18:815, 1984.

267-C   (Braunwald, pp. 1550–1551)

Complete repair by placement of a synthetic prosthesis and resection of aneurysmal segments of the aorta is recommended for any patients with AAA 6 cm or greater in diameter. The management of asymptomatic aneurysms less than 6 cm in diameter remains controversial and depends on the clinical status of the individual patient. In poor-risk patients with aneurysms between 4 and 6 cm, close follow-up and frequent ultrasound examination are warranted. In persons who are otherwise clinically stable and in good health, elective resection of aneurysms between 4 and 6 cm in diameter may be appropriate.[1]

Prior to careful hemodynamic monitoring, "declamping shock" was a difficult problem, characterized by marked hypotension following release of the aortic crossclamp after surgery. This problem has been virtually eliminated in modern surgical care.[2] Similar advances in renal and pulmonary management have relegated complications affecting these organ systems to a much less frequent status. Because patients who do not survive repair of AAA suffer MI 50 per cent of the time,[3] routine coronary angiography and selective coronary bypass surgery prior to aneurysm resection may be appropriate in this population.[4]

The operative risk in the lowest-risk patients from AAA repair is approximately 2 to 5 per cent. If the aneurysm is unstable and has been expanding, mortality is 5 to 15 per cent; in the event of frank rupture, mortality is approximately 50 per cent. Only 5 to 10 per cent of patients survive for 5 years with unrepaired aneurysms larger than 6 cm, compared with more than 50 per cent of those who undergo successful resection and compared with 80 per cent for an age-matched "normal" population.

REFERENCES

1. Gleidman, M.L., Ayers, W.B., and Vestal, B.L.: Aneurysms of the abdominal aorta and its branches: A study of untreated patients. Ann. Surg. 217:1537, 1982.
2. Bush, H.L., Jr., LoGerfo, F.W., Weisel, R.D., Mannick, J.A., and Hechtman, H.B.: Assessment of myocardial performance and optimal volume loading during elective abdominal aortic resection. Arch. Surg. 112:1301, 1977.
3. Hertzer, N.R.: Fatal myocardial infarction following abdominal aortic aneurysm resection. Three hundred forty-three patients followed 6–11 years postoperatively. Ann. Surg. 192:671, 1980.

4. Hertzer, N.R., Bevin, E.G., Young, J.R., O'Hara, P.J., Ruschhaupt, W.F., Graor, R.A., DeWolfe, V.G., and Maljovec, L.C.: Coronary artery disease in peripheral vascular patients. Ann. Surg. 199:223, 1984.

268-E   (Braunwald, pp. 1034–1045 and Table 33–8, p. 1043)

Several clinical features are helpful in distinguishing acute from chronic MR.[1] In acute MR the ECG is usually normal, while in chronic MR abnormalities such as P mitrale, atrial fibrillation and left ventricular hypertrophy are frequently present. The heart size is usually normal in acute MR; cardiomegaly and left atrial enlargement are prominent in chronic MR. An apical thrill is commonly present in chronic MR and frequently absent in acute MR. There are also several differences in the systolic murmurs of acute and chronic MR. In chronic MR the primary location of the murmur is usually at the apex, and in acute MR it is usually at the base of the heart. While the murmur frequently radiates to the axilla in chronic MR, it can radiate to the neck, spine, and top of the head in acute MR depending on the location of the jet. Furthermore, in patients with acute MR who have a normal-sized left atrium the left atrial pressure rises abruptly, frequently leading to pulmonary edema and usually elevated JVP. Because the v wave is markedly elevated in acute MR, the pressure gradient between the left ventricle and atrium declines at the end of the systole. The murmur may not be holosystolic but it may be descrescendo, ending well before A_2. It is also usually lower pitched and softer than the murmur of chronic MR.

REFERENCE

1. Blumenthal, P., et al.: Noninvasive investigations with a diagnosis of mitral valve disease. In Ionescu, M.I., and Cohn, L.H. (eds.): Mitral Valve Disease: Diagnosis and Treatment. London, Butterworths, 1985.

269-B   (Braunwald, p. 1495)

Several forms of cardiac tamponade are evident clinically and can be distinguished by their distinct features. In patients in whom pericardial fluid collects rapidly, such as those who suffer intrapericardial hemorhage from a penetrating heart wound or aortic dissection, the appearance of Beck's triad may be noted. This includes a profound decrease in systemic arterial pressure, concomitant elevation of systemic venous pressure, and a small, quiet heart, as first described by Beck in 1935.[1] Patients who develop tamponade rapidly may show evidence of decreased cerebral perfusion—including stuporous or agitated behavior—as well as an absent or difficult-to-perceive pulsus paradoxus because of the profound hypotension that usually accompanies this scenario.

In patients in whom cardiac tamponade develops at a more gradual rate, dyspnea is often the major complaint. Such patients may appear acutely ill, although not morbidly so, if the tamponade has developed in a chronic manner. Systemic symptoms such as weight loss and profound weakness may also be present. The most common physical finding in a series of 56 medical patients with cardiac tamponade reported by Guberman and colleagues[2] was jugular venous distention, and this was often accompanied by tachypnea, tachycardia, pulsus paradoxus, and hepatomegaly. The presence of pulsus paradoxus is extremely helpful in suggesting the diagnosis of cardiac tamponade. The differential diagnosis of a patient with the triad of pulsus paradoxus, systemic venous distention, and clear lungs includes obstructive pulmonary disease, constrictive pericarditis, restrictive cardiomyopathy, and massive pulmonary embolism.

Low-pressure cardiac tamponade may be seen in patients who are normotensive and in whom the physical examination is normal except for a moderate elevation of jugular venous pressure.[3] This entity has been reported in tuberculous and neoplastic pericarditis and may be associated with severe dehydration. It represents the earliest stages of developing cardiac tamponade in which intrapericardial pressures and right atrial pressures are equalized at a relatively low absolute pressure reading. With rehydration, the clinical picture of tamponade becomes more pronounced.

REFERENCES

1. Beck, C.S.: Two cardiac compression triads. JAMA 104:714, 1935.
2. Guberman, B.A., Fowler, N.O., Engel, P.J., Gueron, M., and Allen, J.M.: Cardiac tamponade in medical patients. Circulation 64:633, 1981.
3. Antman, E.M., Cargill, V., and Grossman, W.: Low-pressure cardiac tamponade. Ann. Intern. Med. 91:403, 1979.

270-D   (Braunwald, pp. 1234–1235)

In general, no precipitating factor is identified in patients with AMI. While heavy exertion may play a role in the development of AMI in some patients, usually there is no direct correlation between physical activity and the onset of AMI. Reduced myocardial perfusion plays a role in precipitating MI in a variety of clinical settings, including acute blood loss secondary to surgical procedures. In addition, increased myocardial oxygen demands such as may occur in the settings of fever, tachycardia, agitation, pulmonary embolism, or hypoglycemia may contribute to the onset of AMI. Patients with Prinzmetal's angina may develop AMI in the territory of the coronary artery, which undergoes spasm. There are considerable data suggesting that emotional stress may precipitate or initiate AMI.[1] In addition, trauma may precipitate a true AMI in two ways. Both myocardial contusion and hemorrhage into the myocardium may actually cause cell necrosis, or the injury may involve a coronary artery, with abrupt occlusion of that vessel and resultant MI. Finally, neurological disturbances such as strokes or transient ischemic attacks have been shown capable of precipitating AMI.[2]

REFERENCES

1. Jenkins, C.D.: Recent evidence supporting psychologic and social risk factors for coronary disease. N. Engl. J. Med. 294:987, 1033, 1976.
2. Norris, R.M.: Myocardial Infarction. New York, Churchill Livingstone, 1982, 322 pp.

271-A *(Braunwald, pp. 3046–3048)*

The echocardiogram shown is from a patient with hypertrophic obstructive cardiomyopathy (HOCM) and illustrates marked systolic anterior motion of the mitral valve with prolonged near contact between the anterior leaflet and the ventricular septum at the arrow. It can also be seen that the ventricular septum is somewhat thickened while the mitral valve leaflets appear normal—without calcification, abnormal fluttering, or failure to oppose in systole. Although a characteristic feature of HOCM is disproportionate septal hypertrophy, generalized LV hypertrophy may also be present. Another feature in many patients with HOCM is a narrowed LV outflow tract, which is formed by the inner ventricular septum anteriorly and the anterior leaflet of the mitral valve posteriorly. When HOCM is associated with obstruction to LV outflow, as in the patient whose echocardiogram is illustrated, there is abnormal systolic anterior motion of the anterior leaflet and occasionally the posterior leaflet of the mitral valve. There is a close relationship between the degree of this abnormal motion and the size of the outflow gradient.

Three explanations have been offered for systolic anterior motion: (1) the mitral valve is pulled against the septum by contraction of the papillary muscles because of the abnormal location and orientation of these muscles due to the hypertrophy; (2) the mitral valve is pushed against the septum because of its abnormal position in the LV outflow tract; and (3) the mitral valve is drawn toward the septum because of the lower pressure that occurs distal to the obstruction as blood is ejected at high velocity through a narrowed outflow tract (Venturi effect). It should be noted that systolic anterior motion may occasionally be found in other conditions, including hypercontractile states, transposition of the great arteries, and infiltration of the septum.

Other common echocardiographic findings in HOCM include a small LV cavity, reduced septal thickening during systole, reduced rate of closure of the mitral valve in mid-diastole, mitral valve prolapse, good systolic function, and a large *a* wave during atrial contraction.

272-D *(Braunwald, pp. 932–936)*

Congenital valvular AS is a relatively common congenital anomaly. It has been estimated to occur in 3 to 6 per cent of patients with congenital cardiovascular defects and is seen much more frequently in males than in females, with a sex ratio of approximately 4:1. Up to 20 per cent of individuals with congenital valvular AS have associated cardiovascular anomalies, of which patent ductus arteriosus and coarctation of the aorta are most frequent. The majority of children with congenital AS develop and grow in a normal manner and are asymptomatic. The diagnosis is therefore usually suspected when a murmur is detected on routine physical examination. When symptoms do occur the most common include fatigability, exertional dyspnea, syncope, and angina pectoris. In general, the presence of symptoms suggests critical stenosis.

Findings on physical examination for children with congenital valvular AS are similar to those in adults. In general, the presence of a fourth heart sound is associated with severe obstruction.

In patients less than 10 years of age, the electrocardiogram provides a more reliable guide to the severity of congenital AS than it does in older patients.[1] The presence of LVH with "strain" generally indicates that severe obstruction is present (see Braunwald, Fig. 30–32, p. 934). Other findings in the younger age group that are associated with severe obstruction include a T-wave axis less than $-40°$, a widening of the angle between the mean QRS and T forces in the frontal plane in excess of 100 degrees, an S wave in V_1 greater than 16 mm, and an R wave in V_5 exceeding 20 mm.

Echocardiography is useful in diagnosing the presence and severity of congenital AS. The most accurate noninvasive approach to quantification of the severity of obstruction is a combination of continuous wave Doppler flow analysis and two-dimensional echocardiography.[2]

Cardiac catheterization in infants and young children with valvular AS is most important for establishing the site and severity, rather than the presence, of the lesion since the malformation is often readily detected by physical examination and noninvasive studies. Catheterization is indicated in children with a clinical diagnosis of AS and the possibility of severe obstruction.[3] The appearance of symptoms that are consistent with AS or that may be related to such a lesion should prompt cardiac catheterization. Management of the child with congenital AS includes antibiotic prophylaxis to prevent infective endocarditis regardless of the severity of aortic valvular obstruction. Participation in competitive sports is usually restricted in patients with milder degrees of obstruction, and strict avoidance of more strenuous physical activity is advisable if severe AS is present.

REFERENCES

1. Braunwald, E., Goldblatt, A., Aygen, M.M., Rockoff S.D., and Morrow, A.G.: Congenital aortic stenosis. I. Clinical and hemodynamic findings in 100 patients. Circulation 27:426, 1963.
2. Robinson, P.J., Wyse, R.K.H., Deanfield, J.E., Franklin, R., and Macartney, F.J.: Continuous wave Doppler velocimetry as an adjunct to cross-sectional echocardiography in the diagnosis of critical left heart obstruction in neonates. Br. Heart J. 52:552, 1984.
3. Friedman, W.F., and Pappelbaum, S.J.: Indications for hemodynamic evaluation and surgery in congenital aortic stenosis. Pediatr. Clin. North Am. 18:1207, 1971.

273-E *(Braunwald, pp. 896–897)*

While the true incidence of congenital cardiovascular malformation is difficult to determine accurately, it has been estimated that approximately 0.8 per cent of live births are complicated by some such disorder. The most common malformation seen is the ventricular septal defect, which is followed in frequency of occurrence by atrial septal defect and patent ductus arteriosus. These data do not take into account the congenital, nonstenotic bicuspid aortic valve or mitral valve prolapse, both of which may be quite prevalent. While the majority of children with congenital heart disease are male, specific defects may show a definite sex predilection. Thus patent ductus arteriosus and atrial septal defects are more common in females, whereas valvular aortic stenosis, congenital aneurysms of the sinus of Valsalva, coarctation of the aorta, tetralogy of Fallot, and transposition of the great arteries are seen more frequently in males. Extracardiac anomalies occur in approximately 25 per cent of infants born with significant cardiac disease and often are multiple.

Approximately one-third of infants with both cardiac and extracardiac anomalies have some established syndrome. For example, maternal rubella during pregnancy may lead to the *rubella syndrome*, which consists of cataracts, deafness, microcephaly, and some combination of patent ductus arteriosus, pulmonic valvular and/or arterial stenosis, and atrial septal defect. Chronic maternal alcohol abuse may lead to the *fetal alcohol syndrome*. This consists of microcephaly, micrognathia, microphthalmia, prenatal growth retardation, developmental delay, and cardiac defects such as ventricular septal defect, which occur in approximately 45 per cent of the affected infants. Maternal systemic lupus erythematosus during pregnancy has been linked to congenital complete heart block but not to any of the specific anatomical abnormalities mentioned.

274-B (Braunwald, pp. 1488–1489)

The scratching, high-pitched pericardial friction rub is pathognomonic of acute pericarditis, and was originally described as "the squeak of leather of a new saddle under the rider" by Laennec's associate Victor Collin. The classic form of this rub has three components: one each due to atrial systole (presystole), ventricular systole, and rapid ventricular filling in early diastole. A prospective analysis of the pericardial friction rub demonstrated that the ventricular systolic component is the loudest and clearest component and is present in almost all cases.[1] The presystolic component is present in approximately 70 per cent of cases, and the rapid diastolic filling component is detected less frequently. This component may therefore be slurred into that of atrial contraction, resulting in a biphasic or "to-and-fro" type of rub.

In the series just referred to, a three-component rub was present approximately 50 per cent of the time. While a single-component rub is least common, it is likely to be the auscultatory form of this finding in patients with atrial fibrillation. It should be noted that the pericardial friction rub may often be evanescent and may have a quality that changes between examinations. The rub must be distinguished from the systolic murmurs of tricuspid or mitral regurgitation, as well as the crunch of air in the mediastinum due to submediastinal emphysema or the artifact of skin rubbing against the stethoscope. Differentiation may be aided in part by the use of mild exercise, which may allow better detection of a classic three-component rub. The appropriate clinical setting and electrocardiographic information will also aid in distinguishing between a pericardial friction rub and other potential auscultatory findings that might be confused with such a rub.

REFERENCE

1. Spodick, D.H.: Pericardial rub: Prospective multiple observer investigation of pericardial friction rub in 100 patients. Am. J. Cardiol. 35:357, 1975.

275-C (Braunwald, pp. 1034–1045 and Fig. 33–13, p. 1037)

The progressive development of mitral regurgitation in this 60-year-old patient following an inferior myocardial infarction (MI) is most consistent with infarction of a posterior papillary muscle. Since papillary muscles are perfused via a terminal portion of the coronary vascular bed, they are particularly vulnerable to ischemia. The posterior papillary muscle, supplied only by the posterior descending branch of the right coronary artery, is more susceptible to ischemia and infarction than the anterolateral papillary muscle, which has a dual blood supply from the diagonal branches of the left anterior descending artery and the marginal branches from the left circumflex artery. Although necrosis of a papillary muscle is a frequent complication of MI, particularly of inferior infarction,[1] frank rupture of a papillary muscle is far less common. Total rupture of a papillary muscle is usually fatal because of the extremely severe and rapid MR that it produces. MR may also occur significantly later in the course of MI, in which case it is usually due to left ventricular dilatation. In this case, dyskinesis of the left ventricle results in an abnormal spatial relationship between the papillary muscles and the chordae tendineae, resulting in MR.

Ruptures of the chordae tendineae are also important causes of MR, although such ruptures bear no special relationship to MI. Common causes of chordal rupture include congenitally abnormal chordae, spontaneous idiopathic rupture, infective endocarditis, trauma, rheumatic fever, and myxomatous degeneration.[2] In idiopathic rupture an increase in mechanical strain of undetermined cause is believed to cause rupture. The posterior chordae rupture spontaneously more frequently than do the anterior chordae.

REFERENCES

1. Balu, V., Hershowitz, S., Masud, A.R.Z., Bhayana, J.N., and Dean, D.C.: Mitral regurgitation in coronary artery disease. Chest 81:550, 1982.
2. Hickey, A.J., Wilcken, D.E.L., Wright, J.S., and Warren, B.A.: Primary (spontaneous) chordal rupture: Relation to myxomatous valve disease and mitral valve prolapse. J. Am. Coll. Cardiol. 5:1341, 1985.

276-C (Braunwald, pp. 1548–1550)

The normal abdominal aorta has a diameter of approximately 2 cm; clinically significant aneurysms measure 4 cm or more. The majority of such aneurysms are asymptomatic and are found either on routine physical examination or during radiographic evaluation for other reasons. A variety of noninvasive methods exist for the diagnosis and accurate sizing of abdominal aortic aneurysms. Among these, physical examination is the *least* accurate. As of this writing, abdominal ultrasound is both the simplest and most accurate method to detect and size abdominal aortic aneurysms. Experience with CT scanning and digital subtraction angiography is still being evaluated. Abdominal aortic angiography may be less accurate in predicting size in some instances because the aneurysm's full width may be masked by the presence of nonopacified thrombus. Aortography is currently used in patients with diagnostic dilemmas, patients with associated renal or vascular disease, or patients who are being prepared for surgical repair of AAA.

Natural history studies of AAA have revealed a critical relationship between aneurysm size and subsequent rupture. Thus, half of all aneurysms that are larger than 6 cm in diameter will rupture within a year of diagnosis, while smaller aneurysms rupture far less frequently, i.e., about 15 to 20 per cent within the first year.[1]

REFERENCE

1. Gleidman, M.L., Ayers, W.B., and Vestal, B.L.: Aneurysms of the abdominal aorta and its branches: A study of untreated patients. Ann. Surg. *217*:1537, 1982.

277-A   *(Braunwald, pp. 1360–1361)*

In 1959 Prinzmetal and colleagues described an unusual syndrome of cardiac pain that occurs almost exclusively at rest and is not precipitated by physical exertion or emotional stress. Furthermore, the syndrome was noted to include ST-segment elevations on the ECG. Clinically, there are features which have subsequently emerged as more typical of Prinzmetal's angina that may distinguish it from classic angina pectoris. Patients with Prinzmetal's angina appear to have a high frequency of abnormal coronary arteriograms, although approximately one-third of the patients have normal coronary arteries. One common clinical feature is clustering of the attacks between the hours of midnight and 8 A.M.[1] Patients studied with 48-hour ambulatory electrocardiograms show more frequent abnormalities in the morning.[2] A high percentage of patients with Prinzmetal's angina are heavy smokers. Furthermore, a subset of these patients appear to have a generalized vasospastic disorder and have increased incidence of both migraine headaches and Raynaud's phenomenon.[3] Patients with Prinzmetal's angina also tend to be younger than those patients with exertion-induced angina, and there is no male predominance as with classical angina.[4]

REFERENCES

1. Yasue, H., Omote, S., Takizawa, A., Nagao, M., Miwa, K., and Tanaka, S.: Cardiac variations of exercise-induced coronary arterial spasm. Circulation 59:938, 1979.
2. Waters, D.D., Miller, D., Bouchard, A., Bosch, X., and Theroux, P.: Circadian variation in variant angina. Am. J. Cardiol. *54*:61, 1984.
3. Miller, D., Waters, D.D., Warnica, W., Szlachcic, J., Kreeft, J., and Theroux, P.: Is variant angina the coronary manifestation of a generalized vasospastic disorder? N. Engl. J. Med. *304*:763, 1981.
4. Antman, E., Muller, J., Goldberg, S., MacAlpin, R., Rubenfire, M., Tabatznik, B., Liang, C., Heupler, F., Achuff, S., Reichek, N., Geltman, E., Kerin, N.Z., Neff, R.K., and Braunwald, E.: Nifedipine therapy for coronary artery spasm. Experience in 127 patients. N. Engl. J. Med. *302*:12, 1980.

278-A   *(Braunwald, pp. 1027–1028)*

The diastolic murmur of MS is a low-pitched rumbling murmur best heard at the apex. This murmur is caused by the increased velocity of blood flow across a narrowed orifice with resulting turbulence. The most useful feature of the murmur with regard to the assessment of the severity of stenosis is the duration of the murmur. In patients with MS the murmur persists as long as the gradient across the mitral valve exceeds approximately 3 mm Hg. Furthermore, persistence of the murmur throughout diastole usually corresponds to a mean transvalvular gradient exceeding 10 mm Hg. The intensity of the murmur is much less closely related to the severity of the stenosis and is determined by factors such as the configuration of the patient's chest, the presence of sinus rhythm, and the compliance of the mitral valve leaflets.

The murmur usually commences shortly after the opening snap and in mild MS quickly fades away to be followed by a presystolic murmur. The diastolic murmur of MS can be distinguished from that of tricuspid stenosis because in MS the murmur is reduced during inspiration, augmented during expiration, and reduced during the strain of the Valsalva maneuver, all of which tend to decrease inflow into the left atrium. The opposite findings occur in tricuspid stenosis.

Several other conditions can mimic the rumbling diastolic murmur of MS including the Austin-Flint murmur heard in aortic regurgitation, due to fluttering of the mitral valve in diastole. In a dilated ventricle or in a hypertrophied ventricle with a restrictive cardiomyopathy, a diastolic murmur due to abnormal diastolic filling may also be present. As mentioned previously, tricuspid stenosis closely mimics the murmur of MS but may be distinguished by several maneuvers. Finally, a left atrial myxoma may impede flow across a normal mitral valve, causing both a diastolic murmur and mitral regurgitation.

279-C   *(Braunwald, pp. 1487–1488)*

The syndrome of acute pericarditis is characterized by an inflammatory process in the pericardium with accompanying chest pain, the presence of a pericardial friction rub, and serial electrocardiographic changes. While the incidence of pericardial inflammation may be as high as 6 per cent in autopsy series, pericarditis is diagnosed less frequently in the clinical setting. In an outpatient setting the most common etiology of pericarditis is presumed viral or idiopathic, while in the inpatient population pericarditis due to trauma, neoplasm, or uremia is more frequently seen. Other relatively common causes of pericarditis include bacterial infection, acute myocardial infarction, and tuberculosis. In addition, a large number of both medical and surgical disorders may lead to pericarditis (see Braunwald, Table 44–1, p. 1488).

Acute pericarditis is accompanied by the pathological changes of acute inflammation, including the presence of polymorphonuclear leukocytes, increased vascularity, and fibrin deposition. Continued evolution of this fibrin deposition may ultimately result in fibrinous adhesions between the pericardial and epicardial layers as well as between the pericardium and adjacent sternum and pleura. The most frequent complaint among patients with acute pericarditis is chest pain that is often localized to the retrosternal area and frequently radiates to both the trapezius ridge and neck. The pain is often aggravated by the supine position, coughing, swallowing, or deep inspiration and may be eased by sitting or leaning forward. This pain may be distinguished from the pain of ischemia in most instances (see Braunwald, Table 44–2, p. 1488). Dyspnea may also accompany acute pericarditis and may be related in part to the need to decrease the depth of respiratory excursions in order to avoid pericardiopleuritic chest pain. Other contributing factors in the development of dyspnea may include the presence of fever or the development of a large pericardial effusion with compression of adjacent bronchi and pulmonary parenchyma.

280-C   (Braunwald, pp. 1239–1241)

While myocardial damage releases a variety of intracellular enzymes into the circulation, specific use of the CPK and LDH enzymes has proven most useful in the diagnosis of AMI. LDH has five isozymes, and type 1 LDH (LDH_1) is the form principally found in the heart. An elevation of serum LDH_1 activity usually precedes elevation of total serum LDH and may occur within 8 to 24 hours after MI.[1] The ratio of LDH_1 to LDH_2 has been employed in the diagnosis of AMI. Specifically, a ratio of LDH_1 to LDH_2 greater than 1.0 is said to be highly specific and sensitive for the diagnosis of AMI. However, current recommendations suggest that routine use of LDH and LDH isoenzyme determinations is not justified and may lead to considerable waste of health care resources.

Serum CPK activity may peak as early as 8 hours after the onset of pain due to AMI or as late as 58 hours after this event. The average peak CPK for AMI occurs approximately *24 hours* after the onset of the event, unless reperfusion due to the administration of thrombolytic therapy or mechanical recanalization has occurred. In the latter cases, peak CPK values usually occur approximately 12 hours after infarction.[2] In addition, the absolute magnitude of the CPK rise following reperfusion is greater than that measured following an infarction of comparable size without reperfusion and thus may render enzyme analysis of infarct size less accurate. False-positive results may occur using total serum CPK values in the setting of patients with muscle disease, alcohol intoxication, diabetes mellitus, skeletal muscle trauma, convulsions, intramuscular injections, pulmonary embolism, or thoracic outlet syndrome or after vigorous exercise.[3]

The use of the CPK-MB isoenzyme has further refined the laboratory diagnosis of AMI. While other forms of injury to cardiac muscle (for example, myocarditis, shock, cardiac surgery) may lead to a false elevation in serum CK-MB activity, the measurement of CK-MB has proven to be very useful in the diagnosis of AMI. In approximately 15 per cent of patients with an apparent AMI, the CK-MB may be elevated despite a normal total CK.[3] While the importance of this finding is not entirely clear, patients in this group in general have a worse prognosis than patients with suspected MI without such a CK-MB elevation. A recent series of recommendations has been proposed for the use of serum enzyme assays in the diagnosis of AMI (see Braunwald, Table 38–3, p. 1240).[4]

REFERENCES

1. Vasudevan, G., Mercer, D.W., and Varat, M.A.: Lactic dehydrogenase isoenzyme determination in the diagnosis of acute myocardial infarction. Circulation 57:1055, 1978.
2. Ong, L., Reiser, P., Coromilas, J., Scherr, L., and Morrison, J.: Left ventricular function and rapid release of creatine kinase MB in acute myocardial infarction: Evidence for spontaneous reperfusion. N. Engl. J. Med. 309:1, 1983.
3. Hong, R.A., Licht, J.D., Wei, J.I., Heller, G.V., Blaustein, A.S., and Pasternak, R.C.: Elevated CK-MB with normal total creatine kinase in suspected myocardial infarction: Associated clinical findings and early prognosis. Am. Heart J. 111:1041, 1986.
4. Lee, T.H., and Goldman, L.: Serum enzyme assays in the diagnosis of acute myocardial infarction. Ann. Intern. Med. 105:221, 1986.

281-B   (Braunwald, pp. 1511–1512)

Purulent pericarditis tends to occur via one of several mechanisms, including contiguous spread from a postoperative infection, an infection related to infective endocarditis, a subdiaphragmatic infection, or hematogenous spread during bacteremia. Of note, direct pulmonary extension from bacterial pneumonia or empyema now accounts for only about 20 per cent of cases of bacterial pericarditis.[1] Several factors may predispose to the development of purulent pericarditis, including a preexisting pericardial effusion from uremic pericarditis as well as the immunosupressed state such as that seen in burns, following immunosuppressive therapy, or with hematological malignancies or the acquired immunodeficiency syndrome. Bacterial pericarditis is usually an acute fulminant illness of short duration that is characterized by high spiking fevers, shaking chills, night sweats, and dyspnea. Typical symptoms of pericarditis may be absent and the process may thus appear for the first time as new jugular venous distention and pulsus paradoxus with the development of cardiac tamponade.

In the patients described by Rubin and Moellering,[1] cardiac tamponade developed acutely in 38 per cent of patients with previously unsuspected bacterial pericarditis. Thus, the key to the diagnosis is a high index of suspicion. However, despite the lower incidence of purulent pericarditis in the antibiotic era, overall survival continues to be very poor, with a mortality of approximately 30 per cent in most series. This poor prognosis is in large part due to the lack of recognition of the entity clinically prior to death. Early complete surgical drainage and appropriate parenteral antibiotic therapy are important parts of the treatment of this devastating disorder. High concentrations of antibiotics may be achieved in pericardial fluid with parenteral therapy; therefore, instillation of antibiotics directly into this space is not warranted. Surgical drainage of the pericardium is essential in almost all patients with this condition.[2]

REFERENCES

1. Rubin, R.H., and Moellering, R.C., Jr.: Clinical, microbiologic and therapeutic aspects of purulent pericarditis. Am. J. Med. 59:68, 1975.
2. Morgan, R.J., Stephenson, L.W., Woolf, P.K., Edie, R.N., and Edmunds, L.H., Jr.: Surgical treatment of purulent pericarditis in children. J. Thorac. Cardiovasc. Surg. 85:527, 1983.

282-A (Braunwald, pp. 1429–1430)

This 16-year-old youth has an examination consistent with hypertrophic obstructive cardiomyopathy. Recommendations of the American College of Cardiology[1] are that competitive sports not be allowed if any of the following clinical features are present: (1) marked ventricular hypertrophy, (2) evidence of significant outflow gradient by echocardiography or catheterization, (3) important supraventricular or ventricular arrhythmias, and (4) history of sudden death in relatives with hypertrophic cardiomyopathy. It is recommended that low-intensity competitive sports be allowed if none of these conditions are present. This boy has evidence for left ventricular hypertrophy on ECG and chest x-ray, a possibly significant outflow gradient by examination, and a history of sudden death in a cousin. Thus, competitive sports would be prohibited. Further workup should obviously be carried out, including echocardiography, and perhaps cardiac catheterization, and ambulatory ECG monitoring should be performed to assess the extent of ventricular arrhythmias.

REFERENCE

1. Maron, B.J., et al.: Task Force III: Hypertrophic cardiomyopathy, other myopericardial diseases and mitral valve prolapse. J. Am. Coll. Cardiol. 6:1215, 1985.

283-D (Braunwald, pp. 915–917)

ASD may be overlooked and only uncommonly results in disability in children or adolescents.[1] The anatomical sites of intraatrial defects include the sinus venosus or high ASD, the ostium secundum ASD, and the ostium primum ASD. The sinus venosus defect is usually associated with and may be a consequence of anomalous connections of the pulmonary veins from the right lung to the junction of the superior vena cava or right atrium.[2] The ostium secundum type of ASD should be distinguished from a patent foramen ovale that may occur in up to 25 per cent of adults; a widely patent foramen ovale may be considered an acquired form of ASD. Ten to 20 per cent of patients with ostium secundum ASD also have prolapse of the mitral valve.[3]

Patients with ASD are usually asymptomatic in early life. Children with ASD occasionally experience exertional dyspnea and easy fatigability, but in general symptoms are not prominent. Children with ASD tend to be somewhat underdeveloped physically and prone to respiratory infections. However, the symptoms and signs of ASD in the adult, such as atrial arrhythmias, pulmonary vascular obstruction, and heart failure, are very uncommon in the pediatric age group. In children, the diagnosis of ASD is most often entertained after detection of a heart murmur on routine physical examination.

REFERENCES

1. Hunt, C.E., and Lucas, R.V., Jr: Symptomatic atrial septal defect in infancy. Circulation 42:1042, 1973.
2. Davea, J.E., Cheitlin, M.D., and Bedynek, J.L.: Venosus atrial septal defect. Am. Heart J. 85:177, 1973.
3. Leachman, R.D., Cokkinos, D.V., and Cooley, D.A.: Association of ostium secundum atrial septal defects with mitral valve prolapse. Am. J. Cardiol. 38:167, 1976.

284-C (Braunwald, pp. 1052–1054)

The LV responds to the sudden production of severe obstruction to outflow by dilatation and reduction of stroke volume. However, in most adults with AS, the obstruction develops slowly over a long period of time, resulting in significant compensatory measures. Fundamentally, LV output is maintained by development of LV hypertrophy. This enables the heart to sustain a large pressure gradient across the aortic valve without reduction in cardiac output, LV dilatation, or development of symptoms. This is due in large part to coexisting hypertrophy of the LA with an increased role for atrial contraction in maintaining appropriate LV filling. This is frequently manifested by the development of large *a* waves in the LA pressure pulse with elevated LV end-diastolic pressure. The latter is also increased by the reduction of diastolic compliance of the LV due to ventricular hypertrophy. However, it is only the patient with LV failure in whom dilatation and an increase in LV end-diastolic volume occur.

285-B (Braunwald, pp. 1242–1244)

The most common findings on chest roentgenography in the patient with AMI are signs of left ventricular failure and cardiomegaly. The presence of the latter usually indicates prior infarction or another form of underlying cardiovascular disease such as chronic hypertension. In general, the presence of cardiomegaly on chest x-ray in this setting is associated with left ventricular dysfunction.[1] The severity of pulmonary vascular congestion and the degree of cardiomegaly on the initial chest film are important predictors in defining groups of patients with AMI who have an increased mortality during the first year after the acute event.

Echocardiography plays an important role in the diagnostic evaluation of patients with AMI. M-mode echocardiography is a sensitive technique for examining the interventricular septum and posterior left ventricular wall in these patients. However, only small segments of the anterior wall may be imaged, and abnormalities of regional wall motion and even left ventricular aneurysm formation may elude diagnosis with this modality.[3] Therefore, the use of two-dimensional echocardiography, which is capable of imaging a large portion of the entire left ventricle, has found increasing popularity. Using this technique, abnormal wall motion may be noted in more than two-thirds of patients with AMI.[4] In addition, this technique is useful in defining relative thinning of infarcted myocardial tissue and in the detection of most of the mechanical complications that occur in AMI. Left ventricular aneurysm and pseudoaneurysm, as well as the detection and localization of ventricular septal defect, and acute mitral regurgitation all may be diagnosed using two-dimensional echocardiography. The diagnosis of left ventricular thrombus, especially in patients with large anterior AMI, may also be made by two-dimensional echocardiography. Doppler echocardiography may be used in conjunction with these techniques. It has found use in defining the degree of mitral or tricuspid regurgitation following AMI as well as in further identifying the site of acute ventricular septal rupture.

REFERENCES

1. Field, B.J., Russel, R.O., Jr., Moraski, R.E., Soto, B., Hood, W.P., Burdenshaw, J.A., Smith, M., Maurer, B.J., and Rackley, C.E.: Left ventricular size and function and heart size in the year following myocardial infarction. Circulation 50:331, 1974.
2. Brattler, A., Karliner, J.S., Higgins, C.B., Slutsky, R., Gilpin, E.A., Froelicher, V.F., and Ross, J., Jr.: The initial chest x-ray in acute myocardial infarction. Prediction of early and late mortality and survival. Circulation 61:1004, 1980.
3. Teicholz, L.E., Kreulen, T., Herman, M.V., and Gorlin, R.: Problems in echocardiographic volume determinations: Echocardiographic-angiographic correlations in the presence or absence of asynergy. Am. J. Cardiol. 37:7, 1976.
4. Parisi, A.F., Moynihan, P.F., Folland, E.D., and Feldman, C.L.: Quantitative detection of regional left ventricular contraction abnormalities by two-dimensional echocardiography. II. Accuracy in coronary artery disease. Circulation 63:761, 1981.

286-C   *(Braunwald, pp. 1122–1126; see also Question 291)*

Infection superimposed on prosthetic valves poses difficult management problems. In general, treatment should involve two drugs with a bactericidal effect on the organism which has been isolated. If the patient appears responsive antibiotics should be continued for 6 to 8 weeks. Late streptococcal endocarditis involving a bioprosthesis is the infection most amenable to intensive antibiotic therapy. Early prosthetic valve endocarditis (less than 60 days following operation) is rarely responsive to medical therapy. The mortality with early prosthetic valve endocarditis is very high, approximating 40 per cent.

There are several *absolute* indications for operation[1]: the presence of congestive heart failure, ongoing sepsis, fungal etiology, valvular obstruction, unstable prosthesis, and recent-onset heart block. *Relative* indications for operation include mild congestive failure, nonstreptococcal etiology, early prosthetic valve endocarditis, embolism, perivalvular leak, vegetations on echocardiography, relapse, and culture-negative endocarditis without clinical response to empiric antibiotic therapy. It should be noted that early failure of therapy necessitates surgical treatment and that the mortality with medical therapy alone in patients with heart failure approaches 100 per cent.

At operation all infected material and tissue and potential sources of emboli should be excised and major hemodynamic abnormalities corrected. In totaling the results in major series, overall mortality of patients with prosthetic valve endocarditis managed with antibiotics was 61 per cent, whereas mortality of those treated surgically (generally a sicker group of patients) was 39 per cent.[1]

REFERENCE

1. Cowgill, L.D., Addonizio, V.P., Hopeman, A.R., and Harken, A.H.: Prosthetic valve endocarditis. Curr. Probl. Cardiol. 11:617, 1986.

287-C   *(Braunwald, pp. 1332–1334)*

Although the calcium channel antagonists differ significantly in structure, they have relatively similar effects on myocardial function. They appear to be beneficial in controlling angina and improving exercise tolerance in patients with chronic stable angina due to coronary atherosclerosis as well as in patients with Prinzmetal's variant angina. The three calcium antagonists currently available in the United States—nifedipine, verapamil, and diltiazem—are all effective in causing relaxation of vascular smooth muscle in both the systemic and coronary arterial beds. There is recent evidence that calcium antagonists may also have antiatherogenic effects in rabbits and monkeys.[1] Several differences are seen in the side effects of calcium channel antagonists. With respect to hypotension, flushing, and headache, nifedipine causes moderate and sometimes severe side effects due to its potent vasodilator effects, considerably more than diltiazem and verapamil at normal doses. Because nifedipine causes the greatest reduction in systemic vascular resistance, it tends to cause less left ventricular dysfunction than either diltiazem or verapamil. However, at high doses, all of these agents may be associated with a fall in cardiac output.

The calcium channel antagonists, unlike the beta blockers, are less likely to affect the heart rate and conduction system. However, verapamil has significant inhibitory effects on AV conduction, and in patients with AV conduction disease may cause P-R interval prolongation. It also decreases the heart rate in patients with sick sinus syndrome. Diltiazem is less likely to do this than verapamil, and nifedipine often raises heart rate. Although all the calcium channel antagonists also reduce gastrointestinal motility, verapamil is significantly more likely to cause gastrointestinal symptoms such as nausea and constipation. Finally, none of the calcium channel antagonists cause bronchoconstriction, which is a significant advantage over the beta blockers.

REFERENCE

1. Henry, P.D.: Atherosclerosis, calcium and calcium antagonists. Circulation 72:456, 1985.

288-E   *(Braunwald, pp. 1509–1511)*

While tuberculous pericarditis is now an uncommon cause of pericarditis in industrialized nations, the disease continues to be an important problem among the disadvantaged and in immunosuppressed patients. Tuberculous pericarditis usually develops by retrograde spread from peritracheal, peribronchial, or mediastinal lymph nodes, or by early hematogenous spread from the primary tuberculous infection. The process is usually chronic. Symptoms may be systemic and nonspecific, and clinical detection of tuberculous pericarditis usually does not occur until the effusive or late constrictive pericarditic stages are reached. The typical pericardial chest pain of acute viral or idiopathic pericarditis is uncommon in tuberculous pericarditis.[1] In addition, typical signs or symptoms of cavitary pulmonary tuberculosis are usually absent.

Typical examination in patients with tuberculous pericarditis usually reveals evidence of chronic cardiac compression, which may mimic heart failure. For example, in one series,[2] 88 per cent of patients had jugular venous extension, 95 per cent had hepatomegaly, and 73 per cent had ascites, whereas a pericardial friction rub was heard in only 18 per cent. While the chest x-ray usually shows an enlarged cardiac silhouette and pleural effusions may be present, the apices and hila of the lung are usually normal. Definitive diagnosis of tuberculous pericarditis is usually difficult because of the low yield of the bacillus in the pericardial fluid, failure of the bacillus to grow on an appropriate medium, and/or the need to observe cultures for a minimum of 8 weeks. The probability of a definitive diagnosis is greatest if both pericardial fluid and a pericardial biopsy are obtained in the effusive stage of the disease.[3]

Initial therapy of tuberculous pericarditis includes hospitalization with bed rest and a three-drug chemotherapy regimen ordinarily consisting of isoniazid, rifampin, and streptomycin or ethambutol. The use of corticosteroids in order to reduce pericardial inflammation has not been shown to reduce the risk of developing constrictive pericarditis and therefore should be reserved for critically ill patients with recurrent large effusions who do not respond to the initial antituberculosis drugs alone.[4]

REFERENCES

1. Hageman, J.T., D'Esopo, N.D., and Glenn, W.W.L.: Tuberculosis of the pericardium: A long-term analysis of forty-four cases. N. Engl. J. Med. 270:327, 1964.
2. Strang, J.I.G.: Tuberculosis pericarditis in Transkei. Clin. Cardiol. 5:667, 1984.
3. Barr, J.F.: The use of pericardial biopsy in establishing etiologic diagnosis in acute pericarditis. Arch. Intern. Med. 96:693, 1955.
4. Rooney, J.J., Crocco, J.A., and Lyons, H.A.: Tuberculosis pericarditis. Ann. Intern. Med. 72:73, 1970.

289-B   (Braunwald, p. 1452)

This 32-year-old woman presents with transient high-grade AV block and syncope. Her history is most consistent with the development of Lyme disease. This disease is caused by a tick-borne spirochete (*Borrelia burgdorferi*), which is distributed throughout the northeast, midwest, and western United States, with many cases found in northeastern resorts such as Nantucket. The disease usually is seen during the summer, beginning with a characteristic skin rash (erythema chronicum migrans), and followed in weeks to months by neurological, synovial, and cardiac involvement.

About 10 per cent of patients with Lyme disease develop evidence of cardiac involvement, with the most common manifestation being variable degrees of AV block. Syncope due to severe AV block occurs occasionally.[1] There may also be transient left ventricular dysfunction, and a positive gallium scan may indicate cardiac involvement. It appears that treatment as soon as possible with tetracycline or erythromycin may improve the prognosis.

Development of rheumatic fever would be unusual without any antecedent febrile episodes or sore throat.

Although systemic lupus erythematosus may cause AV block, it would be unusual for this patient to have a normal physical examination and negative antinuclear antibody. *Trichinella spiralis* infection, which causes the clinical syndrome trichinosis, may occur following ingestion of this helminth in contaminated meat. It rarely causes cardiac disease. In severe cases of trichinosis, there may be congestive heart failure; associated electrocardiographic abnormalities include T-wave abnormalities, prolongation of the QRS complex, diminished QRS voltage, and first-degree AV block. Hemochromatosis, which is related to iron overload, may cause arthritis and joint symptoms, but usually presents with findings of a restrictive or dilated cardiomyopathy and would be unlikely to occur in an otherwise healthy woman.

REFERENCE

1. Steere, A.C., Batsford, W.P., Weinberg, M., Alexander, J., Berger, H.J., Wolfson, S., and Malawista, S.E.: Lyme carditis: Cardiac abnormalities of Lyme disease. Ann. Intern. Med. 93:8, 1980.

290-A   (Braunwald, pp. 1537–1538)

Myocardial contusion is a common occurrence with chest injuries. It has been documented in several series in 7 to 17 per cent of cases of chest trauma. It usually produces no significant symptoms and often goes unrecognized. The most common symptom of myocardial contusion is precordial pain resembling that of myocardial infarction, but pain from musculoskeletal chest trauma can confuse the clinical picture. The ECG is helpful in recognizing contusion, with nonspecific ST-T wave abnormalities or ST-T wave changes of pericarditis being quite common. Although transmural injury with pathological Q waves does occur, it is considerably rarer and is usually masked during the initial presentation by findings of pericarditis. Cardiac muscle enzymes, specifically the CPK-MB band, are very useful, with increases in CPK-MB reported in 17 per cent of patients with chest trauma coming to the Henry Ford Hospital.[1]

Other diagnostic tests include radionuclide imaging; technetium-labeled pyrophosphate shows a positive uptake at sites of myocardial contusion. Two-dimensional echocardiography is useful for documenting regional wall motion abnormalities. ECG monitoring frequently reveals a wide variety of arrhythmias, including most commonly atrial arrhythmias, atrial fibrillation, and atrioventricular and intraventricular conduction defects, as well as sinus node dysfunction and sinus bradycardia.

The development of congestive heart failure is unusual in uncomplicated cases of myocardial contusion and should raise the issue of an associated pathological event. The most common pathological events associated with congestive heart failure in this setting are ruptures of the right or left ventricle or the ventricular septum. These are somewhat rare events and are more common in cases of severe chest wall trauma, especially with motor vehicle accidents.

On the basis of a series of 546 autopsy cases of nonpenetrating injury to the heart, the incidence of rupture of the ventricular septum was estimated to be about 5 per cent, with a similar number of patients experiencing rupture of the atrial septum.[2] In these patients diagnostic catheterization and two-dimensional echocardiography should be performed quickly, with survival often possible following emergency surgery.

REFERENCES

1. Torres-Mirabal, P., Gruenberg, J.C., Brown, R.S., and Obeid, F.N.: Spectrum of myocardial contusion. Am. Surg. 48:383, 1982.
2. Parmley, L.F., Manion, W.C., and Mattingly, T.W.: Nonpenetrating traumatic injury of the heart. Circulation 18:371, 1958.

291-A   (Braunwald, pp. 1122–1126; see also Question 286)

Prosthetic valve endocarditis has been classified as occurring either early (up to 60 days) or late (more than 60 days) after operation.[1] Staphylococci have been reported to be the most common causative organism, responsible for approximately 50 per cent of cases of early prosthetic valve endocarditis. Of these, the largest number were due to *Staphylococcus epidermidis*. This is in contrast to the late appearance of this disease, in which streptococci were the most common causative organisms. It should be noted that *Staphylococcus epidermidis* is resistant to methicillin in more than 90 per cent of cases. Therefore, early prosthetic valve endocarditis should not be treated empirically with antibiotics such as oxacillin and nafcillin; the empiric treatment of choice is *vancomycin* and an aminoglycoside. Active debate continues about whether or not the addition of rifampin is beneficial. Because the organisms associated with early prosthetic valve endocarditis are more resistant to therapy and because patients are frequently debilitated, there is a significantly higher fatality rate than with late disease. Furthermore, early infections in prosthetic valve endocarditis are much more likely to be caused by fungi (10 per cent); fungal endocarditis is associated with a greater than 50 per cent fatality rate.[2]

REFERENCES

1. Dismukes, W.E., Karchmer, A.W., Buckley, M.J., Austen, W.G., and Swartz, M.N.: Prosthetic valve endocarditis. Circulation 48:365, 1973.
2. Cowgill, L.D., Addonizio, V.P., Hopeman, A.R., and Harken, A.H.: Prosthetic valve endocarditis. Curr. Probl. Cardiol. 11:617, 1986.

292-E   (Braunwald, pp. 1264–1266)

A variety of atrioventricular conduction disturbances occur in AMI. First-degree AV block happens in between 4 and 14 per cent of patients with AMI admitted to coronary care units. In almost all patients with first-degree AV block, the disturbance is intranodal (above the bundle of His) and generally does not require specific treatment. Digitalis intoxication may also lead to this conduction disturbance, and may require stopping of the medication. First-degree AV block may also be a manifestation of increased vagal tone and thus may be associated with sinus bradycardia and hypotension which is responsive to atropine in select circumstances.

While second-degree AV block occurs in between 4 and 10 per cent of patients with AMI admitted to coronary care units, about 90 per cent of patients with second-degree AV block have Mobitz type I (Wenckebach block). Mobitz type II second-degree AV block is a rare conduction defect in this setting and appears in a distinctly different clinical setting from that in which Mobitz type I occurs. Mobitz type I second-degree AV block occurs most commonly in patients with inferior myocardial infarction, is usually transient, and rarely progresses to complete AV block. It usually resolves within 72 hours following infarction and does not require specific therapy. In contrast, Mobitz type II block usually occurs below the bundle of His, is associated with a widened QRS complex, and almost always occurs in the setting of anterior infarction. In this situation, Mobitz type II second-degree AV block usually reflects trifascicular block and impaired conduction distal to the bundle of His and therefore frequently progresses to complete heart block. This AV conduction disturbance is generally treated with a temporary demand pacemaker.

Complete AV block (third-degree AV block) may occur in either anterior or inferior infarction. This disturbance occurs in between 5 and 8 per cent of patients with AMI and has a different prognosis based on the location of the inciting infarction. In inferior infarction, complete heart block usually evolves from first-degree and type I second-degree AV block, usually has a stable escape rhythm, and is usually transient, with resolution within a week after infarction.[1] The mortality in this setting is approximately 15 per cent. In contrast, patients with anterior infarction develop third-degree AV block more suddenly, although it is usually preceded by Mobitz type II second-degree AV block. In general, patients in this setting have unstable escape rhythms, wide QRS complexes, and a mortality in the range of 70 to 80 per cent.[2]

REFERENCES

1. Strasberg, B., Pinchas, A., Arditti, A., Lewin, R.F., Sclarovsky, S., Hellman, C., Zafrir, N., and Agmon, J.: Left and right ventricular function in inferior acute myocardial infarction and significance of advanced atrioventricular block. Am. J. Cardiol. 54:985, 1984.
2. Hindman, M.C., Wagner, G.S., JaRo, M., Atkins, J.M., Scheinman, M.M., DeSanctis, R.W., Hutter, A.H., Jr., Yeatman, L., Rubenfire, M., Pujura, C., Rubin, M., and Morris, J.J.: The clinical significance of bundle branch block complicating acute myocardial infarction. 2. Indications for temporary and permanent pacemaker insertion. Circulation 58:689, 1978.

293-C   (Braunwald, pp. 987–988)

The size of VSD and the degree to which pulmonary vascular resistance is altered by increased pulmonic flow from the VSD leads to differing clinical presentations in adults with this lesion. In general, patients with small defects are asymptomatic and are not at risk for the development of pulmonary vascular obstructive disease. However, all patients with VSD are at increased risk for the development of infective endocarditis, which may occur in up to 4 per cent of patients with VSD.[1] This complication usually occurs by the third or fourth decade of life. The infection is usually located in the right ventricle at the site where shunted blood impacts against the ventricular wall.

VSDs in the presence of normal pulmonary artery pressures and pulmonary-to-systemic flow ratios less than 1.5:1 in asymptomatic persons in general do not require surgical closure. Women with VSDs that lead to pulmonary-to-systemic flow ratios less than 2:1 and only modest pulmonary hypertension generally tolerate pregnancy very well. In women with larger left-to-right shunts, however, left ventricular failure may occur during pregnancy. In those who have Eisenmenger complex, pregnancy is extremely poorly tolerated. The development of Eisenmenger complex due to progressive pulmonary vascular disease is one of the most dreaded complications noted in patients with VSD.[2] This usually occurs sometime between the end of the second or during the third decade of life[3] and may be complicated by hemoptysis, chest pain resembling angina, cerebral abscess, parodoxical emboli, and sudden death. Although patients with a VSD and shunt reversal may survive for 5 to 10 years, prognosis is very poor in general and death usually occurs by the fourth decade of life.

REFERENCES

1. Corone, P., Doyon, F., Gaudeau, S., Guerin, F., Vernant, P., Ducan, H., Rumeau-Rouquette, C., and Gaudeau, P.: Natural history of ventricular septal defect: A study involving 790 cases. Circulation 55:908, 1977.
2. Friedman, W.F., and Heiferman, M.F.: Clinical problems of postoperative pulmonary vascular disease. Am. J. Cardiol. 50:631, 1982.
3. Graham, T.P., Jr.: The Eisenmenger syndrome. In Roberts, W.C. (ed.): Adult Congenital Heart Disease. Philadelphia, F.A. Davis, 1987, pp. 567–582.

294-C (Braunwald, pp. 1110–1111)

This patient presents with findings typical of right-sided endocarditis, which almost invariably involves the tricuspid valve. Typical features include the subacute course lasting between 2 weeks and several months, presence of pneumonia and pleural effusions on the chest x-ray, and evidence on examination of tricuspid regurgitation, including c-v waves in the jugular venous pulse and a murmur of tricuspid regurgitation. Because right-sided endocarditis usually involves infection following the use of contaminated needles and syringes, the organisms are atypical. They include the HACEK organisms (Hemophilus, Actinobacillus, Corynebacterium, Eikenella, and Kingella), fungi, and the enterobacteriacea more commonly than the streptococci and staphylococci. There is an associated incidence of left-sided endocarditis in these patients as well, which must be sought carefully during the initial workup.

This particular patient had a Pseudomonas infection, a not uncommon infection associated with significant valvular destruction and frequently, with significant regurgitation. He was treated with appropriate antibiotic therapy, tobramycin and ticarcillin, but after 2 weeks still had persistent evidence of both bacteremia and systemic infection. The chance for cure of infection of the tricuspid valve when it is caused by Pseudomonas and other gram-negative bacteria or fungi may be dramatically improved by surgically removing the valve and not replacing it with a prosthesis.[1] It has been noted that young patients tolerate tricuspid valvulectomy without replacement quite well, provided that there is no associated pulmonary hypertension. This is supported by the experience of Arbulu and Asfaw,[2] who restudied the clinical status of a group of patients with and without prosthetic valve replacement and found no significant differences. Furthermore, in intravenous drug addicts with right-sided endocarditis there is a high incidence of recurrence of intravenous drug abuse and endocarditis. Thus, unless the patient is in refractory congestive heart failure due to left-sided as well as right-sided endocarditis, and unless the patient has pulmonary hypertension, it is recommended that treatment consist of valvulectomy without replacement with a prosthetic valve followed by an additional 4 to 6 weeks of appropriate antibiotic therapy.

REFERENCES

1. Sethia, B., and Williams, B.T.: Tricuspid valve excision without replacement in a case of endocarditis secondary to drug abuse. Br. Heart J. 40:579, 1978.
2. Arbulu, A., and Asfaw, I.: Tricuspid valvulectomy with prosthetic replacement. J. Thorac. Cardiovasc. Surg. 82:684, 1981.

295-A (Braunwald, pp. 1434; p. 1739)

This 57-year-old woman has a history and physical examination suggesting myocardial dysfunction. It appears that her dysfunction is more right-sided than left-sided, with significant pitting edema, elevated jugular venous pressure, and a slightly enlarged liver. Furthermore, there is evidence for AV valvular regurgitation with both tricuspid and mitral valve regurgitant murmurs audible. Several factors in the history and physical examination suggest a diagnosis of hemochromatosis. Specifically, the association of arthritis and diabetes is common in hemochromatosis because of deposition of iron in the pancreas and in synovial tissue. An enlarged liver is also frequently present. Furthermore, her tanned skin may well represent the bronzing that commonly occurs in this disease. Her cardiac examination is consistent with a restrictive cardiomyopathy manifested by AV regurgitation and mild congestive failure.

Hemochromatosis may occur as a familial or idiopathic disorder, or in association with a defect in hemoglobin synthesis resulting in ineffective erythropoesis, in chronic liver disease, and with excessive oral intake of iron over many years. The severity of myocardial dysfunction is proportional to the amount of iron present in the myocardium. Extensive deposits of myocardial iron are invariably associated with cardiac dysfunction, usually chronic congestive heart failure. The clinical manifestations vary but usually involve signs of congestive heart failure and right-sided failure. The diagnosis is aided by finding elevated plasma iron levels, normal or low total iron binding capacity, and markedly elevated transferrin saturation. Cardiac failure is usually progressive and refractory to therapy, although repeated use of the iron-chelating agent desferroxamine may be beneficial, especially in patients presenting earlier in the course of the disease.[1]

Sarcoidosis may cause similar findings, but would be unlikely in a white woman of this age. The lack of pulmonary involvement would also be atypical.

Amyloidosis is another possibility, but significant cardiac amyloidosis is usually associated with immunocyte dyscrasias such as multiple myeloma; it would be unusual in association with rheumatoid arthritis.

A diagnosis of Fabry's disease is possible but less likely. This is an inherited disease of glycosphingolipid metabolism caused by a deficiency of the enzyme ceramide trihexosidase. It is characterized by intracellular accumulation of a neutral glycolipid and prominent involvement of the skin and kidneys. Symptomatic cardiovascular involvement is most common in males rather than females, who are usually asymptomatic carriers. Common findings are systemic hypertension, renovascular hypertension, mitral valve prolapse, and congestive heart failure.

Ischemic cardiomyopathy is possible, especially in the setting of adult onset diabetes, but the presence of a normal electrocardiogram makes this unlikely.

REFERENCE

1. Cutler, D.J., Isner, J.M., Bracey, A.W., Hufnagel, C.A., Conrad, P.W., Roberts, W.C., Kerwin, D.M., and Weintraub, A.M.: Hyperchromatosis heart disease: An unemphasized cause of potentially reversible restrictive cardiomyopathy. Am. J. Med. 69:923, 1980.

296-B   (Braunwald, pp. 988–991)

Classic tetralogy of Fallot is marked by a large VSD in association with infundibular and/or valvular pulmonic stenosis, right ventricular hypertrophy, and an overriding aorta. In all cases, the VSD is located *proximal* to the level of the right ventricular outflow tract obstruction and is therefore associated with elevated right ventricular systolic pressure and right-to-left shunting. This may be contrasted to the situation in patients who have a double-chambered right ventricle and a membranous VSD, so that the septal defect communicates with the low-pressure distal portion of the right ventricle and leads to simple VSD physiology rather than the right-to-left shunting and cyanosis that marks tetralogy of Fallot.

Symptoms and clinical findings of tetralogy of Fallot depend on the severity of right ventricular outflow tract obstruction. In mild right ventricular outflow tract obstruction, a left-to-right shunt is predominant and the patient may remain acyanotic. The condition in patients with right ventricular obstruction severe enough to cause cyanosis usually is recognized during infancy or early childhood; the patients may then undergo palliative or total surgical repair. Patients with uncorrected tetralogy of Fallot who survive into adult life usually have at most moderate obstruction to right ventricular outflow in association with relatively well-preserved pulmonary blood flow. At the other end of the spectrum, if obstruction to right ventricular outflow is complete, a large obligatory right-to-left shunt will be present, and the lungs are then perfused through collaterals that arise from systemic vessels. In these patients there is severe cyanosis, absence of a systolic heart murmur, and presence of a continuous murmur that originates from bronchial collaterals. This variant of tetralogy of Fallot is termed *pseudotruncus arteriosus*.

Because the large VSD allows for decompression of the right ventricle in tetralogy of Fallot, the right ventricular systolic pressure does not exceed that in the aorta, even in the presence of severe obstruction to right ventricular outflow. Congestive heart failure is unusual in patients with tetralogy of Fallot. Instead, a decrease in cardiac reserve in adults with tetralogy of Fallot is more typical. Exertional dyspnea and poor exercise tolerance are present in about one-third of tetralogy of Fallot patients without operation who survive into the third decade of life.[1]

REFERENCE

1. Higgins, C.B., and Mulder, D.G.: Tetralogy of Fallot in the adult. Am. J. Med. 29:837, 1972.

297-C   (Braunwald, pp. 1571–1572)

Showers of microemboli that arise from atherosclerotic plaques in the aortic or major arterial trunks lead to clinical and pathologic changes as the particulate material lodges in small arterial branches. Atheromatous embolism, also known as cholesterol embolism, occurs most commonly following surgery involving manipulation of an atherosclerotic aorta, such as major abdominal vascular procedures, especially resection of abdominal aortic aneurysms. Showers of atherosclerotic emboli may also be provoked by cardiac catheterization, cardiopulmonary bypass, and intraarterial cannulations of any type, and may occasionally occur spontaneously as well. Some studies have suggested a causal relationship between cholesterol embolism and long-term anticoagulant therapy with drugs of the warfarin sodium type. Clinical findings in this disorder may include bilateral lower extremity pain, livido reticularis, and a host of purpuric and ecchymotic lesions in the lower extremities. In addition, abdominal pain may occur.

Two important recognized complications of cholesterol emboli following abdominal aortic surgery are pancreatitis and renal failure due to diffuse microinfarction of the organ in question. The resulting renal failure may be severe and irreversible. Hepatitis is not part of the clinical syndrome. Because showers of cholesterol emboli may be widely scattered, cerebral involvement may occur, and in some instances, visualization of cholesterol particles in the retinal arteries is possible.[1] Unfortunately, there is no specific therapy for cholesterol emboli; specific treatment of the resulting complications of the disorder is the cornerstone of management. The use of anticoagulants to prevent further episodes of embolization remains controversial and does not appear to be of any great value.

REFERENCE

1. Coppello, J.R., Lessell, S., Greco, T.P., and Eisenberg, M.S.: Diffuse disseminated atheroembolism. Arch. Ophthalmol. 102:255, 1984.

298-B *(Braunwald, pp. 1222–1223)*

Statistics compiled by the American Heart Association reveal that approximately one-fourth of all deaths in the United States are due to AMI, and that nearly 1.5 million patients suffer this disorder annually. The majority of deaths associated with AMI occur within the first hour of the event and are attributable to ventricular fibrillation or other arrhythmias. Over 500,000 patients with confirmed AMI are hospitalized yearly in the United States and another group of patients at least as large in number as this are admitted because of suspected AMI. The mortality rate during hospitalization and during the first year following infarction is approximately 12 per cent. Although a decline in the death rate from coronary artery disease has been noted in recent years, the precise explanation for this occurrence is not yet entirely clear. A fall in mortality due to a decrease in the incidence of AMI by 25 per cent has been noted, and a similar fall in the fatality rate associated with each case of myocardial infarction has also been documented.[1] At least some of the latter reduction in mortality is due to the interventions that have been developed over the last several decades for in-hospital care of the patient with AMI, including the development of coronary care units and newer methods of treatment of AMI.

Careful monitoring of cardiac rhythm and prompt treatment of primary arrhythmias in coronary care units have led to a reduction in the incidence of in-hospital deaths from AMI due to arrhythmias. Most deaths in hospitalized patients with AMI presently are caused by left ventricular failure and shock and occur within the first 3 or 4 days following the onset of infarction.[2]

Before the widespread use of coronary care units, treatment of AMI was primarily directed toward allowing healing of the infarct. Subsequently, major emphasis was placed on prevention and aggressive treatment of arrhythmias. Currently, attempts to limit infarct size by restoring perfusion of ischemic tissue, particularly using thrombolytic therapy, have become very important.

REFERENCES

1. Pell, S., and Fayerweather, W.E.: Trends in the incidence of myocardial infarction and in associated mortality and morbidity in a large employed population. 1957–1983. N. Engl. J. Med. 312:1005, 1985.
2. Ong, L., Green, S., Reiser, P., and Morrison, J.: Early prediction of mortality in patients with acute myocardial infarction: A prospective study of clinical and radionuclide risk factors. Am. J. Cardiol. 57:33, 1986.

299-A *(Braunwald, pp. 1318–1319)*

The differential diagnosis of chest pain is difficult because the discomfort of angina due to coronary artery disease is nonuniform, and other disease entities can mimic it. Constant[1] has suggested that physicians should ask specific questions to differentiate nonanginal chest pain from angina. Several characteristics that would tend to rule out ischemic chest pain are listed in question 299; others include a pain lasting less than 5 seconds or more than 20 or 30 minutes, pain precipitated by a single movement of the trunk or arm, and pain associated with tenderness of the chest wall.

Differentiating the discomfort of noncardiac disorders from angina pectoris is possible when the quality of the pain, its duration, precipitating factors, and associated symptoms are taken into consideration (see Braunwald, Table 1–3, p. 4). In general, typical angina usually begins gradually and reaches maximum intensity over a period of minutes before dissipating. The discomfort is usually not sharp but rather is a dull, continuous ache or a squeezing pain. It is usually precipitated by exertion or anxiety and relieved by rest. Associated symptoms frequently include shortness of breath, diaphoresis, and anxiety. Posture can affect the pain of myocardial ischemia; it is often intensified by assuming the horizontal position and relieved by assuming the vertical position.

REFERENCE

1. Constant, J.: The clinical diagnosis of nonanginal chest pain: The differentiation of angina from nonanginal chest pain by history. Clin. Cardiol. 6:11, 1983.

300-A *(Braunwald, pp. 937–938)*

Supravalvular AS is a congenital narrowing of the ascending aorta that may be either diffuse or localized, and originates at the superior margin of the sinuses of Valsalva above the level of the coronary arteries. The clinical picture of supravalvular obstruction usually differs in many ways from that observed in other forms of AS. The lesion may be associated with idiopathic infantile hypercalcemia or may be one finding in the "Williams' syndrome." This condition is marked also by a peculiar elfin facies (see Braunwald, Fig. 30–37 p. 937), mental retardation, auditory hyperacusis, narrowing of peripheral systemic and pulmonary arteries, and abnormalities of dental development. The occurrence of the distinctive elfin facies appearance—even in infancy—should alert the physician to the possibility of a multisystem disease and underlying supravalvular AS.

In general, the major physical findings resemble those observed in patients with valvular AS. Accentuation of the aortic valve closure sound due to elevated pressure in the aorta proximal to the stenosis, and the occurrence of a late systolic continuous murmur that results from coexisting narrowing of peripheral pulmonary arteries, may help distinguish this anomaly from valvular AS. Occasionally, a disparity in upper extremity pulses may be noted, with a higher systolic pressure in the right arm than that in the left. This is caused by streaming of blood from the supravalvular lesion preferentially to the right arm circulation.

Electrocardiography generally reveals LV hypertrophy when obstruction is severe, and chest x-ray rarely reveals poststenotic dilatation of the ascending aorta, in contrast to valvular and discrete subvalvular AS. Echocardiography is the single most valuable technique for localization of the site of obstruction in supravalvular AS. Doppler examination and subsequent retrograde aortic catheterization may determine further the degree of hemodynamic abnormality present. The success of operative repair of this condition depends upon the extent of the abnormality; it is most successful when the obstruction is discrete and there is relatively little accompanying hypoplasia.

301-B   (Braunwald, pp. 1109–1110 and Table 34–4, p. 1109)

The kidneys are frequently involved in endocarditis by a variety of pathological processes. The patient described has subacute endocarditis most likely involving her prosthetic aortic valve. The mild anemia and leukocytosis are consistent with this finding. Urinalysis shows the presence of hematuria. A common lesion in the kidney caused by endocarditis is renal infarction, which occurs in two-thirds of untreated cases. This is consistent with her history of severe right flank pain and the urinary findings. Another common lesion is a focal glomerulonephritis. This complication occurs in up to 50 per cent of untreated cases and 15 per cent of treated ones. It may be also associated with renal failure and the nephrotic syndrome. A diffuse glomerulonephritis occurs in 30 to 60 per cent of untreated cases and in 10 per cent of treated cases.

Renal cortical necrosis is not a primary lesion associated with infective endocarditis but in severe cases will accompany disseminated intravascular coagulation. Renal abscesses may occur with a long course of endocarditis and are most common in association with highly invasive organisms such as *Staphylococcus aureus*. It should be noted that antimicrobial therapy may also be associated with such renal lesions as interstitial nephritis, toxic nephropathy, and acute tubular necrosis.[1]

REFERENCE

1. Feinstein, E.I., Eknoyan, G., and Lister, B.J.: Renal complications of bacterial endocarditis. Am. J. Nephrol. 5:457, 1985.

302-C   (Braunwald, pp. 1011–1012)

In infants and children the important nonobstructive causes of cardiomyopathy are congestive cardiomyopathies, which include the familial and nonfamilial forms of endocardial fibroelastosis (EFE).[1] This classification does not include patients whose myocardial dysfunction is caused by infection, cardiac anomaly, or conditions of increased preload or afterload. Congestive cardiomyopathy in the pediatric age group usually is a disease of infants, with most cases becoming manifested before the age of 1 year.

Pathologically, both primary and secondary forms of EFE have been recognized. In the secondary variety *focal* areas of opaque fibroelastic thickening of the mural endocardium or cardiac valves are observed in association with other types of cardiac malformations. Primary EFE usually involves the entire left ventricle and mitral and aortic valves and is not associated with significant cardiac defects. Primary EFE often occurs in a familial form, although the mode of inheritance has not been defined. Although several pathological mechanisms have been proposed, the most likely one appears to be inadequate subendocardial blood flow. Typically, the LA and LV are dilated with microthrombi found adherent to the endocardium. The aortic and mitral valve leaflets are thickened and distorted, with a murmur of mitral regurgitation audible in approximately 40 per cent of infants. Papillary muscles and chordae tendineae are also part of the fibroelastic process and are shortened and distorted, contributing to the mitral regurgitation.

Clinical features reflect left ventricular dysfunction and congestive heart failure. Infants frequently present with fatigue (during feeding), failure to thrive, cyanosis, wheezing, and cough. Chest x-ray reveals marked generalized cardiomegaly, frequently with pulmonary congestion. Typical ECG findings include left ventricular hypertrophy with inverted T waves in the left precordial leads. Echocardiographic features include a dilated LA and LV, reduced LV ejection fraction, and abnormal mitral valve motion. Differential diagnosis includes anomalous pulmonary origin of the left coronary artery, myocarditis, and glycogen storage diseases. Optimal management includes early and prolonged treatment with digitalis. Results of mitral valve replacement have been disappointing.

REFERENCE

1. Tripp, M.E.: Congestive cardiomyopathy of childhood. In Barness LA (ed): Advances in Pediatrics. Chicago, Year Book Medical Publishers, 1984, pp. 179–203.

303-C   (Braunwald, pp. 1414–1415)

This 26-year-old man presents with atrial fibrillation after New Year's Eve. Furthermore, most of his episodes of atrial fibrillation (AF) have occurred on Mondays. These facts should prompt consideration of the "holiday heart syndrome," which is the occurrence of palpitations, chest discomfort, and syncope following a binge of alcohol consumption. Thus, it is not unreasonable to suspect that this young man had been partying over the New Year's Eve holiday and because of this has developed AF from the holiday heart syndrome.[1]

The most common arrhythmia associated with this syndrome is AF, followed by atrial flutter and frequent ventricular premature contractions. Alcohol consumption may predispose nonalcoholics to atrial fibrillation or flutter. It is suspected that hypokalemia may play a role in the genesis of some of these arrhythmias. The atrial fibrillation usually occurs several hours following the last drink and may be related to the onset of some early withdrawal symptoms, especially sympathetic hyperactivity. The treatment is conservative, with primary focus on decreasing alcohol consumption. In patients with more severe alcoholic disease, AV conduction disturbances (most commonly first-degree heart block), bundle branch block, and left ventricular hypertrophy may be observed. In patients with documented cardiomyopathy and the holiday heart syndrome, the prognosis is poor, with sudden death and ventricular tachyarrhythmia common.

REFERENCE

1. Greenspan, A.J., and Schaal, S.F.: The "holiday heart": Electrophysiologic studies of alcohol effects in alcoholics. Ann. Intern. Med. 98:135, 1983.

304-C *(Braunwald, pp. 1580–1581)*

The clinical presentation of pulmonary embolism may be subtle or may be easily confused with a variety of diagnoses and therefore requires a high index of suspicion. In the Urokinase-Streptokinase Pulmonary Embolism trial (UPET), the most common symptoms reported were dyspnea and pleuritic chest pain, and the most common physical sign was tachypnea, with more than 92 per cent of patients having a respiratory rate greater than 16 breaths/minute.[1]

The use of symptoms and signs alone to identify patients with this condition may be difficult; in one study, symptoms and signs were not often helpful in discriminating between patients with true pulmonary embolism and those with no evidence of it on pulmonary arteriography.[2] Therefore, in patients in whom this diagnosis is suspected clinically the diagnosis must be pursued by obtaining radionuclide scans or by angiography. The differential diagnosis of pulmonary embolism depends in part on the patient population being examined. In an outpatient population, costochondritis, rib fracture, the early stages of pneumonia, and pleurodynia may all enter into the differential diagnosis. In addition, pneumonia, congestive heart failure, myocardial infarction, asthma, chronic obstructive pulmonary disease, and pneumothorax may all enter into the differential diagnosis of pulmonary embolism in outpatients or inpatients.

REFERENCES

1. Bell, W.R., Simon, T.L., and DeMets, D.L.: The clinical features of submassive and massive pulmonary emboli. Am. J. Med. 62:355, 1977.
2. Stein, P.D., Willis, P.W. III, and DeMets, D.L.: History and physical examination in acute pulmonary embolism in patients without preexisting cardiac or pulmonary disease. Am. J. Cardiol. 47:218, 1981.

305-C *(Braunwald, p. 1611)*

This man has the classic findings of the sleep apnea syndrome.[1] These patients frequently present with daytime sleepiness, nighttime snoring with apnea, nocturnal awakenings, difficulties in their jobs, and frequent automobile accidents due to falling asleep at the wheel. Physically, these patients can be distinguished from pickwickian patients, who are invariably very obese. Specific symptoms include paroxysmal nocturnal dyspnea, morning headaches, cardiac arrhythmias (more frequently at night), which are predominantly ventricular arrhythmias, truncal obesity, pulmonary hypertension, nocturnal enuresis, peripheral edema, hypertension, and an elevated hematocrit on laboratory examination.

Although the precise cause of the sleep apnea syndrome is unclear, three types of patterns have been recorded: central apnea, obstructive apnea, and mixed apnea. In central apnea, it appears that there is a decrease in central nervous system sympathetic outflow to the respiratory effort. On the other hand, in obstructive apnea, it seems that the upper airway becomes transiently obstructed, causing airflow to stop despite continuing efforts of the respiratory muscles. These patients experience apneic periods, which can occur between 40 and 100 times per hour. During prolonged periods of apnea, the pO_2 can reach values of 20 to 25 mm Hg with saturations below 50 per cent. Sustained hypoxemia of this type leads to arrhythmias, including sinus bradycardia, sinus arrest, long asystoles, frequent atrial premature beats, and ventricular arrhythmias. Acute elevations of pulmonary capillary wedge pressure during these episodes result in development of pulmonary hypertension and right ventricular hypertrophy.

Treatment can be difficult; however, in general it involves relief of obstruction in patients with obstructive apneas and administration of drugs such as progesterone and tricyclic antidepressants to patients with central apnea.

REFERENCE

1. Burrek, B.: The hypersomnia-sleep apnea syndrome: Its recognition in clinical cardiology. Am. Heart J. 107:543, 1984.

306-A *(Braunwald, pp. 1223–1226)*

In general, patients with AMI who come to autopsy have more than one coronary artery severely narrowed, and between one- and two-thirds of such patients will have a critical obstruction of all three coronary arteries. The remainder are equally divided between those having single-vessel disease and those having two-vessel disease.[1] Most transmural infarctions occur distal to the occlusion of a coronary artery, although total occlusion of a coronary artery is not always associated with MI, largely because of the presence of collateral blood flow. In most series of patients with AMI studied at autopsy or by coronary arteriography, a small number are found to have normal coronary vessels.[2] Possible explanations in these patients include an embolus that has lysed or migrated or a prolonged episode of severe coronary arterial spasm that may have led to myocardial necrosis.

While in the past coronary arteriography was avoided in the acute setting of MI because of potential complications, experience over the last decade has shown that angiography is safe even during the acute phase of MI.[3] Studies in the early hours of AMI have revealed an approximate 90 per cent incidence of total occlusion of infarct-related vessels.[4] Recanalization secondary to spontaneous thrombolysis does indeed contribute to a diminishing incidence of total occlusion in vessels studied in the postinfarction period. The incidence of coronary thrombosis in subendocardial infarction is less well established; however, evidence that thrombosis plays a major role in patients with unstable ischemic syndromes[4] suggests that a similar pathophysiology may exist in the majority of cases of nontransmural AMI.

REFERENCES

1. Buja, L.M., and Willerson, J.T.: Clinicopathologic correlates of acute ischemic heart disease syndromes. Am. J. Cardiol. 47:343, 1981.
2. Betriu, A., Castaner, A., Sanz, G.A., Pare, J.C., Roig, E., Coll, S.,

Magrina, J., and Navarro-Lopez, F.: Angiographic finding 1 month after myocardial infarction: A prospective study of 259 survivors. Circulatin 65:1099, 1982.
3. deFeyter, P.J., van den Brand, M., Serruys, P.W., and Wijns, W.: Early angiography after myocardial infarction: What have we learned? Am. Heart J. 109:194, 1985.
4. DeWood, M.A., Spores, J., Notske, R., Mouser, L.T., Burroughs, R., Golden, M.S., and Lang, H.T.: Prevalence of total coronary occlusion during the early hours of transmural myocardial infarction. N. Engl. J. Med. 303:897, 1980.

307-C   (Braunwald, pp. 942–944)

Valvular PS results from the fusion of the pulmonic valve cusps during mid- to late intrauterine development and is the most common form of isolated RV obstructive heart disease. The severity of the pulmonic obstruction and the degree to which the RV and its outflow tract have developed determine the clinical presentation and course in the newborn with PS. Severe PS is characterized by cyanosis due to right-to-left shunting through the foramen ovale, by cardiomegaly, and by diminished pulmonary blood flow. Thus, hypoxemia and metabolic acidemia are principal clinical disturbances noted in the symptomatic neonate.

Clinical distinction between babies with tetralogy of Fallot or tricuspid or pulmonary atresia and PS is usually possible, since infants with tetralogy generally do not have x-ray evidence of cardiomegaly while those with PS do. Also, infants with tricuspid or pulmonary atresia generally show primarily LV hypertrophy by electrocardiography in contrast to RV hypertrophy observed with critical PS in the neonate. The severity of obstruction is often suggested by the physical findings. Thus, prominent *a* waves in the jugular venous pulse, an S_4, and presystolic pulsations of the liver reflect vigorous atrial contraction and suggest the presence of severe PS. A systolic ejection sound is often heard following the first heart sound at the upper left sternal border. The ejection sound typically is louder during expiration and when it is inaudible or occurs less than 0.08 sec from the onset of the Q wave, severe obstruction is suggested. The electrocardiogram is usually normal in mild PS, whereas moderate and severe PS is associated with right axis deviation and RV hypertrophy.

The severity of obstruction is the most important clinical determinant of subsequent course in PS. In the presence of a normal cardiac output, moderate stenosis is considered to be present if the peak systolic transvalvular pressure gradient is between 50 and 80 mm Hg or the peak systolic RV pressure is between 75 and 100 mm Hg. Reliable localization of the site of obstruction and an assessment of its severity may be obtained by combined continuous wave Doppler and two-dimensional echocardiography.

Cardiac catheterization and angiocardiography may localize the site of obstruction, evaluate its severity, and document the coexistence of other cardiac abnormalities. Patients with mild and moderate PS in general have a favorable course. Approximately three-fourths of such patients reveal unchanged pressure gradients over 4- to 8-year intervals. Percutaneous transluminal balloon valvuloplasty is the initial procedure of choice in patients with valvular PS and moderate to severe degrees of

obstruction.[1] In addition, surgical relief can be accomplished at an extremely low risk if necessary.

REFERENCE

1. Kan, J.S., White, R.I., Jr., Mitchell, S.E., Anderson, J.H., and Gardner, T.J.: Percutaneous transluminal balloon valvuloplasty for pulmonary valve stenosis. Circulation 69:554, 1984.

308-D   (Braunwald, pp. 1093–1095)

The HACEK group of organisms refers to a number of relatively nonpathogenic bacteria that are among the less common causes of endocarditis. The E in HACEK stands for Eikenella. All of these organisms share in common sensitivity to ampicillin, although frequently treatment includes an aminoglycoside as well. The most common of these organisms to cause endocarditis is *Hemophilus influenzae*.

309-D   (Braunwald, pp. 1014–1016)

The child described in the case presentation has several of the classic findings of the mucocutaneous lymph node syndrome of infancy, *Kawasaki's disease*. The syndrome generally presents as a febrile illness in children that occurs before the age of 10 years and usually before the age of 2. Classically these children have fever and ocular and oral manifestations followed in several days by a rash and indurative edema of the hands and feet with palmar and plantar erythema. Finally, after about 2 weeks, cutaneous desquamation occurs.

Diagnostic criteria for Kawasaki's disease include (1) a fever lasting 5 days or more that is unresponsive to antibiotics; (2) bilateral congestion of the conjunctivae; (3) indurative edema of the palms and feet, followed by membranous desquamation of the fingertips; (4) changes in the lips and mouth including dry erythematous and fissured lips with a strawberry tongue and injected oral pharynx; and (5) a polymorphous exanthem of the trunk without crusts or vesicles. Diagnosis is accepted when the first criterion and at least three of the remainder are present.

Multiple organ system involvement has been noted, including arthritis, cerebral spinal fluid pleocytosis, pulmonary infiltrates, and hydrops of the gallbladder. Adenopathy, diarrhea, leukocytosis, thrombocytosis, sterile pyuria and proteinuria, and abnormal liver function are also frequently present. Pathologically, the disease starts as an acute perivasculitis of the small arteries at which time pericarditis, interstitial myocarditis, and endocardial inflammation are seen. It then progresses to a panvasculitis involving the major coronary arteries resulting in aneurysm and thrombus formation, potentially leading to coronary artery thrombosis and myocardial infarction. The syndrome has an associated mortality of 1 to 3 per cent secondary to complications from coronary artery involvement, myocarditis, or pericarditis, with the majority of deaths occurring in the fourth week. Cardiac involvement includes ECG evidence of myocarditis and pericarditis, echocardiographic evidence of poor LV function, cardiomegaly, and pericardial effusion.

High-dose salicylate therapy appears to be useful by preventing platelet thrombus formation and decreasing the development of occluded coronary arteries. Empiric treatment with high-dose intravenous gamma globulin and salicylates has resulted in decreased formation of coronary artery aneurysms.[1] Prognosis is variable; approximately half of the children with coronary aneurysms diagnosed early after the acute phase of the disease subsides have normal-appearing vessels by angiography 1 or 2 years later.[2]

Rubella myocarditis occurs in utero and can cause varying degrees of myocardial damage. Invariably, cardiovascular manifestations of the rubella syndrome, other than myocarditis, dominate the clinical picture.

Coxsackie B infection usually occurs as part of an epidemic myocarditis. The illness is characterized by fever, tachycardia, and symptoms of encephalitis or hepatitis. The characteristic rash and desquamation common to Kawasaki's disease are not present. *Hemophilus influenzae* can cause a purulent pericarditis following upper respiratory infection and croup but is not known to cause myocarditis. *Stevens-Johnson syndrome* is a desquamating skin illness associated with an autoimmune response to a variety of agents involving mucous membranes but does not commonly include cardiac manifestations.

REFERENCES

1. Newburger, J.W., Takahasi, M., Burns, J.C., Beiser, A.S., Chung, K.J., Duffy, C.E., Glode, M.P., Mason, W.H., Reddy, V., Sanders, S.P., Shulman, S.J., Wiggins, J.W., Hicks, R.V., Fulton, D.R., Lewis, A.B., Leung, D.Y.M., Colton, J., Rosen, F.S., and Melish, M.E.: The treatment of Kawasaki syndrome with intravenous gamma globulin. N. Engl. J. Med. 315:341, 1986.
2. Anderson, T., Meyer, R.A., and Kaplan S.: Long-term evaluation of cardiac size and function in patients with Kawasaki disease. J. Am. Coll. Cardiol. 1:714, 1983.

310-A (Braunwald, pp. 1236–1239)

In uncomplicated AMI, subtle changes in the vital signs reflect the underlying pathological process. Most patients with uncomplicated AMI are *normotensive*, although a small group of patients have a mild decrease in systolic blood pressure and an elevation in diastolic pressure due to the reduction in stroke volume that accompanies the usual tachycardia. While the heart rate may vary from marked bradycardia to a variety of tachycardias, most commonly the underlying rhythm in AMI is a mild sinus tachycardia, with a return to a more normal rate following treatment of pain and anxiety. Almost all patients with AMI have ventricular premature beats. Most patients with AMI develop some elevation in temperature, which begins between 4 and 48 hours after the onset of the MI and is probably a nonspecific response to tissue necrosis. Rectal temperatures of 100 to 101°F are usual, and the fever usually abates by the 4th or 5th day following the infarction. The presence of higher fever should prompt the clinician to search for other potential causes of temperature elevation. In uncomplicated AMI, the respiratory rate is often slightly elevated soon after the development of the infarct because of both anxiety and pain. However, it usually returns to

normal upon appropriate treatment. In patients with LV failure, however, the respiratory rate correlates with the severity of underlying congestive heart failure. Many patients with pulmonary edema have respiratory rates exceeding 40/min.

Despite the severity of infarction present, the underlying cardiac examination is often surprisingly unremarkable. The most common finding on palpation is the presence of a presystolic pulsation that is consistent with vigorous atrial contraction in the setting of reduced left ventricular compliance (a palpable S_4). The heart sounds, especially the first heart sound, are frequently muffled.[1] The heart sounds return to normal intensity during recovery. The presence of left ventricular dysfunction or left bundle branch block may lead to paradoxical splitting of the second heart sound. Patients with postinfarction angina may also develop transient paradoxical splitting of the second heart sound due to prolongation of left ventricular ejection during anginal or ischemic episodes. An S_4 is almost always present in patients with sinus rhythm with AMI and reflects atrial contraction against a left ventricle with reduced compliance mentioned above. The presence of an S_3 in AMI is usually a reflection of extensive left ventricular dysfunction and heralds a higher risk of death than that in patients without such a sound.[2] Soft systolic murmurs are also commonly present in patients with AMI and generally reflect mild mitral regurgitation due to papillary muscle dysfunction or left ventricular dilatation.

REFERENCES

1. Stein, P.D., Sabbah, H.N., and Barr, I.: Intensity of heart sounds in the evaluation of patients following myocardial infarction. Chest 75:679, 1979.
2. Riley, C.P., Russell, R.O., Jr., and Rackley, C.E.: Left ventricular gallop sound and acute myocardial infarction. Am. Heart J. 86:598, 1973.

311-D (Braunwald, p. 1170)

The HMG CoA reductase inhibitors are a new class of drugs useful for the treatment of hyperlipoproteinemia. These agents are competitive inhibitors of the enzyme 3-hydroxy-3-methyl glutaryl coenzyme A reductase, the rate-limiting enzyme in cholesterol biosynthesis. By inhibiting this enzyme they reduce cholesterol synthesis and cause a secondary *increase* in the level of hepatic LDL receptors.

Lovastatin, the first of these drugs to gain approval, appears to be quite well tolerated with few side effects, except for infrequent but sustained rises in serum transaminase levels. Therefore, it is recommended that liver function tests be performed every 4 to 6 weeks during the first 15 months of therapy. These drugs may also cause myositis, and an increased incidence of corneal opacities has been noticed. Therefore, a slit-lamp examination is currently recommended before initiation of therapy and yearly thereafter. Because of the ability of HMG CoA reductase inhibitors to increase the number of LDL receptors, they reduce LDL cholesterol very significantly, even in patients who are heterozygotes for familial hypercholesterolemia. They act in an additive manner when used with bile acid sequestrants. These drugs are significantly less effective in patients who are homozygotes for familial hypercholesterolemia, probably because patients with this syndrome have essentially no LDL receptors.

312-E   (Braunwald, pp. 1191–1193)

Myocardial oxygen consumption ($M\dot{V}O_2$) provides an accurate measure of total cardiac metabolism. Over the years, it has been observed that the energy needs of the myocardium cannot be calculated simply from the external work as a product of the developed pressure and stroke volume. In addition, it has been shown that the ratio of the work performed to the oxygen consumed, i.e., the myocardial efficiency, varies widely depending on hemodynamic conditions. Simplistically, the $M\dot{V}O_2$ is determined by the tension time index (which is defined by the area under the LV pressure curve) and the velocity of myocardial contraction. Thus the developed wall tension or stress is an important determinant of $M\dot{V}O_2$. Wall stress can be calculated by LaPlace's law and is related directly to the radius of the heart and the intraventricular pressure but *inversely* related to ventricular wall thickness. Thus, it is an established clinical finding that with increased pressure and volume, there is compensatory wall thickening, which decreases wall stress.[1, 2]

The other major determinant of $M\dot{V}O_2$ is contractility, which is related to the extent of inotropic stimuli and neural influences. Heart rate itself increases contractility and therefore also increases $M\dot{V}O_2$. The maintenance of the active contractile state, which requires continued excitation-contraction coupling, may increase $M\dot{V}O_2$. Finally, $M\dot{V}O_2$ is influenced by the substrate utilized (free fatty acids vs glucose or lactic acid),[3] although this effect is important only in ischemic and failing myocardium. In ischemia there is decreased oxidation of fatty acids with increased utilization of anaerobic substrates resulting in decreased $M\dot{V}O_2$.

REFERENCES

1. Teplick, R., Haas, G.S., Trautman, E., Titus, J., Geffin, G., and Daggett, W.M.: Time dependence of the oxygen cost of force development during systole in the canine left ventricle. Circ. Res. 59:27, 1986.
2. Suga, H., Yamada, Y., Goto, Y., and Igarashi, Y.: Oxygen consumption and pressure volume area of abnormal contractions in canine heart. Am. J. Physiol. 26:H154, 1984.
3. Vik-Mo, H., and Mjos, O.E.: Influence of free fatty acids on myocardial oxygen consumption and ischemic injury. Am. J. Cardiol. 48:361, 1981.

313-B   (Braunwald, pp. 941–942)

Stenoses of the pulmonary artery may be single or multiple and may occur from the main pulmonary artery trunk to the smaller peripheral arterial branches.[1] In general, pulmonary artery stenosis is associated with other cardiovascular defects including ventricular septal defect, tetralogy of Fallot, supravalvular aortic stenosis, and pulmonic valvular stenosis. Perhaps the most impor-

tant cause of significant pulmonary artery stenoses in the newborn is intrauterine rubella infection.[2] Associated cardiovascular malformations in this syndrome include patent ductus arteriosus, pulmonic valve stenosis, and atrial septal defect. Systemic findings may include cataracts, microphthalmia, thrombocytopenia, hepatitis, deafness, and blood dyscrasias.

The clinical features vary, but most infants and children remain asymptomatic.[3] A continuous murmur may be present due to the pulmonary artery stenosis, especially if the lesion is in a main branch pulmonary artery or if an associated anomaly leads to increased pulmonary blood flow. Electrocardiography often demonstrates right ventricular hypertrophy when obstruction is severe.

In the rubella syndrome, left axis deviation with counterclockwise orientation of the QRS complex in the frontal plane is commonly seen. The diagnosis of peripheral pulmonary arterial stenosis may be confirmed by detecting pressure gradients within the pulmonary arterial system at cardiac catheterization. Mild to moderate unilateral or bilateral stenoses do not require surgical relief, and multiple stenoses may not be amenable to correction. Intraoperative or percutaneous balloon angioplasty has been used successfully to treat this disorder.[4]

REFERENCES

1. D'Cruz, I.A., Agustssou, M.M., Bicoff, J.P., Weinberg, M., Jr., and Arcilla, R.A.: Stenotic lesions of the pulmonary arteries. Clinical hemodynamic findings in 84 cases. Am. J. Cardol. 13:441, 1964.
2. Venables, A.W.: The syndrome of pulmonary stenosis complicating maternal rubella. Br. Heart J. 27:49, 1965.
3. Eldredge, W.J., Tingelstad, J.B., Robertson, L.W., Mauck, H.P., and McCue, C.M.: Observations on the natural history of pulmonary artery coarctation. Circulation 45:404, 1972.
4. Rocchini, A.P., Kveselis, D., Dick, M., Crowley, D., Snider, A.R., and Rosenthal, A.: Use of balloon angioplasty to treat peripheral pulmonary stenosis. Am. J. Cardiol. 54:1069, 1984.

314-B   (Braunwald, pp. 1318–1319)

This man has classic findings of chest pain caused by esophageal reflux and spasm. Differentiation of esophageal disorders from ischemic heart disease can be difficult, since the pains are located in similar areas and are frequently associated with emotional stress. However, while ischemic pain may produce substernal burning, certain features, including substernal burning, are more suggestive of esophageal than anginal pain. They include a prolonged, continuous ache, a discomfort that is primarily retrosternal and that does not radiate into the arms, a pain not associated with exercise, and a pain that disturbs sleep. Classically, esophageal disease associated with regurgitation causes "water brash," a taste in the mouth consistent with regurgitation of gastric contents. Frequently, patients with esophageal spasm experience relief with nitroglycerin. Unlike angina, however, esophageal pain is often relieved by milk, antacids, or food.[1]

Esophageal spasm may be documented by performing the Bernstein test, which consists of alternate infusions of dilute acid and normal saline into the esophagus via a nasogastric catheter. In patients with gastroesophageal acid reflux, acid infusion will reproduce the pain within 2 to 4 minutes. It should be noted that ECG changes can occur with gastric reflux and also that coexisting coronary artery disease may be exacerbated by gastroesophageal disorders.

Biliary colic also may be confused with angina pectoris. It is usually caused by a rapid rise in biliary pressure due to obstruction of the cystic or bile ducts. Thus the pain is usually abrupt in onset, steady in nature, and lasts from minutes to hours. It should be suspected when a history of dyspepsia, flatulence, fatty food intolerance, and indigestion is present.

REFERENCE

1. Constant, J.: The clinical diagnosis of nonanginal chest pain: The differentiation of angina from nonanginal chest pain by history. Clin. Cardiol. 6:11, 1983.

315-E (Braunwald, pp. 1164–1165)

Type II hyperlipoproteinemia is defined as an elevation of total plasma cholesterol, predominantly LDL cholesterol. There are two types: in Type IIA triglycerides and VLDL are normal while in Type IIB they are elevated. The most common cause of an isolated elevation of cholesterol and LDL is polygenic hypercholesterolemia, which may account for the condition in as many as 85 per cent of patients shown to have elevated cholesterol levels. Type IIa hyperlipoproteinemia may be due to familial hypercholesterolemia (FH), which is an autosomal dominant disease having a frequency of 1 in 500 for the heterozygote and 1 in one million for the homozygote. Finally, familial combined hyperlipidemia may also present as a Type II phenotype.

All of these patients have protean manifestations clinically. Tendinous xanthomas appearing on the extensor tendons such as the achilles and forearm tendons suggest underlying FH. These patients may have corneal arcus and xanthomas in other areas. Premature development of atherosclerosis is common. However, recurrent pancreatitis is not a commonly associated manifestation of the Type II phenotype. It is much more common in Type I hyperlipoproteinemia and familial hypertriglyceridemia in which chylomicronemia leads to abdominal pain and pancreatitis.

316-C (Braunwald, pp. 902–903)

While the development of congestive heart failure is a common pathological consequence of congenital cardiac lesions, the manifestations of this syndrome in neonates are somewhat different from those observed in the adult population. The advent of fetal echocardiography has allowed the early identification of intrauterine cardiac failure, which is manifested by scalp edema, pericardial effusion, ascites, and decreased fetal movements.

In infants born prematurely, persistent patent ductus arteriosus is the most common cause of cardiac decompensation; other forms of structural heart disease are rare. In the full-term newborn the earliest important causes of heart failure are coarctation of the aorta, hypoplastic left heart, paroxysmal atrial tachycardia, cerebral or hepatic arteriovenous fistula, and myocarditis. While heart failure in newborn infants is most commonly the result of a structural defect, it may occur secondary to severe metabolic abnormalities, such as hypoxemia and acidemia. The signs of pulmonary and systemic venous congestion in infants are somewhat different from those of the older child or adult. Among the most common symptoms and signs of heart failure in the infant are feeding difficulties and failure to gain weight and grow, tachycardia, pulmonary rales and rhonchi, liver enlargement, and cardiomegaly. It is much less common to see peripheral edema and ascites, while gallop rhythms and pleural or pericardial effusions are distinctly rare in infants.

The distinction between left and right heart failure is much less obvious in the infant than it is in the older child or adult. This results from left-to-right shunting in the presence of left heart failure, which leads to concomitant right-sided dysfunction. When right ventricular filling pressure is elevated, it causes a greater apparent reduction in left ventricular compliance in neonates and infants than in adults.

317-B (Braunwald, pp. 1431–1434)

This patient has a history of progressive congestive heart failure. His past medical history is remarkable for mild hypertension, a diagnosis of multiple myeloma, transfusion of one unit of blood monthly, and administration of Leukeran. The most likely diagnosis is cardiac amyloidosis, which is associated with immunocyte dyscrasias, most commonly multiple myeloma, as in this patient.

Amyloidosis of the heart may lead to several clinical syndromes. The most common is congestive heart failure due to systolic dysfunction. Hemodynamic evidence of restriction of ventricular filling is not prominent in these patients. There is frequently cardiomegaly, and progression to death is rapid. A second presentation of cardiac amyloidosis is a restrictive cardiomyopathy with predominant right-sided findings producing a picture similar to constrictive pericarditis. Orthostatic hypotension is a third mode of presentation occurring in about 10 per cent of the cases; it is frequently aggravated by coexisting renal amyloidosis leading to hypovolemia. Finally, abnormalities of cardiac impulse formation and conduction resulting in arrhythmias and conduction disturbances is the least common mode of presentation.

The chest x-ray in this disorder usually shows cardiomegaly, and pleural effusions are common. The ECG is usually abnormal; the most characteristic feature is diminished voltage followed by axis shifts and various conduction disturbances.

Echocardiography most commonly reveals increased thickness of the walls of the ventricles, small ventricular chambers, dilated atria, and impaired left ventricular function. A classic finding, which is infrequently seen, is a granular sparkling texture observed on two-dimensional echocardiography, most typically in the interatrial septum. Treatment of this form of cardiomyopathy is limited, although various efforts are being made to prevent the development of the immune reaction leading to the appearance of amyloid.

REFERENCE

1. Sanchez-Ramos, J.A., Redondo-Sanchez, R., Garcia-Crespo, P., Superby-Jeldres, A., and Schuller-Perez, A.: Cardiac amyloidosis. Cardiovasc. Rev. Rep. 5:524, 1984.

318-D   *(Braunwald, pp. 1198–1200)*

The control of coronary vascular resistance is mediated by neural, metabolic, and myogenic factors as well as by substances released by the endothelium. During states of diminished coronary perfusion, it is likely that adenosine plays a significant role in augmenting perfusion. During periods of relative oxygen deprivation in which the resynthesis of high-energy phosphate compounds by mitochondria is impaired, a relative excess of adenosine monophosphate (AMP) is produced. The enzyme 5'-nucleotidase catalyzes the formation of adenosine from AMP. The adenosine is secreted into the interstitial fluid and appears to cause direct relaxation of smooth muscle cells in the coronary vasculature. The adenosine is then taken up by the myocardial cells, in which it is either phosphorylated to AMP or deaminated to inosine and converted to hypoxanthine. There are many other metabolic products that may be important in vasodilatation, including other nucleotides, prostaglandins (PGI_2, PGE_2), CO_2, hydrogen ions, and less commonly potassium and oxygen.[1]

REFERENCE

1. McKenzie, J.E., Steffen, R.P., and Haddy, F.J.: Relations between adenosine and coronary resistance in conscious exercising dogs. Am. J. Physiol. 242:H24, 1982.

319-D   *(Braunwald, pp. 1345–1350)*

Using angiographic criteria to evaluate prognostic information for patients with chronic stable angina, the two most important variables determined by the CASS were (1) left ventricular function and (2) severity and extent of coronary artery disease. Left ventricular dysfunction is a more important determinant of prognosis than the extent and severity of coronary artery disease,[1] although the two factors are synergistic prognostically. Thus, in patients with one diseased vessel the 4-year survival rate with a 35 to 50 per cent ejection fraction was 91 per cent, while with an ejection fraction below 35 per cent the 4-year survival was 74 per cent. In patients with two diseased vessels, an ejection fraction of 35 to 50 per cent was associated with 83 per cent survival, while an ejection fraction < 35 per cent yielded a 57 per cent survival at 4 years. In three-vessel disease, an ejection fraction of > 50 per cent was associated with an 82 per cent survival, an ejection fraction of 35 to 50 per cent yielded 71 per cent, and an ejection fraction of < 35 per cent was associated with 50 per cent survival.[2] Additional factors that were important prognostically included whether or not the stenosis was in the right coronary artery (better survival) or the left anterior descending coronary artery (worse survival). Also, the extent of stenosis was important, with high-grade stenoses having a worse prognosis.

REFERENCES

1. Sanz, G., Castaner, A., Betriu, A., Magrina, J., Roig, E., Coll, S., Pare, J.C., and Navarro-Lopez, F.: Determinants of prognosis in survivors of myocardial infarction. A prospective clinical angiographic study. N. Engl. J. Med. 306:1065, 1982.
2. Mock, M.B., et al.: Survival of medically treated patients in a coronary artery surgery (CASS) registry. Circulation 66:562, 1982.

320   **A-Y, B-Y, C-Y, D-Y, E-Y**   *(Braunwald, pp. 1228–1230)*

While uncommon, there are a number of nonatherosclerotic causes of AMI. Embolic phenomena may involve the coronary arteries, such as those that may result from endocarditis, either infective or marantic in nature. Such emboli most frequently lodge in the left anterior descending coronary artery. Inflammatory processes can also involve the coronary artery and may occasionally lead to AMI. Kawasaki's disease, necrotizing arteritis, systemic lupus erythematosus, and syphilis can all lead to coronary occlusion by such a mechanism. MI may also result from the coronary arterial involvement in amyloidosis, Hurler's syndrome, pseudoxanthoma elasticum, and homocystinuria. In these cases, coronary mural thickening due to the metabolic disease in question or simultaneous intimal proliferative disease leads to restriction of coronary blood flow. Cocaine abuse has been shown to precipitate AMI in patients with normal coronary arteries, those with a prior history of MI, and those with known coronary spasm. An extensive list of the further potential causes of MI without coronary atherosclerosis may be found in Braunwald, Table 38–1, p. 1229.

321   **A-Y, B-Y, C-Y, D-N, E-Y**   *(Braunwald, p. 989)*

The electrocardiogram in tetralogy of Fallot is characterized by right axis deviation, as well as right ventricular hypertrophy. Older patients with uncorrected tetralogy of Fallot may develop atrial flutter or fibrillation as well. The classic boot-shaped heart that is seen in conjunction with decreased pulmonary blood flow in infants and children with tetralogy of Fallot is less typically seen in adults. A right-sided aortic arch may be apparent on x-ray examination in approximately 30 per cent of patients with tetralogy of Fallot. In adults, especially those who are acyanotic, pulmonary vascularity may be normal or even increased in up to half the patients.

M-mode echocardiography is usually capable of demonstrating the abnormal relationship between the aortic annulus and interventricular septum that exists in this disorder. Two-dimensional echocardiography may give further information regarding the extent and location of infundibular obstruction, the integrity of the pulmonary valve and artery, and the extent of right ventricular hypertrophy, as well as the location of the VSD. Doppler analysis may also be employed to assess blood flow across the VSD as well as quantitate right ventricular outflow tract systolic gradients. More recently, magnetic resonance imaging has been used to diagnose and assess tetralogy of Fallot and the associated cardiac anomalies (see Braunwald, Fig. 31–13, p. 990).

322   A-Y, B-N, C-Y, D-Y, E-N   *(Braunwald, pp. 1360–1362)*

Prinzmetal's angina, or variant angina, is characterized by the development of chest pain and ischemic ECG changes in the absence of an increase in cardiac work or oxygen consumption. Thus, unlike in chronic stable angina (effort-induced), episodes of Prinzmetal's angina occur without increases in heart rate, arterial pressure, or myocardial contractility. Spasm of a proximal coronary artery with resultant transmural ischemia has been convincingly documented arteriographically. This is classically associated with elevation of ST segments. Exercise testing in patients with variant angina is of limited value because there is such a variable response of the patients to exercise. Studies have demonstrated approximately equal numbers of patients who show ST-segment elevation, ST-segment depression, or no change in ST segments during exercise. This reflects the presence of underlying fixed coronary artery disease in some patients and the absence of significant disease in others.

Approximately two-thirds of patients with Prinzmetal's angina will demonstrate severe proximal coronary artery stenosis at coronary angiography. In these patients spasm usually occurs within 1 cm of the stenosis. The other one-third of patients have normal coronary arteries in the absence of ischemia.[1] Patients with normal coronary arteriograms are more likely to have purely nonexertional angina and ST-segment elevations. These patients frequently have an increased incidence of right coronary artery spasm. Patients with no or mild fixed coronary stenoses tend to experience a more benign course than do patients with associated severe obstructive lesions.[2]

A number of provocative tests for coronary spasm have been developed, among which the ergonovine test is one of the most sensitive and useful. *Ergonovine maleate*, an ergot alkaloid, stimulates both alpha-adrenergic and serotonin receptors and therefore exerts a direct constrictive effect on vascular smooth muscle. In patients with Prinzmetal's angina, the sensitivity to this particular vasoconstrictor is heightened. In general, patients with Prinzmetal's angina will develop a sudden and severe vasoconstriction in response to intravenous doses ranging from *0.05 to 0.40 mg*. In normal subjects, doses of this magnitude will cause a uniform, mild vasoconstriction of all the coronary vessels, as opposed to a sudden, dramatic spasm of one coronary artery. Finally, intracoronary acetylcholine has recently been demonstrated to induce coronary spasm in patients with variant angina with high specificity and sensitivity.[4]

REFERENCES

1. Selzer, A., Langston, M., Ruggeroli, C., and Cohn, K.: Clinical syndrome of variant angina with normal coronary arteriogram. N. Engl. J. Med. 295:1343, 1976.
2. Cipriano, P.R., Koch, F.H., Rosenthal, S.J., and Schroeder, J.S.: Clinical course of patients following the demonstration of coronary artery spasm by angiography. Am. Heart J. 101:127, 1981.
3. Winniford, M.D., Johnson, S.M., Mauritson, D.R., and Hillis, L.D.: Ergonovine provocation to assess efficacy of long-term therapy with calcium antagonists in Prinzmetal's variant angina. Am. J. Cardiol. 51:684, 1983.
4. Okumura, K., et al.: Sensitivity and specificity of intracoronary injection of acetylcholine for the induction of coronary spasm. J. Am. Coll. Cardiol. 12:883, 1988.

323   A-N, B-Y, C-Y, D-Y, E-N   *(Braunwald, pp. 917–919)*

Atrioventricular (AV) septal defects include malformations characterized by varying degrees of incomplete development of the atrial septum, the inflow portion of the ventricular septum, and the atrioventricular valves (see Braunwald, Fig. 30–3, p. 900). These anomalies are also known as endocardial cushion defects or atrioventricular (AV) canal defects. AV septal defects may be encountered in association with other congenital abnormalities, including trisomy 21, Ellis–van Creveld syndrome, and asplenia or polysplenia syndromes.

Ostium primum ASDs occur immediately adjacent to the AV valves, either of which may be deformed or incompetent. Most commonly it is only the anterior or septal leaflet of the mitral valve that is displaced and cleft; more often than not the posterior leaflet of the mitral valve and the tricuspid valve are not involved. Ostium primum ASDs lead to large left-to-right intraatrial shunting and have clinical features that are quite similar to those seen in ostium secundum defects.

In addition to similar findings on physical examination, chest x-ray often reveals RA and RV prominence as well as increased pulmonary vascular markings. Left ventriculography performed at the time of cardiac catheterization may reveal the pathognomonic "gooseneck" deformity. This results from the altered relationship between the anterior components of the mitral valve and the right border of the left ventricular cavity as it leads to the aorta.

When a ventricular septal defect accompanies the ostium primum septal defect and a common AV orifice is therefore present, the malformation is known as a complete atrioventricular canal defect. Approximately 35 per cent of patients with common AV canal have accompanying cardiovascular abnormalities including tetralogy of Fallot, double-outlet right ventricle, transposition of the great arteries, total anomalous pulmonary venous connections, left ventricular outflow tract obstruction, pulmonic stenosis, and persistent left superior vena cava. In addition, common AV canal is seen quite commonly in patients with trisomy 21.

324   A-Y, B-Y, C-N, D-Y, E-Y   *(Braunwald, pp. 1266–1268)*

While the use of permanent pacing in survivors of AMI is controversial in some situations, some generalizations can be made regarding this mode of therapy. Patients with inferior infarction without an associated intraventricular conduction defect who experience a transient type II second-degree or complete AV block do *not* appear to require permanent pacemaker therapy. Conflicting data exist regarding the patient with AMI who has both bundle branch block and *transient* high-degree AV block. Some investigators have suggested that prophylactic pacing confers little or no advantage to the long-term survival of such patients.[1] In contrast, a retrospective multicenter study[2] has found that survivors of AMI with bundle branch block and transient high-degree AV block have an increased incidence of recurrent high-degree AV block and sudden death that may be reduced by insertion of a permanent demand pacemaker. Therefore, it seems prudent to consider prophylactic permanent pacemaker therapy in these patients.

One reason for continued controversy regarding permanent pacemaker therapy in patients with AMI is the fact that not all sudden deaths in the post-MI patient population are due to recurrent high-degree AV block. For example, in patients with anteroseptal MI that is complicated by either right or left bundle branch block, there is an increased incidence of late in-hospital ventricular fibrillation.[3] While controversy remains regarding the use of permanent pacemaker therapy in patients with either transient advanced AV block and associated bundle branch block or persistent first-degree AV block and new bundle branch block, it is reasonably well established that patients who have persistent advanced AV block (such as Mobitz II second-degree AV block following AMI) should have permanent pacemakers placed.

REFERENCES

1. Ginks, W.R., Sutton, R., Oh, W., and Leatham, A.: Long-term prognosis after acute inferior infarction with atrioventricular block. Br. Heart J. 39:186, 1977.
2. Hindman, M.C., Wagner, G.S., JaRo, M., Atkins, J.M., Scheinman, M.M., DeSanctis, R.W., Hutter, A.H., Jr., Yeatman, L., Rubenfire, M., Pujura, C., Rubin, M., and Morris, J.J.: The clinical significance of bundle branch block complicating acute myocardial infarction. 2. Indications for temporary and permanent pacemaker insertion. Circulation 58:689, 1978.
3. Wilson, C., and Adgey, A.A.J.: Survival of patients with late ventricular fibrillation after acute myocardial infarction. Lancet 2:214, 1974.

325   A-N, B-Y, C-Y, D-Y, E-N   (Braunwald, p. 1010)

Diphtheria is an acute infectious disease produced by *Corynebacterium diphtheriae*, a gram-positive bacillus. It is characterized by a local inflammatory lesion usually in the upper part of the respiratory tract and by remote effects resulting from the toxin, which affects particularly the heart and peripheral nerves. In the United States diphtheria has been largely eradicated by extensive childhood immunization with diphtheria toxoid. This is given in combination with tetanus toxoid and pertussis vaccine, termed DPT. However, because of recent concern over paralysis associated with the administration of DPT, increasing numbers of children do not receive vaccination. So diphtheria may become a more prominent problem.

Cardiac involvement develops in about two-thirds of patients with diphtheria but is clinically evident in only about 10 per cent of cases. The cardiac involvement is due to the bacterial endotoxin. This appears to cause abnormal fat metabolism in the myocardium with depletion of myocardial carnitine, a cofactor required for the beta-oxidation of fats. Because of this action, triglycerides accumulate in the myocardium and cause fatty degeneration of muscle. The ECG is a fair indicator of the extent of myocardial involvement and also the prognosis. Ventricular fibrillation is a constant threat and is frequently responsible for sudden death. Ninety per cent of patients with atrial fibrillation, ventricular tachycardia, or complete heart block die. Development of right or left bundle branch block is also an ominous sign, associated with a mortality in excess of 50 per cent. Clinically, involvement of the right side of the heart occurs first, and the most common symptom is actually right upper quadrant pain due to hepatic congestion. In children, recovery from the acute episode is usually excellent and associated with a good prognosis. However, in adults there may be permanent cardiac damage including myocardial fibrosis. Recently, parenteral administration of carnitine has been found to reverse diphtheritic cardiac dysfunction partially and to reduce the risk of cardiac death.[1] However, conservative therapy remains the mainstay of management, and includes intravenous penicillin, acute administration of diphtheria antitoxin, digitalis, diuretics, and appropriate antiarrhythmic medications. The value of corticosteroids is debatable.

REFERENCE

1. Ramos, A., Elias, P., Barrucand, L., and DaSilva, J.: The protective effect of carnitine in human diphtheritic myocarditis. Pediatr. Res. 18:815, 1984.

326   A-Y, B-Y, C-N, D-N, E-Y   (Braunwald, pp. 1555–1556)

Aortic dissection affects twice as many men as women, and is seen most commonly in the sixth and seventh decades of life. Over 90 per cent of patients presenting with aortic dissection will complain of severe pain. The pain is usually sudden in onset, most severe at its inception, and may be unbearable; adjectives such as "tearing" and "ripping" are frequently used to describe the discomfort. The discomfort tends to migrate in association with dissection of the hematoma into the aortic wall. The diagnosis is often easily confirmed by physical examination. While patients may appear to be in shock, the blood pressure measured is often elevated, especially in patients with distal dissection. The characteristic physical findings associated with aortic dissection, such as pulse deficits and aortic regurgitation, are more commonly seen in proximal dissection. For example, approximately 50 per cent of patients with a proximal dissection will display some form of a pulse deficit, often involving decrease or loss of pulses associated with the brachiocephalic vessels. Similarly, aortic regurgitation is most commonly seen in association with proximal dissection and occurs in approximately two-thirds of patients.[1]

A variety of clinical conditions in which chest pain consistent with aortic dissection may occur can be confused with this entity, especially if another manifestation such as aortic regurgitation or a neurologic abnormality is associated with the chest discomfort. Included in the differential diagnosis are myocardial infarction, acute aortic regurgitation without dissection, thoracic nondissecting aneurysm, mediastinal tumors, musculoskeletal pain, and pericarditis. The most crucial study in the diagnosis of aortic dissection is aortic angiography, which almost always confirms the diagnosis and is well tolerated, even by the most critically ill patients.

REFERENCE

1. Slater, E.E., and DeSanctis, R.W.: The clinical recognition of dissecting aortic aneurysm. Am. J. Med. 60:625, 1976.

327 A-N, B-Y, C-Y, D-N, E-Y *(Braunwald, pp. 1044–1045)*

Once the decision is made to operate on a patient with predominant mitral regurgitation (MR), several options are available. Excellent results have been obtained with reconstructive procedures that employ a rigid or semi-rigid prosthetic annulus such as the Carpentier ring. Direct suture repair of the valve and replacement, reimplantation, elongation, or shortening of the chordae tendineae as necessary to make the valve nonregurgitant are usually performed. The impetus to repair the mitral valve as opposed to replacement is that many of the hazards of chronic anticoagulation and thromboembolism that accompany use of a mechanical prosthesis are largely eliminated. This procedure can be performed in a wide range of patients, including those with ruptured chordae tendineae, annular dilatation, and even active endocarditis.

However, there are two classes of patients who, in general, should not have a reconstructive procedure. First, patients whose MR originates from myxomatous degeneration (such as occurs in Marfan syndrome) frequently will have progression of underlying disease following reconstruction and will require valve replacement. Second, patients with severe calcification both of the annulus and of the valve, such as elderly persons, do not have enough pliable mitral valve tissue to make a nonregurgitant orifice; these patients are usually more effectively treated with valve replacement.[1]

REFERENCE

1. Kirklin, J.W.: Mitral valve repair for mitral incompetence. Mod. Concepts Cardiovasc. Dis. 56:7, 1987.

328 A-Y, B-N, C-N, D-N, E-N *(Braunwald, pp. 921–923)*

The management of VSD in infants and children begins with elective hemodynamic evaluation between the ages of 3 and 6 years provided that no evidence of pulmonary hypertension is noted. In children with pulmonary systemic flow ratios of less than 1.5:1, surgical treatment is *not* recommended because the risk of infective endocarditis does not exceed the risk of operation.[1] In addition, although the operative repair of VSD has a low morbidity and mortality, postoperative heart block, infection, and other complications do occur occasionally. With larger shunts, elective operation is usually advised before the child enters school in order to minimize any subsequent differences in development between the patient and normal classmates.

The most significant surgically induced abnormality of the conduction system following repair of VSD is complete heart block, which occurs immediately postoperatively in less than 1 per cent of patients. Late-onset complete heart block may occur occasionally, especially in the 10 to 25 per cent of patients whose postoperative ECG findings show complete right bundle branch block with left anterior hemiblock.[2] The presence of the latter pattern defines two populations of patients, those with peripheral damage to the conduction system and those with damage to the bundle of His or its proximal branches.[3] Therefore, the presence of this ECG pattern and accompanying transient heart block in the early postoperative period suggests the need for electrophysiological studies in the postoperative period but may not require permanent pacemaker therapy.

Exercise studies in patients with repair of VSD may uncover late abnormalities in circulatory function despite normal or only moderately elevated pulmonary vascular resistance. An impaired cardiac output response to exercise as well as a markedly abnormal increase in pulmonary arteriovenous pressure gradient may be noted.[4] The precise etiology of these abnormalities remains undefined but may be related to abnormal LV function after closure of the defect and/or to persistent changes in the pulmonary arterioles or to abnormal pulmonary vascular reactivity.

REFERENCES

1. deLeval, M.: Ventricular septal defects. In Stark, J., and deLeval, M. (eds.): Surgery for Congenital Heart Defects. New York, Grune & Stratton, 1983, p. 271.
2. Godman, M.J., Roberts, N.K., and Izukawa, T.: Late postoperative conduction disturbances after repair of ventricular septal defect in tetralogy of Fallot. Circulation 49:214, 1974.
3. Okarama, E.O., Guller, B., Molony, J.D., and Weidman, W.H.: Etiology of right bundle branch block pattern after surgical closure of ventricular septal defects. Am. Heart J. 90:14, 1975.
4. Otterstad, J.E., Simonsen, S., and Erikssen, J.: Hemodynamic findings at rest and during mild supine exercise in adults with isolated uncomplicated ventricular septal defects. Circulation 71:650, 1985.

329 A-Y, B-Y, C-Y, D-N, E-Y *(Braunwald, p. 1266)*

Between 10 and 20 per cent of patients with AMI will sustain block in one or more of the three fascicles of the His-Purkinje system below the AV node. The blood supply of the right bundle branch and the left posterior division of the bundle branch comes from both the left anterior descending and right coronary arteries. The left anterior division of the left bundle branch is supplied by septal perforating branches from the left anterior descending coronary artery alone. Isolated right bundle branch block due to an acute infarction occurs in approximately 2 per cent of patients with AMI and often leads to AV block. The lesion is usually associated with anteroseptal infarction and is associated with a high mortality even if complete AV block does not occur.[1]

Isolated blockade of the left anterior fascicle of the left bundle occurs in between 3 and 5 per cent of patients with AMI and also occurs in an additional 5 per cent of patients in conjunction with right bundle branch block and AMI. Isolated left anterior divisional block confers an increased mortality in the AMI setting, although it is not as great a risk as either left posterior fascicular block or right bundle branch block (see Braunwald, Table 38–10, p. 1232). Because the posterior fascicle of the left bundle branch is larger than the anterior fascicle and is supplied by two arteries, it is less likely to undergo isolated blockade due to AMI. Thus, this lesion occurs in only 1 to 2 per cent of patients with AMI admitted to coronary care units and is associated with an increased mortality, presumably because it occurs in patients with larger infarcts.

Complete AV block is not a frequent complication of either form of isolated divisional blockade. If a new block occurs in two of the three divisions of the conduction system (bifascicular block), the risk of developing complete AV block is quite high, between 20 and 45 per cent. Mortality in these patients is usually due to the presence of severe underlying pump failure secondary to an extensive AMI.

The occurrence of new complete left bundle branch block heralds as high a mortality as right bundle branch block and the other two forms of bifascicular block,[2] although this defect progresses to complete AV block only half as frequently as does right bundle branch block. Interestingly, patients with intraventricular conduction defects, especially right bundle branch block, are more likely to develop ventricular fibrillation late in the hospital course. This is presumed to be secondary to associated cardiac failure and the size of the underlying infarction rather than to the conduction disturbance itself. The existence of bundle branch block or divisional block prior to the development of AMI is less often associated with the development of complete heart block than with blocks acquired during the course of the illness. It should also be noted that the presence of P-R interval prolongation in the setting of bidivisional block may be due to underlying trifascicular block, which progresses to complete heart block in nearly 40 per cent of patients.

In general, the presence of any two of the following variables confers a risk of 25 per cent or higher of developing complete heart block following AMI: first-degree AV block, Mobitz type I second-degree AV block, Mobitz type II second-degree AV block, left anterior fascicular block, left posterior fascicular block, right bundle branch block, and left bundle branch block.[3]

The decision to use temporary pacemaker therapy is often a difficult one and must be tempered by the fact that between 10 and 20 per cent of patients develop pacemaker-related complications.[4] However, the increased risk for the progression to complete heart block in the patient groups just mentioned underscores the importance for the clinician of familiarity with the types of intraventricular block that occur in the AMI setting.

REFERENCES

1. Hindman, M.C., Wagner, G.S., JaRo, M., Atkins, J.M., Scheinman, M.M., DeSanctis, R.W., Hutter, A.H., Yeatman, L., Rubenfire, M., Pujura, C., Rubin, M., and Morris, J.J.: The clinical significance of bundle branch block complicating acute myocardial infarction. I. Clinical characteristics, hospital mortality, and one-year follow-up. Circulation 58:679, 1978.
2. Mullins, C.B., and Atkins, J.M.: Prognoses and management of ventricular conduction blocks in acute myocardial infarction. Mod. Concepts Cardiovasc. Dis. 5:129, 1976.
3. Lamas, G.A., Muller, J.E., Turi, Z.G., Stone, P.H., Rutherford, J.D., Jaffe, A.S., Raabe, D.S., Rude, R.E., Mark, D.B., Califf, R.M., Gold, H.K., Robertson, T., Passamani, E.R., Braunwald, E., and the MILIS Study Group: A simplified method to predict occurrence of complete heart block during acute myocardial infarction. Am. J. Cardiol. 57:1213, 1986.
4. Hynes, J.K., Holmes, D.R., Jr., and Harrison, C.E.: Five-year experience with temporary pacemaker therapy in the coronary care unit. Mayo Clin. Proc. 58:122, 1983.

330   A-Y, B-N, C-N, D-Y, E-N (Braunwald, pp. 1030–1032)

This woman clearly has at least moderately severe MS, and her age and complaint of left-sided chest pain suggest that she may have coexistent coronary artery disease. In addition, her echocardiogram raises the possibility of coexistent aortic stenosis (AS). Therefore, it would be prudent to carry out cardiac catheterization and coronary arteriography to evaluate her coronary artery disease and at the same time to rule out AS and to confirm the presence of significant MS. It would not be good practice in a patient who has symptoms of progressive dyspnea on exertion, arrhythmias, and chest pain to defer further treatment. At cardiac catheterization it is likely that a mitral valve area less than 1.0 cm^2 will be found, in which case surgical treatment should be recommended.

Open commissurotomy and mitral valve repair would be a reasonable suggestion for first-time operation for MS in certain patients. At open commissurotomy, cardiac bypass is established, any thrombi in the left atrium are removed, and then the commissures are incised, the papillary muscles split, and the valves debrided of calcium. This procedure is useful for patients with mild calcific disease and also is helpful in patients with mild to moderate mitral regurgitation. However, this woman is not an ideal candidate for repair for two reasons. First, she has been in atrial fibrillation for many years and has a dilated atrium, which means anticoagulation cannot be avoided following repair. Second, the operation would be technically difficult because of extensive calcification. Therefore, it would be reasonable, if she is to undergo open heart surgery, to carry out mitral valve replacement with a mechanical prosthesis.

Finally, although balloon mitral valvuloplasty[1] has become an attractive intervention in MS, it is still an experimental procedure. In this patient with significant calcification it would be less likely to be successful than in a patient with more moderate or unoperated MS. In addition, the prior surgery may have significantly altered the intraatrial septum, making the balloon valvuloplasty attempt more dangerous, especially during the initial crossing of the foramen ovale. It would therefore be more appropriate to proceed with mitral valve replacement in this patient.

REFERENCE

1. Kveselis, D.A., Rocchini, A.P., Beekman, R., Snider, A.R., Crowley, D., Dick, M., and Rosenthal, A.: Balloon angioplasty for congenital and rheumatic mitral stenosis. Am. J. Cardiol. 57:348, 1986.

331   A-Y, B-Y, C-Y, D-N, E-Y (Braunwald, p. 948)

In general, total correction of tetralogy of Fallot is advised for almost all patients, even in infancy.[1] The successful early correction appears to prevent the consequences of progressive infundibular obstruction and acquired pulmonary atresia, delayed growth and development, and the complications secondary to hypoxemia and polycythemia with bleeding tendencies that arise in this population. It is the size of the pulmonary arteries that is most important in determining candidacy for primary repair of tetralogy of Fallot as opposed to the age or size of the infant or child. Marked hypoplasia of the pulmonary arteries is a relative contraindication for total corrective operation and when present usually leads to a palliative procedure designed to increase pulmonary blood flow by establishing a systemic–pulmonary arterial anastomosis.[2] The total correction of the tetralogy then may be carried out later in childhood or adolescence at lower risk. Such palliative procedures relieve hypoxemia and polycythemia and their attendant complications.

The postoperative period after palliative or corrective surgery is marked by a variety of common complications. A sudden increase in pulmonary venous return may lead to mild to moderate *left* ventricular decompensation, and varying degrees of pulmonic valvular regurgitation may increase right ventricular cavity size.[3] In addition, bleeding problems may frequently be seen, especially in older polycythemic patients. Complete right bundle branch block or left anterior hemiblock is often observed postoperatively. The greatest cause of early and late mortality and poor surgical results is restriction in pulmonary arterial flow due to persistent problems with right-sided outflow tract obstruction. In general, surgical repair leads to relief of symptoms of hypoxemia and the severe exercise intolerance that mark the preoperative period.

REFERENCES

1. Kirklin, J.K., Pacifico, A.D., and Kirklin, J.W.: Tetralogy of Fallot: Principles of surgical managements. Mod. Probl. Paediatr. 22:139, 1983.
2. Kirklin, J.W., Blackstone, E.H., Kirklin, J.K., Pacifico, A.D., Aramendi, J., and Bargeron, L.M., Jr.: Surgical results and protocols in the spectrum of tetralogy of Fallot. Ann. Surg. 198:251, 1983.
3. Naito, Y., Fujita, T., Yagihara, T., Isobe, F., Yamamoto, F., Tanaka, K., Manabe, H., Takahashi, O., and Kamiya, T.: Usefulness of left ventricular volume in assessing tetralogy of Fallot for total correction. Am. J. Cardiol. 56:356, 1985.

332   A-Y, B-N, C-Y, D-N, E-N (Braunwald, pp. 1030–1031)

The M-mode echocardiogram displayed comes from a patient with mitral stenosis (MS). The classic features of MS include thickening of the leaflets, decreased maximal leaflet separation in diastole, and absence of the *a* wave in the setting of normal LV function. Shown in this echocardiogram are redundant echoes consistent with a thickened calcified rheumatic valve. Decreased leaflet separation can be readily seen in diastole. Furthermore, there is minimal reopening during atrial contraction. In normal subjects the posterior leaflet of the mitral valve moves posteriorly during early diastole while in the example shown here it can be seen that the posterior mitral leaflet moves anteriorly, as does the anterior leaflet. Thus, the anterior and posterior leaflets appear to be fused. The LV cavity size and systolic function measured by movement of the septum and the posterior LV wall appear normal, which is characteristic of MS. It

should be noted that determination of mitral valve area is not possible by M-mode echocardiography. However, using two-dimensional echocardiography in the parasternal short-axis view the mitral valve orifice can be observed in cross-section and the innermost portion of the mitral valve orifice planimetered to obtain a measure of the area. Doppler echocardiography, however, is the most accurate noninvasive technique for estimating the transmitral valvular pressure gradient, and for estimating the valve area.

REFERENCE

1. Glover, M.U., Warren, S.E., Vieweg, W.V.R., Ceretto, W.J., Samtoy, L.M., and Hagan, A.D.: M-mode and two-dimensional echocardiographic correlation with findings at catheterization and surgery in patients with mitral stenosis. Am. Heart J. 105:98, 1983.

333   A-Y, B-Y, C-N, D-N, E-Y (Braunwald, pp. 1284–1285)

Left ventricular aneurysm complicates AMI in approximately 12 to 15 per cent of patients who survive the acute insult. Formation of the aneurysm is presumed to occur when intraventricular tension leads to expansion of the noncontracting, infarcted myocardial tissue.[1] In general, an anterior MI complicated by left ventricular aneurysm occurs due to total occlusion of a poorly collateralized left anterior descending artery.[2] The presence of multivessel disease, extensive collaterals, or a nonoccluded left anterior descending artery makes the development of an aneurysm much less likely. Aneurysms occur approximately four times more commonly at the apex and in the anterior wall than in the inferoposterior wall, and in general range from 1 to 8 cm in diameter.[3]

Even when compared with mortality in patients having comparable left ventricular ejection fractions, the presence of a left ventricular aneurysm leads to a mortality that is up to six times higher than that of patients without aneurysm.[4] Death in such patients is often sudden and presumed to be secondary to a high incidence of ventricular tachyarrhythmias that originate from the aneurysmal tissue itself. Diagnosis of aneurysm is best made by echocardiographic study, by radionuclide ventriculography, or at the time of cardiac catheterization by left ventriculography. Interestingly, the classic evidence of aneurysm on electrocardiogram, persistent ST-segment elevation in the area of the infarction, actually indicates a large infarct but does not necessarily imply an aneurysm.[5] In appropriately selected patients, especially those in whom relative preservation of contractile performance of the left ventricle may be achieved, surgical aneurysmectomy may achieve clinical improvement with a relatively low risk of death.

REFERENCES

1. Schuster, E.H., and Bulkley, B.H.: Expansion of transmural myocardial infarction: A patho-physiologic factor in cardiac rupture. Circulation 60:1532, 1979.
2. Forman, M.D., Collins, H.W., Kipelman, H.A., Vaughn, W.K., Perry, J.M., Virmani, R., and Freisinger, G.C.: Determinants of left ventricular aneurysm formation after anterior myocardial infarction: A clinical and angiographic study. J. Am. Coll. Cardiol. 8:1256, 1986.

3. Abrams, D., Edelist, A., Luria, M.H., and Miller, A.J.: Ventricular aneurysm: A reappraisal based on a study in 65 consecutive autopsied cases. Circulation 27:164, 1963.
4. Meizlish, J.L., Berger, H.J., Plankey, M., Errico, D., Levy, W., and Zaret, B.L.: Functional left ventricular aneurysm formation after acute myocardial infarction: Incidence, natural history, and prognostic implications. N. Engl. J. Med. 31:1001, 1984.
5. Lindsay, J., Jr., Dewey, R.C., Talesnick, B.S., and Nolan, N.G.: relation of ST-segment elevation after healing of acute myocardial infarction to the presence of left ventricular aneurysm. Am. J. Cardiol. 54:84, 1984.

334   A-Y, B-Y, C-Y, D-N, E-N (Braunwald, pp. 1501–1502)

Constrictive pericarditis usually results from progressive scarring and thickening of the pericardium with subsequent obliteration of the pericardial space due to an inflammatory process in the pericardium. The end-stage constricted pericardium is a fibrotic, thickened, adherent structure in which the visceral and parietal layers have become fused. This stiffened structure restricts diastolic filling and therefore leads to elevation and equalization of diastolic pressures in all four chambers of the heart. In general, cardiac filling occurs only early in diastole when the intracardiac volume is less than that defined by the stiffened pericardium. Because of the elevation of systemic venous pressure in this disorder, this early diastolic filling occurs more rapidly than in normal patients. Therefore, the characteristic dip-and-plateau wave form, in which rapid early diastolic filling is followed by an abrupt halt in filling leading to a plateau phase, is commonly seen in constriction. A prominent y descent results from the rapid early diastolic filling, and a clear x descent is usually present as well, leading to the characteristic "M" or "W" configuration of the venous wave form seen in this disorder. This may be compared with cardiac tamponade, in which the diastolic phase of venous return is blunted due to the presence of cardiac compression throughout the cardiac cycle. This results in a venous pressure tracing that shows a diminished or absent y descent and a predominant x descent.

335   A-N, B-Y, C-Y, D-Y, E-Y (Braunwald, p. 1474)

It has recently been recognized that certain families appear to have an autosomal dominant transmission of recurrent myxomas. In addition, some patients with familial myxoma have a syndrome that involves a complex of abnormalities, including lentigines or pigmented nevi or both, primary nodular adrenal cortical disease with or without Cushing's syndrome, myxomatous mammary fibroadenomas, testicular tumors, and pituitary adenomas with gigantism or acromegaly. Patients who have two or more components of this complex usually present at a relatively young age. Either of two mnemonics are applied to their disease: NAME syndrome (nevi, atrial myxoma, myxoid neurofibroma, and ephelides) or LAMB syndrome (lentigines, atrial myxoma, and blue nevi). Approximately 7 per cent of all myxomas are found in persons with familial myxoma or the aforementioned complex of findings. These patients, in comparison to others, tend to be younger, have multiple myxomas of chambers other than the left atrium, and are more likely to have postoperative recurrence of myxoma.[1]

REFERENCE

1. McCarthy, P.M., Piehler, J.M., Schaff, H.V., Pluth, J.R., Orszulak, T.A., Vidaillet, H.J., Jr., and Carney, J.A.: The significance of multiple, recurrent, and "complex" cardiac myxomas. Thorac. Cardiovasc. Surg. 91:389, 1986.

336   A-Y, B-Y, C-N, D-N (Braunwald, p. 1286)

The development of angina in the postinfarction period is a complication that requires immediate evaluation. When postinfarction angina is accompanied by ST- and T-wave changes in the area where the infarction originally occurred, it may be due to occlusion of an initially patent vessel, reocclusion of a recanalized vessel, or coronary spasm in that location.[1] The presence of postinfarction angina means increased short-term and long-term mortality for the AMI patient.[2] In general, patients who develop spontaneous postinfarction angina early following the acute event should have cardiac catheterization and coronary arteriography to evaluate the need for and possibility of coronary angioplasty or, if necessary, coronary artery bypass graft surgery.[3]

It is difficult to distinguish postinfarction angina from extension of the underlying infarction. Infarct extension occurs in about 8 per cent of patients with AMI during the first 10 days.[4] Infarct extension is characterized by severe and prolonged chest discomfort, persistent ECG changes, and the reappearance of CK-MB in the patient's serum. Infarct extension leads to an increase in in-hospital mortality in the AMI setting. It appears to be more common in patients with diabetes, a previous MI, and an early-peaking CK-MB curve, and in obese females who have experienced a nontransmural infarction as their initial event.[5]

REFERENCES

1. Koiwaya, Y., Torii, S., Takeshita, A., Nakagaki, O., and Nakamura, M.: Post-infarction angina caused by coronary arterial spasm. Circulation 65:275, 1982.
2. Schuster, E.H., and Bulkley, B.H.: Early postinfarction angina. Ischemia at a distance and ischemia in the infarct zone. N. Engl. J. Med. 305:1101, 1981.
3. Epstein, S.E., Palmeri, S.T., and Patterson, R.E.: Evaluation of patients after acute myocardial infarction. Indications for cardiac catheterization and surgical intervention. N. Engl. J. Med. 307:1467, 1982.
4. Muller, J.E., Rude, R.E., Braunwald, E., Hartwell, T.D., Roberts, R., Sobel, B.E., Ritter, C., Parker, C.B., Jaffe, A.S., Stone, P.H., Raabe, D.S. Jr., Willerson, J.T., Robertson, T., and the MILIS study group: Myocardial infarct extension: Occurrence, outcome, and risk factors in the Multicenter Investigation of Limitation of Infarct Size. Ann. Intern. Med. 108:1, 1988.
5. Marmor, A., Sobel, B.E., and Roberts, E.: Factors presaging early recurrent myocardial ("extension"). Am. J. Cardiol. 48:603, 1981.

337   A-N, B-Y, C-N, D-Y, E-Y (Braunwald, p. 1507)

Because of the progressive nature of constrictive pericarditis, the majority of patients become symptomatic and come to medical attention due to weakness, peripheral edema, and/or ascites. The treatment for constrictive pericarditis is complete resection of the pericardium, including excision of the pericardium from the anterior and inferior surfaces of the RV as well as the diaphragmatic and anterolateral surfaces of the LV, extending upward to the great vessels and to or across the atrioventricular grooves. This procedure has been performed more successfully using an approach via median sternotomy rather than left thoracotomy and in patients who have had cardiopulmonary bypass to allow greater mobility of the heart.[1] In most series, the average operative mortality has ranged between 10 and 15 per cent, with a clear correlation between the degree of the functional disability before the operation and the survival following repair. Other factors that have an adverse influence upon overall outcome include diuretic use, renal insufficiency in the preoperative period, and a history of radiation pericarditis.[2]

It is generally agreed that patients should undergo pericardiectomy soon after the development of symptoms. Between 14 and 28 per cent of patients in the immediate postoperative period will develop a low-output syndrome. This occurs more commonly in patients with a marked degree of preoperative disability and high RV end-diastolic pressures, indicative of severe constriction.[3] Symptomatic improvement is seen in approximately 90 per cent of survivors of pericardiectomy, and 5-year survivals are in the 74 to 84 per cent range.

Patients with presumed tuberculosis pericarditis should receive a course of antituberculosis therapy before operation, which may be continued for 6 to 12 months after pericardiectomy if the diagnosis is confirmed. The time course for symptomatic improvement following pericardiectomy varies. Some patients may experience immediate decreases in symptomatology, while others may have a delayed or partial response that requires weeks or months for resolution of elevated jugular venous pressures and abnormal filling pressures.[4]

REFERENCES

1. Copeland, J.G., Stinson, E.B., Griepp, R.B., and Shumway, N.E.: Surgical treatment of chronic constrictive pericarditis using cardiopulmonary bypass. J. Thorac. Cardiovasc. Surg. 69:236, 1975.
2. Siefort, F.C., Miller, C.D., Oesterle, S.N., Oyer, P.E., Stinson, E.B., and Shumway, N.E.: Surgical treatment of constrictive pericarditis: Analysis of outcome and diagnostic error. Circulation 72(Suppl. II): 264, 1985.
3. McCaughlin, B.C., Schaff, H.V., Piehler, J.M., Danielson, G.K., Orszulak, T.A., Puga, F.J., Pluth, J.R., Connolly, D.C., and McGoon, D.C.: Early and late results of pericardiectomy for constrictive pericarditis. J. Thorac. Cardiovasc. Surg. 89:340, 1985.
4. Viola, A.R.: The influence of pericardiectomy on the hemodynamics of chronic constrictive pericarditis. Circulation 48:1038, 1973.

338 **A-Y, B-N, C-N, D-Y, E-Y** *(Braunwald, pp. 1442–1443)*

Many viruses can cause an associated myocarditis. The myocarditis characteristically develops after a lag period of several weeks following initial systemic infection, which suggests that the myocarditis is due to an immunological response. Coxsackie viruses, in particular Coxsackie B, are the agents most frequently associated with viral myocarditis. Echovirus, which is similar to the Coxsackie virus, is also associated with myopericarditis, frequently during the course of an acute pleurodynia-like illness.

Myocardial involvement during the course of mumps is rare, occurring in less than 10 per cent of adults affected with this virus, and even less frequently in children. Similarly, infectious mononucleosis is rarely associated with significant myocarditis. Neither variola nor vaccinia is associated with myocarditis. One-third of patients dying of influenza have associated myocarditis, indicating that cardiovascular involvement may be important in the mortality rate of this viral illness. Cardiac involvement occurs 1 to 2 weeks after the onset of the illness, manifested by signs and symptoms of congestive heart failure and pericarditis. Other viral illnesses in which myocarditis occurs include poliomyelitis and viral hepatitis, and illnesses involving the human immunodeficiency virus.

339 **A-Y, B-N, C-Y, D-Y, E-Y** *(Braunwald, pp. 1582–1583)*

While perfusion lung scanning is generally a useful diagnostic test in screening for pulmonary embolism, a number of ambiguities associated with this procedure limit its usefulness. The designations "low," "moderate," "high," and "indeterminate" for perfusion lung scans are widely used, but these categories have not been standardized by a national body or organization. In addition, while prospective studies comparing ventilation-perfusion lung scans with pulmonary angiograms have been carried out, the results have usually been challenged due to potential selection biases in the patient populations studied. A recently completed prospective investigation of the diagnosis of pulmonary embolism will attempt to provide this comparison in approximately 1000 patients. However, at the time of this writing the results of this analysis have not yet been released.

In general, patients with perfusion defects that are segmental or greater in size and with accompanying normal chest x-rays or normal ventilation scintigrams in the same areas as the perfusion defects have a high likelihood of embolism. Such high probability scans have been accurately correlated with positive pulmonary angiographic studies in between 66 and 86 per cent of cases.[1] The presence of chest x-ray abnormalities in the regions of the perfusion defect makes the designation of "indeterminate" probability necessary and not infrequently limits the usefulness of the perfusion lung scan. Low probability scans, in contrast, in which subsegmental and nonsegmental perfusion defects that may match ventilation defects are present, often are seen in conjunction with normal angiographic findings. In patients with low probability scans pulmonary angiography generally is not warranted, unless there is a high level of clinical suspicion.[2] In general, pulmonary angiography is reserved for patients with moderate probability or indeterminate lung scans or those in whom clinical suspicion remains high regardless of the perfusion lung scan findings.

REFERENCES

1. Hull, R.D., Hirsch, J., Carter, C.J., Raskob, G.E., Gill, G.J., Jay, R.M., Leclerc, J.R., David, M., and Coates, G.: Diagnostic value of ventilation-perfusion lung scanning in patients with suspected pulmonary embolism. Chest 88:819, 1985.

2. Cheely, R., McCartney, W.H., Perry, J.R., Delaney, D.J., Bustad, L., Wynia, V.H., and Griggs, T.R.: The role of non-invasive tests versus pulmonary angiography in the diagnosis of pulmonary embolism. Am. J. Med. 70:17, 1981.

340   A-Y, B-N, C-Y, D-Y, E-Y *(Braunwald, pp. 1157–1158)*

There has been a great deal of controversy over the levels of plasma cholesterol which are thought to be excessive for age and sex. A cholesterol consensus conference was held at the National Institutes of Health in 1984 to review the available data and establish new guidelines for defining hypercholesterolemia.[1] This panel concluded that the available evidence established beyond reasonable doubt that blood cholesterol levels in most Americans are undesirably high, in large part because of a high dietary intake of calories saturated with fat and cholesterol. They therefore recommended treatment of individuals with blood cholesterol levels above the 75th percentile of the current American reference values. Thus, the level of cholesterol at which treatment is deemed necessary was significantly lowered. On the basis of age-adjusted statistics, cholesterol values between the 75th and 90th percentiles were: for ages 20 to 29 values between 200 and 220, for ages 30 to 39 values between 220 and 240, and over the age of 40 values between 240 and 260. They further recommended that it was desirable for cholesterol concentrations of individuals *over the age of 30* to be *under 200 mg/dl* and for those under the age of 30 to be under 180 mg/dl. Thus, in the examples listed, a 19-year-old man with a cholesterol reading of 200 mg/dl would be in the 90th percentile and should be treated. A 30-year-old man with a reading of 200 is between the 50th and 75th percentile, a 45-year-old with a reading of 260 would be in the 90th percentile, as would a 60-year-old woman with the same reading, and a 30-year-old woman with a reading of 215 would be in the 90th percentile. Although diet frequently achieves only a 5 to 10 per cent reduction in cholesterol, this would be associated with a 10 to 20 per cent decrease in cardiovascular mortality.

REFERENCE

1. Consensus Conference Statement: Lowering blood cholesterol to prevent heart disease. J.A.M.A. 253:2080, 1985.

341   A-Y, B-Y, C-Y, D-N, E-Y *(Braunwald, pp. 1293–1294 and Fig. 38–46, p. 1294)*

In general, assessment of the patient recovering from acute MI in the weeks following the event may be accomplished by a combination of exercise testing and ambulatory ECG monitoring.[1] Before discharge, a submaximal exercise test is useful for screening for both ischemia and arrhythmias, which may identify such abnormalities even in patients who do not demonstrate such problems during their hospital course. It should be noted, however, that a maximal stress test, performed 4 to 6 weeks following such a submaximal test, will identify a number of additional patients with residual myocardial ischemia.[2] In either event, the presence of marked ST-segment abnormalities, the appearance of angina or dyspnea at low levels of exercise, and a fall in blood pressure during exercise are all associated with a poor prognosis.

One-year mortality is adversely and independently affected by two factors: (1) LV ejection fraction of less than 40 per cent and (2) the presence of electrical instability, defined as frequent, multiple, or complex ventricular extrasystoles.[3] Patients with ventricular ectopy during their hospital stay, or those with documented depressed LV dysfunction, are excellent candidates for ambulatory ECG monitoring before discharge. However, routine, uncomplicated MI in the absence of recurrent ischemia or documented LV dysfunction does not require routine ambulatory ECG monitoring. In patients in whom an assessment of LV function has not been obtained, the use of radionuclide ventriculography to measure ejection fraction may be of benefit. While this test is not routinely performed in the postinfarction patient, the presence of a marked fall in left ventricular ejection fraction during exercise should prompt the clinician to obtain coronary arteriography to assess the presence of residual myocardium at ischemic risk.

REFERENCES

1. Madsen, E.B., Hougaard, P., and Gilpin, E.: Dynamic evaluation of prognosis from time-dependent variables in acute myocardial infarction. Am. J. Cardiol. 51:1579, 1983.
2. Starling, M.R., Crawford, M.H., Kennedy, D.T., and O'Rourke, R.A.: Treadmill exercise tests predischarge and 6 weeks post myocardial infarction to detect abnormalities of known prognostic value. Ann. Intern. Med. 94:721, 1981.
3. Moss, A.J., Bigger, J.T., Case, R.B., Gillespie, J., Goldstein, R., Greenberg, H., Krone, R., Marcus, F.I., Odoroff, C.L., and Oliver, G.C.: Risk stratification and prognostication after myocardial infarction. J. Am. Coll. Cardiol. 1:716, 1983.

342   A-N, B-Y, C-N, D-Y, E-N *(Braunwald, pp. 1050–1057)*

The valve depicted in *A* is a stenotic aortic valve with three cusps. This is the most common form of aortic stenosis in the elderly and is an acquired type of aortic stenosis. If the valve illustrated were bicuspid (in which the cusps are situated anteriorly and posteriorly with commissures on either side), it would be a congenital defect. In acquired aortic stenosis, years of normal mechanical stress on the valve are thought to result in degenerative calcification. It is likely that the valve illustrated had suffered damage secondary to rheumatic fever because fusion of the commissures and development of calcific nodules on the cusps as shown are typical of rheumatic valvular disease. Because the apposition of the valve leaflets is otherwise good, it is unlikely that this individual had significant aortic regurgitation. Endocarditis would be unlikely to result in aortic stenosis of this type. Both diabetes mellitus and hypercholesterolemia increase the risk of aortic valve calcifications. Patients with tricuspid aortic valves with commissural fusion are excellent candidates for balloon valvuloplasty as shown in the accompanying photograph (*B*), which demonstrates reopening of the valve following balloon valvuloplasty (in this case, in vitro).

343   A-Y, B-Y, C-N, D-Y, E-N *(Braunwald, p. 1396)*

Prior to any patient's embarking on an exercise program, a careful clinical examination is necessary; the severity and duration of specific underlying disorders may require special attention. In general, the presence of a poorly controlled systemic disease, an unstable condition, or any acute illness carries an unacceptable risk with exertional activities. Several specific cardiovascular contraindications to exercise exist. Among these are resting blood pressure greater than 200/110 mm Hg, unpaced third-degree heart block, left ventricular outflow tract obstruction, cardiomyopathy, unstable ischemic syndromes including myocardial infarction, significant arrhythmias, active myocarditis within the last year, recent thromboembolic disorders, and aortic dissection.[1] It should be noted that while patients with underlying disorders of a more chronic nature may require special attention, such disorders rarely prohibit the patient from undertaking any physical exertion. Thus, patients with conditions such as diabetes, renal disease, anemia, obstructive lung disease, and orthopedic disabilities may perform rehabilitation programs with appropriate supervision.

Cardiac rehabilitation is especially useful in patients who have undergone recent coronary artery bypass grafting, although those who do exhibit sternal instability after such a procedure should be prohibited from performing exercise involving the upper extremities or trunk.[2] The specific medical regimen that the patient brings to the rehabilitation program should also be known so that potential side effects of underlying medications may be taken into consideration. For example, individuals on anticoagulation must be observed carefully to avoid local trauma, and insulin-dependent diabetics must be made aware that their insulin requirements may decrease with the exercise program. It should be noted that even though beta blockers alter the heart rate for given exercise intensities, the net effect of training is preserved in patients on such medications.[3]

REFERENCES

1. Council on Scientific Affairs: Physician-supervised exercise programs in rehabilitation of patients with coronary heart disease. J.A.M.A. 245:1463, 1981.
2. Metier, C.P., Pollock, M.L., and Graves, J.E.: Exercise prescription for the coronary artery bypass graft surgery patient. Journal of Cardiac Rehabilitation 6:85, 1986.
3. Beta blockers and exercise: A symposium. *In* Harrison, D.C. (ed.) Am. J. Cardiol. 55:167D-171D, 1985.

344   A-N, B-N, C-Y, D-N, E-Y *(Braunwald, pp. 1380–1387)*

In the past decade, the technology of PTCA for coronary arterial stenoses has evolved to the point that complex distal and multiple lesions may be treated. Lesions that involve coronary bifurcations may be approached using either two wires or two angioplasty balloons in order to prevent the occurrence of a "snow plow" occlusion of the side branch, which may complicate 14 per cent of such dilatations.[1] In addition, totally occluded coronary arteries may be reopened with PTCA, especially if the occlusion is relatively fresh. Approximately 75 per cent of occlusions of less than 3 months' duration may be reopened, whereas fewer than 50 per cent of occlusions that are older than 3 months of age are successfully dilated.[2]

While the procedure is more difficult, PTCA for multivessel coronary artery disease has really evolved as an alternative to bypass surgery. In general, PTCA in a patient with multivessel disease is designed to dilate all lesions with a 70 per cent or greater stenosis. In cases in which a stenosis remains that is 70 per cent or more in a vessel that is not dilated, a significantly greater chance for the development of recurrent angina exists (see Braunwald, Fig. 40–9, p. 1384). While a carefully controlled comparison between PTCA and bypass surgery has been begun, known as the Bypass Angioplasty Revascularization Intervention (BARI), this trial has not as of this writing been completed. No conclusions are possible regarding the *relative* efficacies of these two therapeutic options at this time. In addition to its application to more difficult anatomical problems, PTCA has also been used recently in unstable angina. Fifty to 75 per cent of patients with unstable angina may be anatomically suitable for PTCA, and this technique may also be used in the early postinfarction period.[3]

REFERENCES

1. Meier, B., Gruentzig, A.R., King, S.B., Douglas, J.S., Hollman, J., Ischinger, T., Aueron, F., and Galan, K.: Risk of side branch occlusion during coronary angioplasty. Am. J. Cardiol. 53:10, 1984.
2. Kereiakes, D.J., Selmon, M.R., McAuley, B.J., McAuley, D.B., Sheehan, D.J., and Simpson, J.B.: Angioplasty of total coronary occlusion: Experience in 76 consecutive patients. J. Am. Coll. Cardiol. 6:526, 1985.
3. De Feyter, P.J., Serruys, P.W., Van den Brand, M., Balakumaran, K., Mochtar, B., Soward, A.L., Arnold, A.E.R., and Hugenholtz, P.G.: Emergency coronary angioplasty in refractory unstable angina. N. Engl. J. Med. 313:342, 1985.

345   A-Y, B-Y, C-N, D-N, E-N *(Braunwald, pp. 1490–1491)*

Initial management of acute pericarditis should begin with an attempt to detect any underlying causes of the inflammatory process which might be amenable to specific therapy. Patients who have pain and fever during an acute phase of pericarditis should be placed on bed rest, since activity may lead to an increase or worsening of symptoms. In general such patients should be hospitalized, to exclude the possibility of an associated MI as well as to watch for the development of tamponade and to rule out any possibility that the pericarditis is due to an acute pyogenic process.

Treatment of the chest pain associated with pericarditis usually begins with a nonsteroidal antiinflammatory agent such as aspirin or indomethacin. If patients fail to respond to such measures after 48 hours and pain remains severe, corticosteroid therapy may be employed using larger doses of prednisone, such as 60 to 80 mg daily in divided doses over 5 to 7 days. If symptoms subsequently abate during this time, the steroids may be tapered. Antibiotic therapy is reserved for patients who have documented purulent pericarditis. Oral anticoagulants should *not* be administered during the acute phase of pericarditis of any cause because of the increased possibility of resulting hemopericardium. Patients with acute pericarditis who require anticoagulant therapy for the presence of a prosthetic heart valve, for example, should be given intravenous heparin as their anticoagulant therapy in order to allow for prompt reversal with protamine should any difficulties arise. Such patients require close monitoring with both physical examination and echocardiography in order to detect the early development or accumulation of pericardial fluid.

346   A-Y, B-Y, C-N, D-N, E-Y *(Braunwald, pp. 1026–1029)*

The clinical and hemodynamic features of MS of any given severity are dictated largely by levels of cardiac output and pulmonary vascular resistance. Several clinical features nonetheless are commonly present in all patients. First, women tend to be affected more commonly than men. S_1 is usually loud, unless sufficient calcification and fibrosis have occurred to decrease the mobility of the valve. This is in contrast to mitral regurgitation in which the first heart sound is usually diminished. An S_3 is rarely heard in pure MS since ventricular filling is slow and the LV wall has normal compliance. The presence of S_3 is an indication of coexisting cardiomyopathy or regurgitant lesion. The left ventricle in MS usually has normal or slow filling due to the impaired flow of blood across the stenotic mitral valve. Thus, a presystolic lift or a presystolic wave is highly unlikely to be found on physical examination in MS. The LV is rarely hyperdynamic and is usually normal in size.

The hallmark of MS is the presence of a presystolic murmur in patients in sinus rhythm because transvalvular blood flow is accelerated by atrial contraction. Such a murmur may also occur in patients with atrial fibrillation due to increased blood flow velocity across a mitral valve orifice that begins to narrow after the onset of LV contraction. Conditions other than MS that may mimic the crescendo presystolic murmur include aortic regurgitation, in which an Austin-Flint murmur may extend to S_1. In a hypertrophied restrictive ventricle the combination of S_3 and S_4 may be loud enough to simulate a presystolic murmur. In both tricuspid stenosis and left atrial myxoma a narrowed orifice may contribute to a crescendo presystolic murmur.

347   A-Y, B-Y, C-N, D-Y, E-N *(Braunwald, pp. 1498–1499)*

Preparation of patients for pericardiocentesis should include administration of intravascular fluids to allow for volume expansion and thus to delay the appearance of right ventricular diastolic collapse and subsequent hemodynamic deterioration. The major risk of percutaneous cardiocentesis is laceration of the heart or great vessels. The use of a subxyphoid approach under fluoroscopic guidance in the catheterization laboratory has greatly decreased the likelihood of such complications. In the large series describing the Stanford experience,[1] pericardial fluid was obtained in more than 80 per cent of patients studied. Of note, the probability of successfully obtaining such fluid was directly proportional to the size of the pericardial effusion present. Fluid was obtained in 93 per cent of patients with effusions present both anteriorly and posteriorly on echocardiogram but in only 58 per cent of those with an isolated small posterior effusion.

Cardiac tamponade associated with malignant effusions or with prior radiation therapy can often be managed using pericardiocentesis in combination with local or systemic chemotherapy and may therefore allow patients with end-stage disease to avoid the stress of major surgery. Certain situations make pericardiocentesis either more complicated or less likely to succeed. These include acute traumatic hemopericardium in which blood continues to enter the pericardial space rapidly, small pericardial effusions such as those that are solely posterior, the presence of clot and fibrin in the pericardial space, and the presence of a loculated effusion.

REFERENCE

1. Krikorian, J.G., and Hancock, E.W.: Pericardiocentesis. Am. J. Med. 65:808, 1978.

348   A-Y, B-N, C-N, D-Y, E-Y *(Braunwald, pp. 1342–1345)*

Improved long-term success in coronary artery bypass surgery has been associated with use of the internal mammary artery (IMA). The primary reason for the increased utilization of this vessel is that many studies have shown that the IMA is remarkably free of atheroma at baseline, and has a markedly diminished capacity to develop intimal hyperplasia, unlike saphenous vein grafts. Thus the patency of the IMA graft averages about 90 per cent at 1 year. Recent data have shown that after 7 to 10 years the patency of such grafts is 85 to 95 per cent.[1] Furthermore, the long-term survival of patients with IMA grafts is better for a given LV function than for patients who have received only saphenous vein grafts. Although the diameter of the IMA is considerably smaller than of a saphenous vein graft, it is more closely matched to the coronary artery. Although total flow through an IMA graft is less than through a vein graft, the velocity of flow may be greater because of the smaller diameter of the IMA.

Long-term patency of grafts is determined by multiple factors. Primary among these are the extent of coronary arterial run-off as determined by the diameter of the coronary artery into which the graft is inserted and the size of the distal vascular bed, and to a lesser degree the severity of coronary atherosclerosis distal to the site of insertion of the graft. With regard to vein grafts, in some studies it has been shown that the flow rates shortly after operation are prognostic. In optimal cases, blood flow averages 70 ml/min while those in which the flow is less than 45 ml/min and especially less than 25 ml/min are more frequently associated with graft closure.[2] Future efforts will be directed to inhibiting the mechanisms responsible for intimal hyperplasia and development of atherosclerosis in vein grafts.

REFERENCES

1. Grondin, C.M., Campeau, L., Lesperance, J., Enjalber, T.M., and Bourassa, M.G.: Comparison of late changes in internal mammary artery in saphenous vein grafts in two consecutive series of patients 10 years after operation. Circulation 70(Suppl. I): 208, 1984.
2. Grondin, C.M., Lapage, G., Castoguay, Y.R., Meere, C., and Grondin, P.: Aortocoronary bypass graft. Initial blood flow through the graft, and early postoperative patency. Circulation 44:815, 1971.

349   A-Y, B-N, C-N, D-Y, E-Y (Braunwald, p. 1489)

Acute pericarditis is believed to cause an actual current of injury by a superficial myocardial or epicardial inflammatory process and leads to electrocardiographic changes that may be extremely useful in confirming the diagnosis. Four stages of abnormalities of the ST segments and T waves may be distinguished in classic acute pericarditis (see Braunwald, Fig. 44–5 and Table 44–3, p. 1489). The first stage of ECG changes is virtually diagnostic of acute pericarditis. This change includes ST-segment elevation, in which the segment is concave upward; this occurs in all leads except aV_r and V_1.[1] The T waves during this stage are usually upright. PR-segment depression occurs early in acute pericarditis in approximately 80 per cent of patients.[2] The return of ST segments to baseline, accompanied by T-wave flattening, comprises stage II and usually is seen before the occurrence of T-wave inversion. This should be contrasted with the early evolution of T-wave changes in acute MI. The third electrocardiographic stage of acute pericarditis is characterized by inversion of the T waves, so that the T-wave vector is directed opposite to that of the ST segment. The fourth and final stage represents reversion of the T-wave changes to normal and may occur between weeks and months following the acute event.

While all four stages are detected in approximately half of patients with acute pericarditis, about 90 per cent of patients will demonstrate some electrocardiographic abnormalities that allow characterization of an acute chest pain episode as pericarditis. It should be noted that stage I changes of pericarditis must be differentiated from normal early repolarization. In this regard, an ST-segment:T-wave ratio greater than 0.25 in lead V_6 has been noted to be more consistent with acute pericarditis while a ratio less than 0.25 is more suggestive of normal early repolarization.[3]

REFERENCES

1. Surawicz, B., and Lasseter, K.C.: Electrocardiogram in pericarditis. Am. J. Cardiol. 26:471, 1970.
2. Spodick, D.H.: Diagnostic electrocardiographic sequences in acute pericarditis: Significance of PR segment and PR vector changes. Circulation 48:575, 1973.
3. Ginzton, L.E., and Laks, M.M.: The differential diagnosis of acute pericarditis. Circulation 65:1004, 1982.

350   A-Y, B-Y, C-N, D-Y, E-N (Braunwald, p. 1055 and Fig. 33–28, p. 1058)

Although AS in adults has a long latent period some symptoms eventually develop, most commonly in the sixth decade of life. The most frequent symptoms consist of angina pectoris, syncope, and heart failure. When symptoms become manifested, prognosis for untreated AS is poor; survival curves show that the interval from the onset of symptoms to the time of death is approximately 5 years for patients with angina, 3 years in those with syncope, and 2 years in patients with heart failure.[1] Angina is present in approximately two-thirds of patients with critical AS and associated with coronary artery disease in approximately 50 per cent. In these patients angina may be due to associated coronary artery disease, but in general it is caused by a combination of increased oxygen needs of the hypertrophied myocardium and a reduction of oxygen delivery due to excessive compression of the coronary vessels during diastole.

Syncope is usually orthostatic and occurs most commonly following exertion. Most commonly it is due to reduced cerebral perfusion caused by systemic vasodilatation in the presence of a fixed cardiac output. Sudden death occurs with increased frequency in patients with critical AS and almost invariably in those who have been previously symptomatic. Asymptomatic patients frequently present during an episode of transient atrial fibrillation. Because of the decrease in diastolic compliance of the hypertrophied ventricle these patients are critically dependent upon the atrial contraction to deliver appropriate preload and to maintain cardiac output. Thus, when atrial fibrillation (AF) develops, these patients may have impaired filling of the LV with a decrease in cardiac output and tolerate AF poorly. Also, an increased ventricular rate during AF further compromises diastolic filling of coronary arteries leading to impaired cardiac performance.

REFERENCE

1. Frank, S., Johnson, A., and Ross, J., Jr.: Natural history of valvular aortic stenosis. Br. Heart J. 35:41, 1973.

351   A-Y, B-Y, C-N, D-Y, E-Y (Braunwald, pp. 1354–1355)

Coronary arteriographic findings in patients with unstable angina have generally shown the same distribution of disease as in patients with chronic angina pectoris, although there is usually a higher incidence of severe obstructive three-vessel disease and left main coronary artery disease.[1] The left anterior descending coronary artery is the most commonly affected vessel in patients with unstable (as well as chronic stable) angina.[2]

It has recently become clear that the morphology and histology of coronary artery lesions associated with unstable angina are characteristic of this clinical syndrome. In stable angina, stenoses usually have smooth borders, an hourglass shape, and no intraluminal lucencies. In contrast, patients with unstable angina often exhibit lesions with irregular borders which are likely to rupture and intraluminal lucencies that represent partially occlusive thrombus.[3]

It is clear that eccentric lesions with filling defects represent "active" coronary lesions. In patients with known coronary anatomy who were restudied after an episode of unstable angina, it appeared that acute progression of a previously insignificant lesion had occurred in most instances with appearance of an eccentric lesion.[4] Thus it is clear that unstable angina represents an acute progressive illness of the coronary artery, both clinically and histopathologically associated with an increased incidence of thrombosis, plaque hemorrhage, and vasospasm. Therapeutic efforts should be directed at all three of these pathogenic processes.

REFERENCES

1. Alison, H.W., Russell, R.O., Jr., Mantle, J.A., Kouchoukos, N.T., and Rackley, C.E.: Coronary anatomy and arteriography in patients with unstable angina pectoris. Am. J. Cardiol. 41:204, 1978.
2. Roberts, W.C., and Virmani, Z.: Quantitation of coronary arterial narrowing in clinically isolated unstable angina pectoris: An analysis of 22 necropsy patients. Am. J. Med. 67:792, 1979.
3. Ambrose, J.A., Winters, S.L., Arora, R.R., Eng, A., Riccio, A., Gorlin, R., and Fuster, V.: Angiographic evolution of coronary artery morphology in unstable angina. J. Am. Coll. Cardiol. 7:472, 1986.
4. Moise, A., Theroux, P., Taeymans, Y., Descoings, B., Lesperance, J., Waters, D.D., Pelletier, G.B., and Bourassa, M.G.: Unstable angina and progression of coronary atherosclerosis. N. Engl. J. Med. 309:685, 1983.

352   A-Y, B-N, C-N, D-N, E-Y (Braunwald, pp. 1521–1522)

Distinction is made between acute postinfarction pericarditis occurring during the first week following acute myocardial infarction (AMI) and the Dressler, or postmyocardial infarction, syndrome. This usually occurs 2 to 3 weeks following infarction and may appear from a week to several months following infarction. Original reports of this syndrome indicated that it occurred in approximately 4 per cent of patients following AMI, although more recent series indicate that the incidence has decreased substantially.[1] This syndrome is of unknown etiology and is marked by an acute febrile illness with associated pericarditis and pleuritis. Some evidence exists for an autoimmune mechanism, and a role for antimyocardial antibodies has been suggested in the past; however, the cause of this disorder remains unknown. Some investigators have concluded that the development of myocardial antibodies is not specific for this condition.[2]

The pericardium in this disorder undergoes a nonspecific inflammation which is usually diffuse in nature and characteristically leads to fibrin desposition. Clinical features of this disorder usually include a severe febrile illness characterized by malaise and dramatic chest pain with or without pleurisy. The chest discomfort may be severe enough on presentation to cause consideration of recurrent MI. Physical examination usually discloses a pericardial friction rub, and chest x-ray often reveals an enlarged cardiac silhouette. Electrocardiographic changes typical of acute pericarditis are frequently present as well, although the ECG may not be as helpful in patients who have sustained permanent ST-segment and T-wave abnormalities due to the recent MI.

The syndrome tends to be self-limited but may recur. Observation in a hospital setting is usually warranted to monitor for the possible development of pericardial effusion and/or cardiac tamponade, as well as to clearly distinguish between the chest discomfort of Dressler's syndrome and recurrent ischemia. Discontinuation of oral anticoagulants and therapy with aspirin or a nonsteroidal antiinflammatory agent of choice are both recommended.

REFERENCES

1. Lichstein, E., Arsura, E., Hollander, G., Greengart, A., and Sanders, M.: Current incidence of postmyocardial infarction (Dressler's) syndrome. Am. J. Cardiol. 50:1269, 1982.
2. Liem, K.L., ten Veen, J.H., Lie, K.I., Feltkamp, T.E.W., and Durrer, D.: Incidence and significance of heart muscle antibodies in patients with acute myocardial infarction and unstable angina. Acta Med. Scand. 206:473, 1971.

353   A-Y, B-Y, C-N, D-Y, E-Y (Braunwald, p. 1420)

Asymmetric septal hypertrophy most commonly refers to the presence of an abnormally thickened intraventricular septum compared with the left ventricular free wall, which is frequently familial and associated with disarray of ventricular septal myocardial fibers. However, echocardiographically, disproportionate septal hypertrophy may be documented in several other situations. In neonates and infants the predominance of the right ventricle relative to the left ventricle may result in the appearance of an enlarged ventricular septum.[1] This usually disappears by the age of 1 to 2 years. However, in individuals with other etiologies for right ventricular pressure overload, such as pulmonic stenosis or primary pulmonary hypertension, there may be persistent septal hypertrophy. Abnormal thickness of the septum relative to the free wall may also occur in coronary artery disease; for example, following infarction of the free wall there may be compensatory hypertrophy of the septum and inferior wall.[2] Other conditions that may present similar patterns of disproportionate septal hypertrophy include lentiginosis, Turner's syndrome, hyper- and hypothyroidism, hyperparathyroidism, and Friedreich's ataxia.[1, 3] Although beriberi may be associated with dilated cardiomyopathy, it is not usually associated with asymmetric septal hypertrophy.

REFERENCES

1. Larter, W.E., Allen, H.D., Sahn, D.J., and Goldberg, S.J.: The asymmetrically hypertrophied septum. Further differentiation of its causes. Circulation 53:19, 1976.
2. Maron, B.J., Savage, D.D., Clark, C.E., Henry, W.L., Vlodaver, Z., Edwards, J.E., and Epstein, S.E.: Prevalence and characteristics of disproportionate ventricular septal thickening in patients with coronary artery disease. Circulation 57:250, 1978.
3. Wilson, R., Gibson, T.C., Terrien, C.M., Jr., and Levy, A.M.: Hyperthyroidism and familial hypertrophic cardiomyopathy. Arch. Intern. Med. 143:378, 1983.

354   A-Y, B-N, C-Y, D-N (Braunwald, pp. 1542–1543)

Penetrating chest wounds, whether due to gunshots or stabbings, frequently involve damage to cardiac structures. All of these injuries are associated with significant bleeding into the pericardial space, as well as intramyocardial hemorrhage. Thus, post-traumatic pericarditis symptoms are common. Although these are not functionally limiting, they are nonetheless associated with a pericardial type of pain. Because the ventricles are larger than the atria, they are more commonly involved in penetrating wounds. However, survival is better with injuries to the ventricles than the atria. Wounds involving thin-walled structures such as the atria and pulmonary artery rarely seal off spontaneously and therefore are associated with more bleeding and volume loss. Because of this acute complication, delay in performing a thoracotomy in patients with rapidly developing tamponade and excessive pericardial bleeding is ill-advised. A late complication of penetrating chest wounds is rupture of the interventricular septum, although frequently these defects are of minor hemodynamic significance. Laceration of the coronary artery is also a common occurrence with penetrating chest wounds, and because of its anterior location, the left coronary artery is most commonly involved. Following laceration of a coronary artery, myocardial infarction frequently develops even if rapid reanastomosis is performed.

355   A-Y, B-N, C-Y, D-N, E-N (Braunwald, pp. 1327–1330)

Nitrates are important agents for treatment of ischemic heart disease. They directly relax vascular smooth muscle by activating intracellular guanylate cyclase and causing an increase in cyclic guanosine monophosphate, which triggers smooth muscle relaxation. It is also possible that nitrates may activate the vasodilator prostaglandin system (PGI_2). Nitrates act directly on smooth muscle and therefore do not require an intact endothelium. The vasodilating effect of nitrates is present in both arteries and veins but appears to predominate in the venous circulation. The decrease in venous tone lessens the return of blood to the heart and reduces preload and ventricular dimensions, which in turn diminishes wall tension. As well as decreasing wall tension and myocardial oxygen demand, nitrates also increase oxygen supply by dilating coronary arteries. This dilatation is also present in vessels containing atherosclerotic plaques, presumably because the pathological atherosclerotic changes are eccentric and normal vascular smooth muscle, which can respond to nitrates, is present in a portion of the plaque. Quantitation of the direct vasodilatory effect of nitrates on coronary vessels has been performed by intracoronary administration and a direct effect of varying magnitude has been universally demonstrated.

356   A-Y, B-N, C-Y, D-Y, E-N (Braunwald, pp. 1106–1107)

This woman presents with a classic history for the development of an intracardiac abscess involving the aortic valvular ring. The following criteria have been found to be of value in the diagnosis of abscess of the valvular ring: (1) infection of the aortic valve, (2) recent appearance of regurgitation, (3) presence of pericarditis, (4) atrioventricular block, and (5) short duration of symptoms followed by rapid severe disability and death.[1] This woman's case satisfies several of these criteria including

early postoperative development of a diastolic murmur, most likely due to aortic regurgitation and the development of first-degree atrioventricular block.

Treatment of these patients usually involves early operation because of the inability of antibiotics to eradicate the infection. Nonetheless, initial antibiotic management should cover the organisms known to be involved in early prosthetic valve endocarditis. Since there is a high incidence of *Staphylococcus epidermidis*, empirical therapy should include vancomycin and aminoglycosides. Nonetheless, *Staph. aureus* is the most common cause of cardiac abscess in early prosthetic valvular endocarditis and would be the most likely organism to be isolated from blood cultures.

The appearance of right bundle branch block is unlikely in this setting. In general, bundle branch block occurs with infections that are located in the lower part of the interventricular septum, such as those associated with mitral valve infection. However, these infections usually cause *left* rather than right bundle branch block.[2]

REFERENCES

1. Arnett, E.N., and Roberts, W.C.: Valve ring abscess in active infective endocarditis. Frequency, location and clues to clinical diagnosis from the study of 95 necropsy patients. Circulation 54:140, 1976.
2. Gopalakrishna, K.V., Kwan, K., and Shah, A.: Metastatic myocardial abscess due to group F streptococci. Am. J. Med. Sci. 274:329, 1977.

357   A-N, B-N, C-Y, D-N, E-Y (Braunwald, pp. 1127–1128)

Patients at risk for endocarditis in general include those with congenital heart disease both before and after operation, with mitral valve prolapse who have significant mitral regurgitation, with rheumatic valvular heart disease and other acquired forms of valvular disease, with hypertrophic obstructive cardiomyopathy, with a history of infective endocarditis, with transvenous pacemakers, with ventriculoatrial shunts for hydrocephalus, and renal dialysis patients with shunts. Patients at particularly high risk are those with prosthetic valves, conduits, patches, and surgically created shunts. Patients who ordinarily do *not* require prophylaxis are those with isolated ostium secundum ASD, patients more than 6 months after repair of such a defect without a patch, patients more than 6 months after ligation of a patent ductus arteriosus, and patients following coronary artery bypass surgery.

The prophylactic antibiotic regimen is determined by the organisms likely to be encountered and also by the potential risk. Thus, patients with prosthetic valves, conduits, patches, and shunts are at much higher risk and should receive an intravenous antibiotic regimen whenever possible.[1]

REFERENCE

1. Kaplan, E.L., and Anthony, B.F.: Prevention of bacterial endocarditis. Circulation 56:139A, 1977.

358   A-N, B-Y, C-Y, D-N, E-N (*Braunwald, pp. 1422–1423*)

In patients with hypertrophic obstructive cardiomyopathy (HOCM) the physical examination may be quite variable. However, the apical precordial impulse is usually abnormally prominent. Because of decreased diastolic compliance, a prominent presystolic apical impulse is frequently felt, which correlates with the presence of a prominent *a* wave in the jugular venous pulse. A more characteristic but less frequently recognized abnormality is a triple apical impulse, a third impulse being a late systolic bulge associated with end-systolic contraction. A systolic murmur along the lower left sternal border is frequently present. The murmur of mitral regurgitation in association with systolic anterior motion of the mitral valve is also common. However, the murmur of aortic regurgitation is very rare without coexisting aortic valve disease or following an episode of infective endocarditis. An S_3 is frequently audible because these patients are usually young and because there is rapid ventricular filling.

It is important to emphasize the features of physical examination that permit differentiation of HOCM from fixed aortic valve disease. The character of the carotid pulse is the most useful feature in this regard.[1] In aortic stenosis there is obstruction to left ventricular emptying from the beginning of systole, causing the carotid upstroke to be slowed and of low amplitude (pulsus parvus et tardus). With HOCM, however, initial ejection of blood from the left ventricle is unimpeded and in fact is more robust than usual. Therefore, the arterial upstroke initially is brisk, followed by a more sustained plateau, giving rise to the classic "spike-and-dome" configuration.

REFERENCE

1. Maron, B.J., Wolfson, J.K., Ciro, E., and Spirito, P.: Relation of electrocardiographic abnormalities and patterns of left ventricular hypertrophy identified by two-dimensional echocardiography in patients with hypertrophic cardiomyopathy. Am. J. Cardiol. 51:189, 1983.

359   A-Y, B-Y, C-N, D-Y, E-N (*Braunwald, p. 1212*)

Among the various mechanisms potentially responsible for tissue damage following ischemia and reperfusion are oxygen-derived free radicals. Under normal conditions, oxygen free radicals are not normally found in the cell in significant concentrations. These molecules are characterized by an odd number of electrons, which makes them chemically reactive. There are three principal oxygen radicals: the superoxide anion ($\cdot O_2^-$), hydrogen peroxide (H_2O_2), and the hydroxyl radical ($\cdot OH$). During severe ischemia, several mechanisms appear to increase the production of oxygen radicals: dissociation of intramitochondrial electron transport, ischemia-induced calcium influx activating arachidonic acid metabolism, ischemia converting the normal myocardial enzyme xanthine dehydrogenase to xanthine oxidase (which in the presence of xanthine produces oxygen radicals), and activation of complement with accumulation of neutrophils, which release oxygen radicals.[1, 2]

These radicals damage cell membranes by a variety of mechanisms, impair cell enzymes, and contribute to cell death. The superoxide anion can be dismutated to hydrogen peroxide by the superoxide dismutase enzymes. Hydrogen peroxide then may be converted via catalase and other peroxidases to O_2 and thereby deactivated. However, the superoxide anion can also, in the presence of iron, be converted to the hydroxyl radical, which is a potent oxidizing species. Thus, interventions directed at preventing oxygen-derived free radical injury have focused on administration of superoxide dismutase to convert these radicals to hydrogen peroxide followed by antioxidant treatment to convert the H_2O_2 to oxygen. Furthermore, administration of xanthine oxidase inhibitors to prevent this enzyme's action has been suggested. Finally, limiting iron availability and iron-containing enzyme availability to convert the superoxide anion to the hydroxyl radical has also been suggested. Currently, several clinical trials are under way to investigate the efficacy of these measures to limit oxygen free radicals in terms of myocardial protection during reperfusion.

REFERENCES

1. Hammond, B., and Hess, M.L.: The oxygen free radical system: Potential mediator of myocardial injury. J. Am. Coll. Cardiol. 6:215, 1985.
2. Rossen, R.D., Swain, J.L., Michael, L.H., Weakley, S., Giannini, E., and Entman, M.L.: Selective accumulation of the first component of complement and leukocytes in ischemic canine heart muscle. Circ. Res. 57:119, 1985.

360   A-Y, B-Y, C-N, D-Y, E-N (*Braunwald, p. 1317*)

The classic teaching with regard to the etiology of angina is that the pain is related to an increase in myocardial oxygen demands, most commonly brought about by physical activity. Thus, a variety of factors which increase metabolic demands—such as fever, thyrotoxicosis, tachycardia from any cause, severe anemia, and physical exertion in the presence of underlying fixed coronary artery disease—result in an increase in oxygen demand and an inability in the presence of fixed and limited oxygen supply to meet myocardial oxygen needs. However, it has become increasingly evident that angina may also be caused by transient reductions of oxygen supply as a consequence of coronary vasoconstriction.[1] There is a reciprocal relationship between the severity of dynamic and organic obstruction required to cause myocardial ischemia. Thus, in the occasional patient with no organic lesions, only severe dynamic obstruction such as occurs with Prinzmetal's angina can cause myocardial ischemia and result in angina. On the other hand, in patients with subcritical severe fixed obstructions, a minor increase in dynamic constriction results in myocardial ischemia.

These changes in coronary vascular tone are particularly prominent in patients with so-called variable-threshold angina. These patients frequently have "good days," in which they are capable of substantial physical activity, and "bad days," when owing to alterations in coronary artery tone insignificant stimuli can cause large changes in dynamic obstruction. Patients with variable-threshold angina frequently complain of angina precipitated by cold temperature, emotion, and meals and also of angina occurring at rest or nocturnally.[2] Hemodynamic observations in these patients show that an increase in either peripheral resistance or coronary artery resistance probably explains the dynamic nature of their ischemia. Thus, it has been shown that cold induces direct coronary vasoconstriction as well as increasing peripheral resistance. Similarly, these patients are more prone to develop angina in the morning than in the afternoon, which correlates with the angiographic finding of smaller coronary artery diameter in the morning.[3]

In contrast, patients with fixed-threshold angina usually have a very characteristic level of physical activity (a reflection of myocardial oxygen consumption) required to precipitate angina. These patients have very reproduceable pressure-rate products that result in angina and/or electrocardiographic evidence of ischemia. In general, patients with fixed-threshold angina benefit from drugs that decrease maximum heart rate, such as beta blockers, while those with variable angina do better with agents directed at reducing coronary artery tone, such as calcium channel blockers and nitrates. At this time there are no clear data indicating whether or not a higher incidence of MI or worse outcome occurs in patients with variable-threshold angina.

REFERENCES

1. Epstein, S.E., and Talbot, T.L.: Dynamic coronary tone in precipitation, exacerbation and relief of angina pectoris. Am. J. Cardiol. 48:797, 1981.
2. Schiffer, F., Hartley, L.W., Schulman, C.L., and Abelmann, W.H.: Evidence for emotionally induced coronary artery spasm in patients with angina pectoris. Br. Heart J. 44:62, 1980.
3. Yasue, H.: Pathophysiology and treatment of coronary arterial spasm. Chest 78:216, 1980.

361   A-N, B-Y, C-N, D-N, E-Y (Braunwald, pp. 1431–1434)

Amyloidosis may occur in one of three clinical pathological forms: acquired systemic amyloidosis, organ-limited amyloidosis, and localized deposition. Three forms of acquired systemic amyloidosis are commonly described: those associated with an immunocyte dyscrasia (e.g., multiple myeloma), reactive (e.g., due to chronic infectious or inflammatory conditions), and heredofamilial. Three different forms of heredofamilial disorder exist, depending upon the principal organ system involved: nephropathic, neuropathic, and cardiopathic. An organ-limited form of amyloidosis common with aging is also seen, termed senile amyloidosis. Cardiac amyloidosis of a significant extent is almost unique to the immunocyte dyscrasias. In reactive amyloidosis such as occurs with rheumatoid arthritis, tuberculosis, and endocarditis, clinically significant cardiac involvement is uncommon.[1] In these cases, myocardial deposits are typically small and perivascular and usually do not result in significant myocardial dysfunction. In familial amyloidosis, cardiac involvement is seen only in the cardiopathic form and even here it usually occurs only late in the course of the disease. In senile amyloidosis cardiac involvement is

common but usually not significant, most often including small atrial deposits and deposits in the aorta. Cardiac amyloidosis occurs more commonly in men than in women, and is rare before the age of 30 years. Even in the familial form, the onset of clinical cardiac disease usually is not noted before the age of 35.

REFERENCE

1. Glenner, G.C.: Amyloid deposits and amyloidosis: The beta-fibrilloses. N. Engl. J. Med. 302:1283 and 1333, 1980.

362   A-Y, B-N, C-N, D-Y, E-Y (Braunwald, pp. 1342–1353)

Before it can be recommended that a patient with chronic stable angina undergo coronary bypass surgery, certain criteria must be met. The most widely accepted indication for coronary bypass surgery for stable angina pectoris is significant disability from symptoms despite optimal medical care. The results of several studies, including the CASS and the Veterans Administration Cooperative study, have provided prognostic information for all classes of patients with coronary artery disease. These studies indicate that patients with left main coronary artery stenosis of greater than 60 per cent have improved survival with surgery. These studies have also shown that patients with critical three-vessel disease (> 70 per cent stenoses) who demonstrate either resting LV dysfunction or inducible ischemia with poor exercise tolerance also have better long-term survival with surgery than with medical therapy. Patients with normal resting LV ejection fractions and three-vessel disease show no significant difference in their long-term survival with surgical as compared with medical therapy. This is probably due to the fact that the 5-year survival for patients in this category is more than 90 per cent. Finally, patients with one critical stenosis, but with evidence for poor exercise tolerance and significant inducible ischemia, also do better with surgical than with medical treatment.

Thus the sum of the mass of myocardium damaged and at risk is the critical factor in evaluating a patient for surgery as opposed to medical therapy, all other factors being equal. Extenuating circumstances include failure of medical treatment to control symptoms and the presence of significant left main coronary artery stenosis.

363-A   (1, 2, and 3 are correct) (Braunwald, pp. 1212–1216)

During reperfusion of ischemic myocardium, significant additional myocardial injury occurs due to a variety of mechanisms. Myocytes that appear to be ischemic upon reperfusion often suddenly develop ultrastructural changes of irreversible cell death, including explosive cell swelling and widespread architectural disruption, as if an acceleration of normal ischemic damage were occurring. It appears that reperfusion predominantly accelerates necrosis of irreversibly injured myocardium,[1] although during reperfusion there is significant cell swelling with resulting vascular compression. This may damage some reversibly injured cells.

Two mechanisms are thought to be responsible for

reperfusion-induced injury. The reintroduction of oxygen to ischemic cells causes formation of oxygen-derived free radicals. These radicals disrupt cell membranes, impair enzyme function, and may result in cellular calcium overload. The increase in cell calcium then impairs mitochondrial function, disabling energy production and resulting in loss of cell integrity. Thus interventions directed at preventing formation of oxygen free radicals may be helpful in preventing reperfusion injury.

Because of the microvascular damage present in severely ischemic myocardium, hemorrhage is likely to occur upon reperfusion. Some areas of the myocardium are so severely ischemic that there is an absence of reflow, termed the "no-reflow phenomenon." These areas appear to result from ischemia-induced microvascular damage and myocardial contracture of such severity as to be nonreperfusable. However, the no-reflow phenomenon does not appear to enhance myocyte death, because the zone of reflow is always contained within areas in which myocytes are already necrotic at the time of onset of reperfusion.[2]

REFERENCES

1. Jennings, R.B., Sommers, H.M., Smyth, G.A., Flack, H.A., and Linn, H.: Myocardial necrosis induced by temporary occlusion of a coronary artery in the dog. Arch. Pathol. 70:68, 1960.
2. Braunwald, E., and Kloner, R.A.: Myocardial reperfusion: A double-edged sword? J. Clin. Invest. 76:1713, 1985.

364-A   (1, 2, and 3 are correct) (*Braunwald, pp. 1030–1031; 1042*)

Doppler echocardiography is the usual noninvasive procedure for quantitating and assessing the presence of both stenotic and regurgitant lesions of several valves. Figure *A* is an example of a continuous wave Doppler echocardiogram in combined mitral stenosis (MS) and mitral regurgitation (MR). In Figure *B*, pulsed wave Doppler measurement of normal mitral valve flow is displayed. Diastolic flow toward the transducer (above the baseline) is present; an early diastolic peak and an end-diastolic peak resulting in "M" configurations similar to the mitral valve pattern on M-mode echocardiography may be noted. Normally, no systolic flow signals are detected on Doppler examination of the mitral valve. The mitral valve peak diastolic velocity normally is less than 1.3 meters/sec. MS results in high diastolic velocity (usually exceeding 1.5 meters/sec). The difference in diastolic pressure between the LA and LV is increased and the rapidity of LA emptying is reduced in patients with mitral stenosis, as shown in *A*. This reduced rate of pressure equalization appears as a slower decline of the velocity signals during diastole.

The diagnosis of MR by pulsed wave Doppler examination consists of the detection of the systolic turbulence when the probe is in the LA. In the example shown in Figure *A*, it can be seen that there is a high-velocity signal moving away from the transducer as indicated by the signal below the baseline with a velocity of 4.4 meters/ sec. Doppler echocardiography is quite sensitive for detecting MR that is due to rheumatic deformity which causes thickening and calcification of the edges of the valve leaflets and a wide regurgitant jet directed to the left atrium parallel to the long axis of the heart. In contrast, the regurgitant signals of mitral valve prolapse, papillary muscle dysfunction, or prosthetic valve dysfunction are more difficult to detect, since these lesions cause small localized jets that "hug" the left atrial wall. Color-flow imaging may be more successful in detecting these forms of MR.

Assessment of MR by echocardiography is at best semiquantitative. The systolic jet of mild MR is detected only immediately above the mitral valve leaflet. As MR becomes more severe the turbulence becomes greater in the LA and can be detected further back in the LA. It should be noted that because the pressure gradient between the LV and LA in systole is much greater than between the LA and LV in diastole, signals produced by MR occur at a much higher flow velocity than those produced by MS.

365-A   (1, 2, and 3 are correct) (*Braunwald, pp. 1115–1116*)

Two-dimensional echocardiography has been very useful in demonstrating the presence of vegetations during endocarditis. Amsterdam and colleagues[1] demonstrated that two-dimensional echocardiography detects 50 to 80 per cent of cases of infective endocarditis. Factors important for the detection of valvular vegetations include the size of the lesion (3 mm or larger), its location, duration of the disease for at least 2 weeks (vegetations are usually not seen before this), the presence of abscess of the myocardium or valvular ring, and aneurysm of the sinus of Valsalva. Echocardiography is also useful in identifying rupture of the ventricular septum, flail leaflets, and fluttering of the mitral valve during diastole. Doppler echocardiography is of particular value in detecting early valvular regurgitation and assessing its severity.

Stewart et al.[2] divided patients into two groups on the basis of identifiable vegetations on echocardiography. Those in whom one or more vegetations were demonstrated were found to be at higher risk for developing complications such as emboli, congestive heart failure, and the need for surgery than those in whom echocardiography demonstrated no vegetations. The ability of echocardiography to demonstrate vegetations is related primarily to the size of the lesions. Fungal endocarditis is much more likely to yield echocardiographically visible vegetations than is bacterial endocarditis. In endocarditis caused by the less virulent organisms—especially *Streptococcus viridans*—vegetations documented by echocardiography are quite rare. Although it is typical for successful therapy to result in a decrease in the size of a vegetation, successful therapy may be associated with an increase or no change in the size of vegetations. In fact, in right-sided endocarditis it is not uncommon for vegetations to persist for years following curative therapy.[3]

REFERENCES

1. Amsterdam, E.A.: Value and limitations of echocardiography in endocarditis. Cardiology 71:229, 1984.

2. Stewart, J.A., Silimperi, D., Harris, P., Wise, N.K., Fraker, T.D., and Kisslo, J.A.: Echocardiographic documentation of vegetative lesions in infective endocarditis. Clinical implications. Circulation 61:374, 1980.
3. Neimann, J.L., Fischer, M., Kownator, S., and Faivre, G.: Echocardiographic follow-up of vegetations in infectious endocarditis. Arch. Mal. Coeur 75:1329, 1982.

366-E   (1, 2, 3, and 4 are correct) (Braunwald, pp. 951–952)

Clinical manifestations of Ebstein's anomaly of the tricuspid valve are variable because the spectrum of pathology varies widely and because of variations in the presence of associated malformations. The most common important associated cardiac defect is pulmonic stenosis or atresia. In addition, ostium primum atrial septal defect, ventricular septal defect, and physiologically corrected transposition of the great arteries all sometimes accompany Ebstein's anomaly.

The usual clinical manifestations of Ebstein's anomaly in infancy are cyanosis, a cardiac murmur, and congestive heart failure. However, beyond infancy the onset of symptoms may be insidious and the most common complaints tend to be exertional dyspnea and fatigue as well as cyanosis. Approximately one-fourth of patients suffer episodes of paroxysmal supraventricular tachycardia. Evidence of tricuspid regurgitation and wide splitting of the first and second heart sounds are characteristic features of the cardiac examination. Electrocardiographic abnormalities in Ebstein's anomaly may include right bundle branch block and the Wolff-Parkinson-White (WPW) syndrome. The latter case is usually type B WPW, with a left bundle branch block pattern and predominant S waves in the right precordial leads. The risk of paroxysmal supraventricular tachycardia appears to be increased in patients with the WPW pattern on their ECGs.[1] In addition, the ECG may show giant P waves, a prolonged P-R interval, and a prolonged terminal QRS depolarization with variable degrees of right bundle branch block.

Radiographic studies usually demonstrate right atrial enlargement in the presence of a small right ventricle. M-mode echocardiography demonstrates increased right ventricular dimensions, paradoxical ventricular septal motion, and an increase in tricuspid valve excursion. These findings may be seen in other forms of right ventricular overload. However, more specific findings for Ebstein's anomaly include a delay in tricuspid valve closure relative to mitral closure and a decrease in the E-F slope of the tricuspid valve, an abnormal anterior position of the tricuspid valve during diastole, and tricuspid valve echoes detected when the transducer is placed laterally. Leftward and inferior displacement of the tricuspid valve and its abnormal position in relation to the mitral valve may be demonstrated by two-dimensional echocardiography (see Braunwald, Fig. 30–59, p. 952). Doppler examination may detect the presence of tricuspid regurgitation.

At cardiac catheterization an intracavitary ECG recorded proximal to the tricuspid valve shows a right ventricular type of complex, while the pressure recorded is that of the right atrium, demonstrating the presence of an "atrialized" portion of the right ventricle (see Braunwald, Fig. 30–60, p. 952). It is common for significant arrhythmias to occur during catheterization, since the heart is unusually irritable in this condition. Selective right ventricular angiography may show the position of the displaced tricuspid valve, the size of the right ventricle, and the configuration of the outflow portion of the right ventricle, further confirming the diagnosis.

REFERENCE

1. Kastor, J.A., Goldreier, B.N., Josephson, M.E., Perloff, J.K., Scharf, D.L., Manchester, J.H., Schelbourne, J.C., and Hirshfield, J.W., Jr.: Electrophysiologic characteristics of Ebstein's anomaly of the tricuspid valve. Circulation 52:987, 1975.

367-C   (2 and 4 are correct) (Braunwald, pp. 411–412; 1197–1198; 1253)

The clinical history presented is consistent with myocardial ischemia, most likely involving the right coronary artery and the inferior wall. The sudden decrease in chest discomfort associated with reductions in heart rate and blood pressure are consistent with coronary artery reperfusion. In this case it appeared that reperfusion caused activation of the Bezold-Jarisch reflex, which is a reflex that leads to bradycardia and hypotension.[1] The afferent limb of this reflex involves the vagus nerves and its efferent limb, coronary parasympathetic components. A similar phenomenon can be demonstrated experimentally by intracoronary injection of veratrum alkaloids as well as other metabolically active substances documenting the direct reflex arc from the coronary artery itself.

The term Anrep effect, also called "homeometric autoregulation," is applied to a positive inotropic effect following abrupt elevation of systolic aortic and left ventricular pressures. This effect occurs during the first minutes after aortic pressure is abruptly elevated, with the end-diastolic pressure then tending to fall as stroke volume and stroke work recover. Homeometric autoregulation is most marked in the anesthetized state. A variety of observations support the concept that the phenomenon is related, at least in part, to recovery from transient subendocardial ischemia. Thus, the Anrep effect would have been associated with an increase rather than a reduction in systolic pressure. A ruptured abdominal viscus would not be associated with a sudden decrease in chest pain.

REFERENCE

1. Jarisch, A., and Zotterman, Y.: Depressor reflexes from the heart. Acta Physiol. Scand. 16:31, 1948.

368-B   (1 and 3 are correct) (Braunwald, p. 1436)

Löffler's endocarditis is a cardiac syndrome associated with eosinophilia, occurring in temperate climates. The typical patient with Löffler's endocarditis is a male in his 40's who has had persistent eosinophilia with greater than 1500 eosinophils/mm³ for at least 6 months, with evidence of organ involvement.[1] Cardiac involvement is seen in approximately 75 per cent of patients with hypereosinophilia. The combination of hypereosinophilia and cardiac involvement is also part of the Churg-Strauss syndrome, which can be differentiated by the coexisting presence of asthma, nasal polyposis, and necrotizing vasculitis.

The pathology of Löffler's endocarditis involves biventricular mural endocardial thickening with histological findings demonstrating an acute inflammatory eosinophilic myocarditis, thrombosis, fibrinoid change and inflammation of intramural coronary vessels, mural thrombosis, and fibrotic thickening. Clinically, patients have weight loss, fever, cough, skin rash, and congestive heart failure. Cardiomegaly is present early in the course, even in the absence of congestive heart failure, and the murmur of mitral regurgitation is common. Systemic embolism is frequent and may lead to neurological and renal dysfunction. Laboratory examination is remarkable for an elevated erythrocyte sedimentation rate and an increased eosinophil count. The echocardiogram frequently demonstrates localized thickening of the posterobasal LV wall with absent or remarkably limited motion of the posterior leaflet of the mitral valve. The hemodynamic consequences of the dense endocardial scarring are those of a restrictive cardiomyopathy with abnormal diastolic filling leading to a restrictive picture with "square root sign." A characteristic feature is the presence of largely preserved systolic function, with near-obliteration of the apex of the ventricles when studied angiographically. Medical treatment of Löffler's endocarditis is moderately effective, with administration of both steroids and hydroxyurea improving survival substantially.

REFERENCE

1. Olsen, E.G., and Spry, C.J.: Relation between eosinophilia and endomyocardial disease. Prog. Cardiovasc. Dis. 27:241, 1985.

369-C   (2 and 4 are correct) (*Braunwald, pp. 1027–1029; 1064–1067; and 1077*)

This woman with rheumatic heart disease presents an interesting problem. It is clear that she has mitral stenosis (MS) based on the opening snap, loud S_1, and holodiastolic rumbling murmur, but it is unclear what coexisting valvular disease she may have. Many patients with severe MS have an early blowing diastolic murmur along the left sternal border and a normal pulse pressure. In 90 per cent of these patients the murmur is due to aortic regurgitation (AR), and it is usually of little clinical importance. However, approximately 10 per cent of patients with MS have severe rheumatic AR. This can usually be recognized by the peripheral signs of AR such as widened pulse pressure, water hammer pulses, and signs of LV enlargement of x-ray and ECG.

In patients with multivalvular disease, a proximal valvular lesion often masks a distal lesion. Thus, significant AR may be missed in patients with severe MS. The widened pulse pressure in particular may be absent in the presence of severe MS. Furthermore, the Austin-Flint murmur may be mistaken for the diastolic rumbling murmur of MS. These two murmurs may be distinguished

at the bedside by means of amyl nitrite inhalation, which diminishes the Austin-Flint murmur but augments the murmur of MS. Isometric handgrip and squatting augment both the diastolic murmur of AR and the Austin-Flint murmur but have little effect on the diastolic rumbling murmur of MS. In this patient the responses to amyl nitrite and handgrip are consistent with the presence of an Austin-Flint murmur.

The fact that the ECG in the patient described shows evidence of left ventricular hypertrophy and left-axis deviation in addition to left atrial enlargement is inconsistent with simple MS and suggests either AR or aortic stenosis (AS). The presence of the murmur of AR makes the latter the more likely diagnosis. There is no evidence for tricuspid stenosis or mitral regurgitation.

Further evaluation to confirm the diagnosis would probably include echocardiography and cardiac catheterization. Diastolic fluttering of the anterior leaflet of the mitral valve is an important clue to the presence of AR. Furthermore, a two-dimensional Doppler echocardiographic examination would be helpful because the Doppler is relatively sensitive (greater than 90 per cent detection) for AR.

Patients such as this woman are most effectively treated by combined aortic and mitral valve replacement. This is usually associated with a higher risk and poorer survival than replacement of one of these two valves.[1] Kirklin reported a 5-year survival rate of 70 per cent for double-valve replacement compared to 80 per cent for single-valve replacement.[2] In general, patients with more dilated ventricles, especially those with a combination of AR and MR, fared worse than did those patients with the other combinations.

REFERENCES

1. Baxley, W.A., and Soto, B.: Hemodynamic evaluation of patients with combined mitral and aortic prostheses. Am. J. Cardiol. 45:42, 1980.
2. Kirklin, J.W., and Barratt-Boyes, B.G.: Combined aortic and mitral valve disease with or without tricuspid valve disease. *In* Cardiac Surgery. New York, John Wiley and Sons, 1986, pp. 431–446.

370-C   (2 and 4 are correct) (*Braunwald, pp. 1026–1028*)

The opening snap (OS) of the mitral valve appears to be caused by a sudden tensing of the valve leaflets after the valve cusps have completed their opening excursion. The OS is usually heard in valves that have not become completely calcified and therefore is accompanied by an accentuated S_1. The mitral OS follows A_2 by 0.04 to 0.12 second and the A_2-OS interval varies *inversely* with the left atrial pressure.[1] A short A_2-OS interval (less than 0.08 sec) is a reliable indicator of tight MS and usually signifies significant left atrial pressure elevation. However, the reverse is not the case, since a long A_2-OS interval may be present in significant MS. This may occur when the time interval between the actual opening of the mitral valve and the OS is prolonged due to valvular calcification.

The A_2-OS interval can be altered by various maneuvers. Specifically, differentiation of tricuspid stenosis (TS) from MS can be aided by the fact that both the diastolic murmur and the OS of TS are accentuated during inspiration and reduced during expiration, while little change or the opposite occurs in MS. Furthermore, sudden standing with the resultant decrease in venous return causes a lowering of left atrial pressure and therefore widens the A$_2$-OS interval.[2] This maneuver is particularly useful in distinguishing the A$_2$-OS from a split S$_2$, which narrows on standing. However, the most reliable maneuver is exercise. This causes the A$_2$-OS interval to narrow, particularly in moderate or severe MS as there is a rapid elevation of the left atrial pressure resulting in the OS moving toward A$_2$.

REFERENCES

1. Ebringer, R., Pitt, A., and Anderson, S.T.: Hemodynamic factors influencing opening snap interval in mitral stenosis. Br. Heart J. 32:350, 1970.
2. Surawicz, B.: Effect of respiration and upright position on the interval between the two components of the second heart sound and that between the second sound and mitral opening snap. Circulation 16:422, 1957.

371-C (2 and 4 are correct) *(Braunwald, pp. 1497, 1501)*

Cardiac catheterization has proved extremely useful in establishing the presence and hemodynamic importance of pericardial effusion and tamponade. A number of characteristic cardiac catheterization findings confirm the diagnosis of cardiac tamponade. Simultaneous recordings of intrapericardial and RA pressure tracings reveal that they are virtually identical and track together; except in instances of low-pressure cardiac tamponade, both are elevated as well. The RA pressure tracing displays a prominent systolic *x* descent and a small or absent systolic *y* descent in cases of cardiac tamponade. RV diastolic pressures are equal to RA and intrapericardial pressures and do not display the characteristic dip-and-plateau configuration that is seen in constrictive pericarditis (see Braunwald, p. 1506). The systolic pressures demonstrated on RV and pulmonary artery tracings are the summed result of the pressure developed by the RV and the intrapericardial pressure and are therefore often moderately elevated in the range of 35 to 50 mm Hg. The pulmonary capillary wedge pressure and the LV diastolic pressure are also often elevated and are equal to intrapericardial, RA, and RV diastolic pressures when simultaneous recordings are performed. It should be noted that in patients with severe underlying LV dysfunction, LV diastolic pressure may exceed that of the equalized intrapericardial and RA pressures.[1]

REFERENCE

1. Reddy, P.S., Curtiss, E.I., O'Toole, J.D., and Shaver, J.A.: Cardiac tamponade: Hemodynamic observations in man. Circulation 58:265, 1978.

372-C (2 and 4 are correct) *(Braunwald, pp. 1445–1448)*

Chagas' disease is caused by the protozoan *Trypanosoma cruzi*. The major cardiovascular findings are exten-

sive myocarditis with congestive heart failure. Typically, the disease becomes evident 20 to 30 years after the initial infection. Chagas' disease is prevalent in Central and South America, where approximately 10 to 20 million people are infected.

The disease is characterized by three phases: acute, latent, and chronic. During the acute phase, the disease is transmitted to humans by the bite of a reduviid bug, commonly called the kissing bug. Following inoculation, protozoa multiply and migrate widely through the body, and then enter a latent phase. Interestingly, about 30 per cent of infected individuals develop findings of chronic Chagas' disease, but many individuals with high parasite burdens do not develop the disease. Furthermore, it is not unusual to be unable to detect parasites in patients dying of Chagas' disease, so that an autoimmune mechanism for cardiac dysfunction appears to be involved.

Classic findings at autopsy include lesions of the cardiac nerves with evidence of cardiac parasympathetic denervation. There is usually cardiac enlargement with dilatation and hypertrophy of cardiac chambers. The left ventricular apex is often thin and bulging, resembling an aneurysm. Thrombus formation is frequent and may occupy much of the apex.

Clinically, chronic progressive heart failure, predominantly right sided, is the rule in advanced cases. There is usually severe cardiomegaly, with the most common ECG abnormalities being *right bundle branch block* and left anterior hemiblock. T-wave abnormalities and atrioventricular block are also seen with some frequency. Ventricular arrhythmias are a prominent feature of chronic Chagas' disease.

Diagnosis is made using a complement-fixation test (Machado-Guerreiro test). At this time, no clinically effective treatment is available, although immunoprophylaxis with a vaccine is hoped for in the near future.

373-A (1, 2, and 3 are correct) *(Braunwald, pp. 1414–1417)*

The consumption of alcohol may result in myocardial damage by three mechanisms: most commonly a direct effect of alcohol or its metabolites; a nutritional effect, occasionally with thiamine deficiency leading to beriberi heart disease; and rarely, toxic effects due to additives in the alcoholic beverage, such as cobalt.[1–3] It has become clear that even in the presence of normal nutritional status, alcohol can cause significant cardiomyopathy.[3] Alcohol results in acute as well as chronic depression of myocardial contractility and may produce acute demonstrable cardiac dysfunction even in normal individuals. It appears that prior cigarette consumption and coexisting hypertension augment the cardiomyopathic effects of alcohol.

The mechanism of cardiac depression produced by alcohol remains unclear. In several studies, alcohol and its metabolite acetaldehyde have been shown to interfere with a number of myocardial cellular functions including transport and binding of calcium, mitochondrial respiration, lipid metabolism, protein synthesis, and myofibrillar ATPase.[1] Alcohol also is associated with systemic electrolyte imbalances (*hypokalemia*, hypophosphatemia, and hypomagnesemia), which may also play a role in alcohol-induced damage.

The gross and microscopic pathological findings of alcoholic cardiomyopathy are nonspecific and are similar to those observed in idiopathic dilated cardiomyopathy.

REFERENCES

1. Reagan, T.J.: Alcoholic cardiomyopathy. Prog. Cardiovasc. Dis. 27:141, 1984.
2. Cardiovascular beriberi (editorial). Lancet 1:1287, 1982.
3. Lange, L.G., and Sobel, B.E.: Myocardial metabolites of ethanol. Circ. Res. 52:479, 1983.

374-A   (1, 2, and 3 are correct) *(Braunwald, pp. 1268–1269)*

The ECG demonstrates atrial fibrillation with a moderately rapid ventricular response, a common arrhythmia that occurs in between 10 and 15 per cent of patients with AMI. This should be contrasted with atrial flutter, which is a far less common atrial arrhythmia associated with AMI and which occurs in only 1 to 3 per cent of patients in this setting. While atrial fibrillation in patients with AMI is usually transient and occurs more commonly in patients with LV failure, it is seen more frequently following anterior infarction and appears to be caused by left atrial ischemia in most cases.[1] Atrial fibrillation is more common during the first 24 hours following infarction than later. It appears to be associated with an increased mortality, in part because it commonly involves extensive anterior wall infarction. The rapid ventricular response and loss of atrial contribution to ventricular filling both may lead to a significant reduction in cardiac output.

In patients who are hemodynamically stable, the use of digitalis or verapamil to slow ventricular response has proved useful. However, electrical cardioversion is the treatment of choice in patients with clinical and/or hemodynamic evidence of decompensation. The management of atrial fibrillation in patients with AMI is often complicated by frequent recurrence, especially when left atrial dilatation due to LV failure is the inciting event.

REFERENCE

1. Hod, H., Lew, A.S., Keltai, M., Cereek, B., Geft, I.O., Shah, P., and Ganz, W.: Early atrial fibrillation during evolving myocardial infarction: A consequence of impaired left atrial perfusion. Circulation 75:146, 1987.

375-C   (2 and 4 are correct) *(Braunwald, pp. 1154–1157)*

For many years, a statistical correlation has been noted between the level of serum cholesterol and the risk of coronary artery disease. However, the "cholesterol hypothesis," which states that reducing cholesterol levels will actually decrease the risk of developing coronary artery disease, has been difficult to prove. A number of studies have provided supportive evidence that this hypothesis is indeed true, including a VA study done at the Wadsworth Hospital in Los Angeles,[1] a World Health Organization trial,[2] and the Oslo study.[3] All of these showed to varying extent that dietary and drug interventions resulted in significant reductions in nonfatal and fatal myocardial infarctions.

However, the Coronary Primary Prevention Trial (CPPT)[4] for the first time demonstrated that lowering cholesterol, in particular low-density lipoprotein (LDL), decreases the likelihood of developing coronary artery disease. The patients were randomized to receive either placebo or the bile acid sequestrant cholestyramine. The recommended dosage of drug was 24 gm/day; however, only a minority of participants took the drug at full dosage. Use of the drug resulted in a lowering of total cholesterol by approximately 9 per cent and a reduction in LDL cholesterol by about 12 per cent. This was associated with a decrease in the frequency of coronary events of 19 per cent. Furthermore, a graded effect was observed; that is, the level of reduction in cholesterol and the amount of medication taken correlated with the decrease in coronary disease. As a rough rule of thumb, a 1 per cent reduction in cholesterol reduced the risk of developing coronary disease by 2 per cent. Also, secondary endpoints such as angina pectoris, positive exercise tolerance tests, and the number of coronary bypass operations decreased in parallel. Although the treatment group exhibited a reduction in cardiovascular-related deaths, it also exhibited an increase in noncardiovascular-related deaths. An overall effect on mortality was therefore not demonstrated. It is possible that a decrease in overall mortality may be observed in trials with longer terms. Such long-term trials are now in progress.

REFERENCES

1. Dayton, S., and Pearce, M.L.: Diet high in unsaturated fat. A controlled clinical trial. Minn. Med. 52:1237, 1969.
2. Committee of Principal Investigators: WHO Clofibrate Trial. WHO cooperative trial on primary prevention of ischemic heart disease using clofibrate to lower serum cholesterol: Mortality follow-up report. Lancet 2:379, 1980.
3. Hjermann, I., Holme, I., Byre, K., and Leren, P.: Effect of diet and smoking on the incidence of coronary heart disease: Report from the Oslo study group of a randomized trial in healthy men. Lancet 2:1303, 1981.
4. Lipid Research Clinics Program: The Lipid Research Clinics coronary primary prevention trial results. I. Reduction in incidence of coronary heart disease. II. The relationships of reduction in incidence of coronary heart disease to cholesterol lowering. J.A.M.A. 251:351, 1984.

376-B   (1 and 3 are correct) *(Braunwald, p. 924)*

In the majority of preterm infants under 1500 gm of birth weight, PDA persists for a prolonged period of time, and in approximately one-third of these infants a large shunt leads to significant cardiopulmonary deterioration.[1] Noninvasive evaluation may reveal evidence of significant right-to-left shunting before the appearance of physical findings suggesting ductal patency. Physical examination may reveal bounding peripheral pulses, an infraclavicular and interscapular systolic murmur (which occasionally is heard as a continuous murmur), a hyperactive precordium, hepatomegaly, and recurrent episodes of apnea and bradycardia with or without respirator dependency. On chest x-ray an increase in the cardiothoracic ratio is seen on sequential radiographs and may be accompanied by increased pulmonary arterial markings, perihilar edema, and ultimately generalized pulmonary edema. Echocardiography may demonstrate increases in LV end-diastolic and LA dimensions. Cardiac catheterization is rarely necessary.

Management of the premature infant with a PDA depends upon the clinical presentation of the disorder. In an asymptomatic infant intervention is usually unnecessary since the PDA will almost always undergo spontaneous closure and will not require surgical ligation and division. Infants with respiratory distress syndrome and signs of a significant ductal shunt usually are unresponsive to medical measures to control congestive heart failure and require closure of the PDA for survival. This usually may be accomplished pharmacologically, utilizing indomethacin to inhibit prostaglandin synthesis and achieve constriction and closure of the ductus.[2] Approximately 10 per cent of infants are unresponsive to indomethacin and require surgical ligation.

REFERENCES

1. Friedman, W.F.: Patent ductus arteriosus in respiratory distress syndrome. Pediatr. Cardiol. 4(Suppl 2):3, 1983.
2. Gersony, W.M., Peckham, G.J., Ellison, R.C., Miettinen, O.S., and Nadas, A.S.: Effects of indomethacin in premature infants with patent ductus arteriosus: Results of a national collaborative study. J. Pediatr. 102:895, 1983.

377-C   (2 and 4 are correct) (Braunwald, pp. 1426–1427)

The most common physiological abnormality in hypertrophic obstructive cardiomyopathy (HOCM) is not systolic but rather diastolic dysfunction. Thus, HOCM is characterized by abnormal stiffness of the left ventricle during diastole, which results in impaired ventricular filling. This abnormality in diastolic relaxation results in elevation of the left ventricular end-diastolic pressure with associated elevations of left atrial, pulmonary venous, and pulmonary capillary pressures. Usually, the left ventricle is actually hypercontractile with a normal or supernormal ejection fraction. Although the generation of a pressure gradient due to subaortic obstruction would ordinarily imply that left ventricular ejection is slowed or impeded at some point during systole, actually there are rapid ventricular emptying and normal or even high ejection fractions. Hemodynamic studies have shown that the majority of flow (at least 80 per cent) is unusually rapid in patients with HCOM and is completed earlier in systole than normal, regardless of whether gradients are absent, provokable, or present. Thus, the symptoms in general are due to difficulty with diastolic filling rather than with systolic ejection. While there is a strong temporal and quantitative relationship between mitral valve systolic anterior motion and the subaortic gradient, symptoms do not necessarily correlate with the size of the gradient. Furthermore, there are significant variations on a daily basis in the extent of both the gradient and symptoms. Exertional and postexertional syncope and angina occur in some patients and are probably caused, at least in part, by systolic obstruction.

378-B   (1 and 3 are correct) (Braunwald, p. 1049)

The auscultatory findings of the MVP syndrome are determined by the volume of the LV. The mitral valve begins to prolapse when the decrease in LV volume during systole reaches a critical point at which the mitral valve leaflets no longer coapt; at this instant the click occurs and the murmur commences. Thus, any maneuver that decreases LV volume will result in an earlier occurrence of prolapse during systole so that the click and onset of the murmur move closer to S_1. Conversely, any maneuver which increases LV volume will move the click and murmur toward S_2 and the murmur may actually disappear. Thus, during the straining phase of the Valsalva maneuver, upon sudden standing, and early during the inhalation of amyl nitrite, LV volume decreases and the click and murmur occur earlier in systole. Conversely, a sudden change in posture from standing to prone, leg raising, squatting, isometric exercise such as handgrip, and slowing of the heart rate with propranolol all increase LV volume and delay the click and murmur. When the onset of the murmur is delayed, both its duration and intensity are diminished because of a reduction in the severity of MR. However, with some maneuvers there is a discrepancy between the changes in the intensity and duration of the murmur. For example, following amyl nitrite the click occurs earlier and usually becomes softer, while the murmur becomes softer immediately but then after about 15 seconds becomes louder as a result of the reflex overshoot of blood pressure.

379-B   (1 and 3 are correct) (Braunwald, p. 1363)

Ischemic chest pain is frequently *not* a reliable or sensitive marker of transient acute myocardial ischemia as measured by ambulatory electrocardiography. It has been shown that despite reduction in coronary flow many patients with ECG abnormalities consistent with transient myocardial ischemia have no symptoms. Among patients with angina at rest and demonstrated decreases in coronary sinus oxygen saturation (reflecting changes in coronary blood flow), pseudonormalization of previously inverted or flat T waves occurred in a majority of instances of ischemia (77 per cent), ST-segment elevation in some (20 per cent), and ST-segment depression in a few (2 per cent).[1] In this study, in those instances of transient ischemia associated with chest pain (10 of 37 patients), the pain always occurred 50 to 120 seconds *after* the onset of ST–T wave changes. It is now recognized that patients with either stable or unstable angina have a high incidence of ischemic ECG changes without accompanying symptoms when continuous ECG monitoring is performed.[2] In patients with chronic stable angina, ST-segment depression on ambulatory monitoring occurs more frequently than do symptoms of angina.

REFERENCES

1. Chierchia, S., Brunellis, C., Simonetti, I., Lazzari, M., and Maseri, A.: Sequence of events in angina at rest: Primary reduction in coronary blood flow. Circulation 61:759, 1980.
2. Cecchi, A.C., Dovellini, E.V., Marchi, F., Pucci, P., Santoro, G.M., and Fazzini, P.F.: Silent myocardial ischemia during ambulatory electrocardiographic monitoring in patients with effort angina. J. Am. Coll. Cardiol. 1:934, 1983.

380-D   (4 is correct) (*Braunwald, pp. 1056–1059*)

In calculating aortic valve area in patients with combined AR and AS, it is important to use a measure for cardiac output that represents the *total* left ventricular output. Both the cardiac output measured by the Fick method, which is obtained by measurement of pulmonary artery saturation and pulmonary mixed venous oxygen saturation, and the output measured by the dye dilution method measure the *effective* cardiac output delivered to the body, i.e., the *forward* cardiac output. However, these measurements do *not* include the regurgitant flow that moves back and forth across the aortic valve. Thus, forward output alone will be smaller than total cardiac output and will give an inappropriately small measurement of the aortic valve area. Therefore, in order to accurately calculate valve area by the Gorlin formula, it is important to measure carefully the angiographic LV cardiac output (LV stroke volume times heart rate).

381-E   (1, 2, 3, and 4 are correct) (*Braunwald, pp. 1569–1570*)

Traumatic injuries of the aorta, including complete aortic rupture, are most commonly associated with sudden high-speed deceleration injuries that result from motor vehicle accidents or other severe jolting injuries. Because they occur in the setting of other serious injuries and rarely have specific symptoms or signs, aortic injuries may be extremely difficult to diagnose without a high index of suspicion. Approximately two-thirds of patients with aortic rupture have clear-cut evidence of accompanying thoracic trauma, including chest or cardiac contusions, multiple rib fractures, hemorrhagic pleural effusions, and pulmonary contusions.[1] The specific physical examination for this injury, however, may be relatively unrevealing. A syndrome of "acute coarctation" with upper extremity hypertension, dereased blood pressure in the lower extremities, precordial systolic murmur, and a pulse lag between the radial and femoral arteries is nearly pathognomonic for the diagnosis but occurs relatively uncommonly. In general, the diagnosis is best suspected from the chest x-ray, which is abnormal in more than 90 per cent of patients with traumatic aortic rupture. These abnormalities are due to the collection of blood and its continual leakage from the injury and are manifested in specific changes in mediastinal contour, and in the spatial relations of the intrathoracic structures (see Braunwald, Fig. 46–23, p. 1569).

The diagnosis of traumatic aortic rupture may be confirmed by the use of CT scanning with contrast injection; in patients about whom some doubt remains, thoracic aortography may be performed. While up to 90 per cent of patients with aortic rupture will die instantly, those patients who do reach the hospital alive with this injury have survival rates that approach 70 per cent in various series.[2] Survivors may have progressive hemorrhage at the site of the aortic tear and thus early, emergency surgical therapy is crucial to survival.

REFERENCES

1. Sturm, J.T., Billiar, T.R., Dorsey, J.S., Luxenberg, M.G., and Perry, J.F.: Risk factors for survival following surgical treatment of traumatic aortic rupture. Ann. Thorac. Surg. 39:418, 1985.

2. Atkins, C.W., Buckley, M.J., Daggett, W., McIlduff, J.B., and Austen, W.G.: Acute traumatic disruption of the thoracic aorta. A ten-year experience. Ann. Thorac. Surg. 31:305, 1981.

382-A   (1, 2, and 3 are correct) (*Braunwald, pp. 993–994*)

The size of the patent ductus arteriosus (PDA) and the ratio of pulmonary to systemic vascular resistance determine the pathophysiological consequences of this disorder. A large PDA leads initially to increased pulmonary blood flow with subsequent enlargement of the pulmonary arterial circuit, left atrium, left ventricle, and descending aorta, and eventually the development of congestive heart failure.[1] The development of pulmonary arterial hypertension may herald the onset of bidirectional or reversed shunting through the ductus. If this occurs, differential cyanosis may develop with a relatively acyanotic right upper extremity and cyanotic lower extremities because of the persistence of the PDA, the onset of Eisenmenger's syndrome, and right-to-left shunting through the ductus.

The physical findings in a patient with a large left-to-right shunt through a PDA include vigorous peripheral arterial pulses, a wide arterial pulse pressure, and a hyperdynamic precordium. On auscultation, a high-pitched continuous murmur may be heard, which is loudest at the left upper sternal border or in the infraclavicular area. If the shunt is large, the increased flow across the mitral valve may create a diastolic flow rumble. When pulmonary vascular resistance rises, the left-to-right shunt is diminished and the continuous murmur may be replaced by a rough systolic murmur with an accentuated pulmonary component of the second heart sound.

The ECG in this disorder shows either a normal pattern or if the PDA is large, the development of left ventricular hypertrophy with strain[2]; right ventricular hypertrophy may be present with pulmonary hypertension. Most commonly, sinus rhythm is present. The chest x-ray usually reveals dilatation of the proximal pulmonary arteries and pulmonary plethora if the shunt is moderate to large in size. The M-mode echocardiogram is nonspecific in PDA and in general shows only left atrial, left ventricular, and aortic enlargement. Two-dimensional echocardiography, however, may allow diagnosis by direct visualization of the ductus. Doppler analysis may further aid in quantifying the magnitude of the left-to-right shunt as well as the pulmonary artery pressure.

REFERENCES

1. Campbell, M.: Natural history of patent ductus arteriosus. Br. Heart J. 30:4, 1968.
2. Fisher, R.G., Moodie, D.S., Sterba, R., and Gill, C.C.: Patent ductus arteriosus in adults. Long-term follow-up: Nonsurgical versus surgical treatment. J. Am. Coll. Cardiol. 8:280, 1986.

383-B   (1 and 3 are correct) (*Braunwald, pp. 1016–1020*)

Approximately 2 per cent of the pediatric population has elevations of systemic blood pressure. Three points in particular with regard to hypertension in infants and children should be noted: (1) The causes of hypertension in infants and children differ markedly from those in adults. Both infants and children more commonly have secondary than primary (essential) forms of hypertension. Renal disease is by far the most common form of secondary hypertension. Examples of sources of renal hypertension in infants and children include unilateral hydronephrosis, unilateral pylonephritis, unilateral tumors, unilateral multicystic kidney, unilateral renal occlusion, renal artery stenosis, fibromuscular renal artery dysplasia, and nephritis due to acute poststreptococcal disease, anaphylactoid purpura, or disseminated lupus erythematosus. (2) The offspring of hypertensive patients are known to have an increased susceptibility to blood pressure elevation. (3) Children with elevated blood pressure require the same surveillance and treatment as those required in adults.

To measure blood pressure correctly, the inner rubber bag should be wide enough to cover two-thirds of the limb and three-fourths of the circumference of the upper arm while leaving the antecubital pulse free. A cuff that is too small is likely to produce spuriously *high* readings. Blood pressure increases with age; in 2-year-olds the 50th percentile is approximately 95/60 mm Hg while at age 10 the 50th percentile is 110/70.[1]

The workup for hypertension in infants and children should focus on identifying secondary causes of hypertension.[2] Since renal disease is the most common cause, typical tests should include urinalysis, complete blood count, serum electrolytes, blood urea nitrogen, serum creatinine, echocardiogram, ECG, and chest x-ray. Recently, it has been shown that echocardiograms allow careful delineation of changes in myocardial function at an early age and can be used to follow children with both mild hypertension and children of parents with significant hypertension. This can then be used to decide whether or not to initiate therapy at any particular point. Obviously in children, even more so than in adults, treatment of borderline hypertension (between 5 and 10 mm Hg beyond the 90th percentile value for age) is an issue because of difficulties with compliance and potential long-term side effects of chronic treatment. In general, drug therapy is initiated if diastolic blood pressure is greater than 85 mm Hg in children younger than 12 years, and greater than 90 mm Hg in children older than 12. If left ventricular hypertrophy is evident by echocardiogram, drug therapy is advisable even with lower diastolic pressures. An oral thiazide diuretic is usually the initial drug of choice. Converting enzyme inhibitors such as captopril and enalapril and the calcium channel blockers are drug choices that may be better tolerated.

REFERENCES

1. Colan, S.D., Fujii, A., Borow, K.M., MacPherson, D., and Sanders, S.P.: Noninvasive determination of systolic, diastolic and end-systolic blood pressure in neonates, infants, and young children: Comparison with central aortic measurements. Am. J. Cardiol. 52:867, 1983.
2. Rocchini, A.P.: Childhood hypertension: Etiology, diagnosis and treatment. Pediatr. Clin. North Am. 31:1259, 1984.

384-A (1, 2, and 3 are correct) *(Braunwald, pp. 1537–1538)*

The treatment of myocardial contusion is quite similar to that of acute myocardial infarction (AMI). Therefore, a period of bed rest of approximately 3 days is recommended, followed by progressive ambulation based on consideration of the patient's clinical symptoms. The chest pain is readily treated with a variety of analgesics, including the nonsteroidal antiinflammatory agents. Patients should *not* be anticoagulated because this may precipitate or exacerbate intramyocardial or intrapericardial hemorrhage. Such hemorrhage is a particular problem in these patients, since undiagnosed lacerations of the pericardium and/or the RV which clot spontaneously, may rebleed in the presence of systematic anticoagulation and cause cardiac tamponade. Finally, because of the large variety of arrhythmias that occur in patients with myocardial contusion, they should be monitored. The prognosis for patients who survive the initial injury is excellent, primarily because they are usually relatively young, and unlike patients with AMI secondary to coronary atherosclerosis, their coronary arteries are usually normal.

385-B (1 and 3 are correct) *(Braunwald, pp. 1558–1560)*

Initial therapy for acute aortic dissection includes immediate admission to an intensive care unit, where careful hemodynamic monitoring is carried out. The earliest therapeutic goals include elimination of pain as well as reduction of systolic arterial pressure. This correlates directly with the degree of stress on the vascular wall which is exerted by LV ejection. The most common pharmacological approach is the simultaneous use of the vasodilator sodium nitroprusside to lower arterial pressure and of a beta-adrenoreceptor blocking agent to reduce wall stress acutely. In patients in whom sodium nitroprusside is poorly tolerated or ineffective, trimethaphan, a ganglionic blocking agent, may be used instead. Lowering of arterial pressure and reduction of left ventricular ejection force allows for temporary stabilization in appropriate surgical candidates, and is the treatment of choice for those patients in whom surgery is not indicated. Following stabilization by such measures, definitive angiography to establish a diagnosis of the extent of the dissection should be performed. The appearance of a life-threatening complication such as aortic rupture, aortic regurgitation, cardiac tamponade, and compromising of a vital organ mandates immediate surgical therapy.

The general consensus regarding definitive subsequent therapy for aortic dissection has evolved over the last several decades. It may be summarized as follows: surgical results are in general superior to medical results in acute proximal dissection, while medical therapy is the preferred treatment in cases of uncomplicated acute distal dissection[1] (see Braunwald, Table 46–1, p. 1559). Patients with distal aortic dissection are in general older and have increased operative risk due to the coincident presence of severe ischemic heart disease or pulmonary disease. Medical therapy in this population has proved quite effective and differs sharply with the natural history of patients with proximal aortic dissection, in whom every minute progression may lead to devastating complications and consequences.

REFERENCE

1. Doroghazi, R.M., Slater, E.E., DeSanctis, R.W., Buckley, M.J., Austen, W.G., and Rosenthal, S.: Long-term survival of patients treated with aortic dissection. J. Am. Coll. Cardiol. 3:1026, 1984.

386-C   (2 and 4 are correct) *(Braunwald, pp. 1385–1386)*

In approximately 4 per cent of patients undergoing PTCA, the dilatation may lead to abrupt occlusion of the treated vessel within 30 minutes. Certain lesions are more likely to lead to this outcome—particularly long, eccentric, or curved stenotic segments.[1] Approximately half the arteries in which abrupt occlusion occurs may be reopened by repeat PTCA.[2] However, the other half require emergency surgical intervention and in general display both clinical and electrocardiographic evidence of myocardial ischemia as well as some degree of MI. Such patients comprise a significant portion of the 0.4 per cent mortality that has been reported in association with elective PTCA.[3] The management of abrupt occlusion has been improved in recent years with the development of special perfusion or "shunt" catheters (see Braunwald, Fig. 40–15, p. 1386).[4] These may allow perfusion of the distal coronary bed while surgical preparations are made and the patient is transported to the operating suite. Such catheters thus serve as temporary intracoronary stents. The placement of more permanent vascular stents or the use of thermal welding in this and other settings is undergoing investigation as of this writing.

REFERENCES

1. Dorros, G., Cowley, M.J., Simpson, J., et al.: Percutaneous transluminal coronary angioplasty: Report of complications from the National Heart, Lung and Blood Institute PTCA Registry. Circulation 67:723, 1983.
2. Hollman, J., Gruentzig, A.R., Douglas, J.S., King, S.B., Ischinger, T., and Meier, B.: Acute occlusion after percutaneous transluminal angioplasty—new approach. Circulation 68:725, 1983.
3. Bredlau, C.E., Roubin, G.S., Leimgruber, P.P., Douglas, J.S., King, S.B., and Gruentzig, A.R.: In-hospital morbidity and mortality in elective coronary angioplasty. Circulation 72:1044, 1985.
4. Hinohara, T., Simpson, J.B., Phillips, H.R., Behar, V.S., Peter, R.H., Kong, Y., Carlson E.B., and Stack, R.S.: Transluminal catheter reperfusion: A new technique to reestablish blood flow after coronary occlusion during percutaneous transluminal coronary angioplasty. Am. J. Cardiol. 57:684, 1986.

387-A   (1, 2, and 3 are correct) *(Braunwald, pp. 1577–1578; Schafer, A.I.: The hypercoagulable states. Ann. Intern. Med. 102:814, 1985.)*

The primary hypercoagulable states may be defined by specific laboratory abnormalities and are suggested clinically when thrombosis occurs at an early age, at unusual anatomical sites, in a recurrent fashion without apparent precipitating factors, or when a family history of thrombosis exists. Antithrombin III deficiency is probably the most common of the primary hypercoagulable states and

is marked clinically by the occurrence of recurrent pulmonary emboli and deep venous thrombosis (DVT). Antithrombin III is the major inhibitor of thrombin in the circulation. Protein C, which consumes factors Va and VIIIa and stimulates fibrinolysis (as well as protein S, a cofactor for activated protein C), may predispose to recurrent venous thromboembolic disease if decreased or absent in the circulation. The "lupus anticoagulant" is most commonly associated with a prolongation of the partial thromboplastin time, but paradoxically leads to an increased risk of venous thromboembolic disease. Either defective release of tissue plasminogen activator or an excess of tissue plasminogen activator inhibitor may also lead to a defective fibrinolytic state, which is associated with venous thrombosis. While oral contraceptive use is associated with coronary emboli and deep venous thrombosis, the association is clinical and without specific laboratory abnormalities and is therefore considered a *secondary* hypercoagulable state.

388-B   (1 and 3 are correct) *(Braunwald, pp. 698 and 1271)*

The rhythm displayed is an example of accelerated idioventricular rhythm (AIVR), which is commonly defined as a ventricular escape rhythm with a rate between 60 and 100 beats/min. This rhythm is frequently referred to as "slow ventricular tachycardia" and may be seen in up to 20 per cent of patients with AMI, most commonly in the first 2 days after the acute infarction. In addition, AIVR is the most common arrhythmia noted following reperfusion of an occluded coronary artery by fibrinolytic therapy.[1] Approximately one-half of all episodes of AIVR are initiated by the occurrence of a premature beat; the other half of episodes are caused by sinus slowing or gradual speeding of a ventricular pacemaker with the emergence of an AIVR as an escape rhythm.[2] In general, episodes of AIVR are of short duration and may show variation in rate. Unlike more rapid forms of ventricular tachycardia, episodes of AIVR are in general thought not to affect prognosis in the setting of AMI.[1] It should be noted, however, that AIVR can occasionally accelerate to a more rapid ventricular tachycardia, which may require treatment. If an AIVR emerges which compromises hemodynamic function in any manner, treatment by accelerating the sinus rate with atropine or atrial pacing or by suppressing the ventricular pacemaker with lidocaine may be undertaken. However, no definitive evidence exists that AIVR by itself may lead to an increase in the incidence of either ventricular fibrillation or mortality.[3]

REFERENCES

1. Cercek, B., and Horvat, M.: Arrhythmias with brief, high-dose intravenous streptokinase infusion in acute myocardial infarction. Eur. Heart J. 6:109, 1985.
2. Lichstein, E., Ribas-Mineolier, C., Gupta, P.K., and Chadda, K.D.: Incidence and description of accelerated idioventricular rhythm complicating acute myocardial infarction. Am. J. Med. 58:192, 1975.
3. Bigger, J.T. Jr., Dresdale, R.J., Heissenbuttel, R.H., Weld, F.M., and Wit, A.L.: Ventricular arrhythmias in ischemic heart disease: Mechanism, prevalence, significance and management. Prog. Cardiovasc. Dis. 19:255, 1977.

389-A (1, 2, and 3 are correct) (*Braunwald, pp. 1421–1427*)

Among the characteristic features of hypertrophic obstructive cardiomyopathy (HOCM) is the variability of the left ventricular outflow gradient. Therefore, it is important when evaluating such a patient to perform a variety of dynamic maneuvers to bring out the murmur. Three basic mechanisms may be utilized to alter the systolic murmur, which reflects the severity of the obstruction: (1) increased contractility, (2) decreased preload, (3) decreased afterload. Increases in contractility and decreases in preload or afterload all tend to augment the murmur in the outflow tract. Perhaps the most helpful maneuver is sudden standing from a squatting position. Squatting results in an increase in venous return and an increase in aortic pressure, which increases the ventricular volume, diminishes the gradient, and decreases the intensity of the murmur. Sudden standing following this has the opposite effects and results in accentuation of the gradient and murmur. Similarly, during the strain phase of the Valsalva maneuver the murmur increases, owing to decreased preload and afterload. Other interventions that increase contractility, such as premature atrial contraction with post-extrasystolic potentiation, exercise, tachycardia, hypovolemia, and use of isoproterenol and digitalis, all increase the gradient and the murmur. Amyl nitrite, which markedly diminishes preload and afterload, will also increase the gradient and murmur.

A decrease in the gradient may result from any intervention that increases preload or decreases contractility. Thus, the Müller maneuver, i.e., a deep inspiration against a closed glottis, which is the opposite of the Valsalva maneuver, results in a lessening of the dynamic obstruction to LV outflow by increasing preload and afterload. Similarly, during the overshoot phase of the Valsalva maneuver, there is an increase in preload and afterload and a decrease in the murmur. Other interventions that tend to decrease the murmur include phenylephrine, beta-adrenoceptor blockade, and isometric handgrip.

390-B (1 and 3 are correct) (*Braunwald, pp. 1398–1399*)

Formulation of the target exercise intensity for each patient must take into consideration individual physical changes during exercise, symptoms, and the patient's perceived level of exertion. It is important to remember that the patient's training intensity should never exceed the point at which ischemia occurs. In general, a cardiac patient should train at between 50 and 75 per cent of maximal oxygen uptake, although in some situations a relative load of 40 per cent may be sufficient.[1] Conveniently, a wealth of information indicates that a heart rate of between 70 and 85 per cent of maximal capacity corresponds directly to the 50 to 75 per cent levels of maximal oxygen uptake that are required for training.[2] Of note, this relationship of heart rate to oxygen uptake is essentially constant for persons regardless of age and prior cardiac history.

Several methods exist for the estimation of a "target" heart rate that can be used to regulate physical activity intensity during exercise training. The simplest technique involves computation of the target heart rate zone as that which is 70 to 85 per cent of the maximal heart rate achieved during an earlier test. More complicated methods allow consideration of the variability of the resting heart rate as well as the symptom-limited relative functional aerobic capacity. However, in practice persons rarely maintain an exact target heart rate, demonstrating instead a variability of approximately 5 per cent above and below target heart rate values. Therefore, simpler techniques for estimating exercise intensity are probably acceptable and may even be preferable to the more complex methods alluded to.

REFERENCES

1. Exercise prescription for cardiac patients. *In* Blair, S.N., Gibbons, L.W. Painter, P., Pate, R.R., Taylor, C.B., and Wall, J. (eds.): American College of Sports Medicine Guidelines for Exercise Testing and Prescriptions. 3rd ed. Philadelphia, Lea and Febiger, 1986, pp. 53–71.
2. Franklin, B.A., Hellerstein, H.K., Gordon, S., and Timmis, G.C.: Exercise prescription for the myocardial infarction patient. Journal of Cardiopulmonary Rehabilitation 6:62, 1986.

391-B (1 and 3 are correct) (*Braunwald, pp. 1426–1429*)

Treatment of hypertrophic obstructive cardiomyopathy (HOCM) is difficult because many cardiac drugs affect contractility, preload, and afterload. These effects may produce beneficial results in some instances and adverse consequences in others. The mainstays of therapy have been beta-adrenoceptor blockers, which appear to prevent the increase in outflow obstruction accompanying exercise while not altering resting gradients. Beta blockade also inhibits the chronotropic response, thus limiting the demand for increased myocardial oxygen delivery. The calcium channel antagonists, such as verapamil, diltiazem, and nifedipine, are also efficacious. These drugs most likely improve function by depressing myocardial contractility, although the vasodilator effects of these agents would *not* be helpful in HOCM. Verapamil appears to improve diastolic filling by causing improved relaxation, rather than by changes in left ventricular diastolic stiffness; at any given diastolic volume, filling pressure is reduced.[1] Several complications have been observed with verapamil therapy including hemodynamic compromise—so that therapy should be carefully monitored.

Disopyramide, an antiarrhythmic drug, has produced symptomatic improvement in some patients with HOCM, presumably as a consequence of depression of left ventricular systolic performance.

Diuretics should be used carefully and sparingly in patients with HOCM, since reduction of intravascular volume may reduce ventricular size and increase the systolic pressure gradient, as well as cause a reduction in cardiac output and blood pressure. This is a particular problem in elderly patients with hypertensive, hypertrophic cardiomyopathy[2] who have small ventricular volume and limited stroke volume.

REFERENCES

1. Bonow, R.O., Ostrow, H.G., Rosing, D.R., Cannon, R.O. 3d, Lipton, L.C., Maron, B.J., Kent, K.M., Bacharach, S.L., and Green, M.V.: Effects of verapamil on left ventricular systolic and

diastolic function in patients with hypertrophic cardiomyopathy. Pressure-volume analysis with a non-imaging scintillation probe. Circulation 68:1062, 1983.
2. Topol, E.J., Traill, T.A., and Fortuin, N.J.: Hyperactive hypertrophic cardiomyopathy of the elderly. N. Engl. J. Med. 312:277, 1985.

392-B   (1 and 3 are correct) *(Braunwald, pp. 1364–1366)*

This 52-year-old man has the classic findings associated with a large anterior MI complicated by development of an LV aneurysm. The frequency of development of LV aneurysms after AMI depends on the incidence of transmural MI and congestive heart failure in the population studied. Over 80 per cent of LV aneurysms are located anterolaterally near the apex, with approximately 5 to 10 per cent located posteriorly. Most anterior aneurysms are true aneurysms, whereas nearly half of posterior aneurysms are false aneurysms, also known as pseudoaneurysms. These represent localized myocardial rupture in which the hemorrhage is limited by pericardial adhesions, with no myocardium present in the wall. About three-fourths of patients with aneurysms have multivessel coronary artery disease. Approximately 50 per cent of patients with moderate or large aneurysms will present with symptoms of heart failure, with or without associated angina. Thirty per cent have severe angina alone, and approximately 15 per cent have symptoms related to ventricular arrhythmias. Thrombi are found in about 50 per cent of patients with LV aneurysms, and embolic events occur with some frequency, usually within the first 4 to 6 months following infarction. Thus, it is prudent to administer anticoagulants, usually warfarin compounds, during this time period.

The most sensitive technique for diagnosis is biplane ventriculography. Although persistent ST-segment elevation on the ECG, a bulge on the cardiac silhouette, radionuclide ventriculography, and two-dimensional echocardiography all can suggest ventricular aneurysms, they rarely provide accurate assessment of the effect of the aneurysm on systolic function. Normal systolic motion of the interventricular septum is of importance in evaluating the function of residual myocardium because patients with impaired septal motion have a less favorable outcome following aneurysm surgery compared with patients who exhibit residual septal motion.[1]

The treatment of choice in symptomatic patients is aneurysmectomy, which is indicated in patients with congestive heart failure, refractory ventricular tachycardia, recurrent thromboembolism, and refractory angina. It is helpful, if possible, to wait approximately 6 months after the MI for the aneurysm to mature, at which point there is sufficient scar tissue to allow adequate surgical repair. The prognosis for patients with aneurysmectomy is significantly better than for those without, with an improvement of at least one New York Heart Association functional class in 70 to 80 per cent of the patients as well as improvement in the ejection fraction.

REFERENCE

1. Mullen, D.C., Posey, L., Gabriel, R., Singh, H.M., Flemma, R.J., and Lepley, D., Jr.: Prognostic considerations in the management of left ventricular aneurysms. Ann. Thorac. Surg. 23:455, 1977.

393-A   (1, 2, and 3 are correct) *(Braunwald, pp. 1410–1417)*

This 55-year-old man has congestive heart failure. There are several possible etiologies for his left ventricular dysfunction based on the clinical history. These include coronary artery disease exacerbated by his cigarette smoking and hypertension, primary hypertensive disease with evidence on chest x-ray and ECG for left ventricular hypertrophy, and alcohol-induced cardiomyopathy. Chronic excessive consumption of alcohol may itself cause hypertension. It has been observed clinically that the toxic effects of alcohol are more dramatic in hypertensive individuals and those with left ventricular hypertrophy. Alcoholic heart disease causes abnormalities of both systolic and diastolic function.[1] Two basic patterns have been observed: left ventricular dilatation with impaired systolic function and left ventricular hypertrophy with diminished compliance and normal or increased contractile performance. Left ventricular size is substantially increased in both. Frequently, these individuals have atrial fibrillation and ventricular arrhythmias as well as congestive heart failure. Angina pectoris does not usually occur unless there is concomitant coronary artery disease or aortic stenosis. Physical examination usually reveals elevated diastolic pressure, secondary to excessive peripheral vasoconstriction. There is frequently cardiomegaly, and S_3 and S_4 gallop sounds are common. An apical systolic murmur consistent with mitral regurgitation due to papillary muscle dysfunction is also found frequently, as in this individual.

The natural history of alcoholic cardiomyopathy depends on the drinking habits of the patient. Total abstinence in the early stages of the disease frequently leads to resolution of the manifestations of congestive heart failure and the return of the heart size to normal. Continued alcohol consumption leads to further myocardial damage and fibrosis with development of refractory heart failure. Thus, the key to treatment is complete abstinence. In this particular individual, who presented relatively early in the course of the illness, it is important that he curtail his drinking. It is also important to prescribe thiamine for the small possibility that thiamine deficiency may be contributing to the heart failure (see also Braunwald, pp. 786–787).

REFERENCE

1. Dancy, M., Leech, G., Bland, J.M., Gaitonde, M.K., and Maxwell, J.D.: Preclinical left ventricular abnormalities in alcoholics are independent of nutritional status, cirrhosis, and cigarette smoking. Lancet 1:1122, 1985.

394-A   (1, 2, and 3 are correct) *(Braunwald, pp. 1183–1196)*

Blood flow to the myocardium is determined by the perfusion pressure gradient and the vascular resistance of the appropriate myocardial bed. This is influenced by factors extrinsic to the bed (particularly compressive forces within the myocardium) and by metabolic, neural, and humoral factors intrinsic to the bed. Intramyocardial pressure is determined primarily by the ventricular pressure throughout the cardiac cycle. Because the ventricular pressure is so much higher in systole than it is in diastole, myocardial compressive forces acting on intra-myocardial vessels are much greater during this phase of the cardiac cycle. Therefore, the endocardium, which is subjected to higher systolic pressures, has a smaller systolic flow than the subepicardium. However, total flow is greater in the subendocardium than the subepicardium because there is enhanced basal vasodilatation in the subendocardium.[1] Interventions that reduce the perfusion gradient during diastole, when the majority of subendocardial flow occurs, lower the ratio of subendocardial to subepicardial flow and may cause the subendocardium to become ischemic. Thus, an increase in ventricular end-diastolic pressure such as occurs with stenotic lesions or a decrease in diastolic time as occurs with an increase in heart rate will decrease subendocardial flow disproportionately. Since the subendocardium has higher metabolic demands and hence lower basal vascular tone, the reserve for vasodilatation is less than in the subepicardium. Therefore, as perfusion is reduced, the deeper layers of the myocardium become ischemic sooner than the more superficial ones.

The subendocardium is susceptible to ischemia due to the combination of limited reserve of vasodilatation, extrinsic compression from the higher wall stress to which it is subjected, and the increased metabolic demands. This susceptibility accounts for the ST-segment depression on the ECG that is observed with episodes of transient ischemia.

REFERENCES

1. Klocke, F.J.: Coronary blood flow in man. Prog. Cardiovasc. Dis. 19:117, 1976.
2. Sabbaha, H.N., and Stein, P.D.: Effect of acute regional ischemia on pressure in the subepicardium and subendocardium. Am. J. Physiol. 242(Heart Circ. Physiol. 11): H240, 1982.

395-A (1, 2, and 3 are correct) *(Braunwald, pp. 1589 and 1778)*

Available data strongly suggest that tPA will have a major role in the treatment of pulmonary embolism. Initial interest in this agent was stimulated by experimental findings by Collen and colleagues of decreased hemorrhage and more fibrin-specific thrombolysis in rabbit and canine models of venous thrombosis. Clinical studies of the short-term efficacy and safety of acutely administered recombinant tissue plasminogen activator in acute pulmonary embolism have recently been carried out.[1, 2] In this study, 44 of 47 patients with angiographically documented pulmonary embolism had significant clot lysis within 2 to 6 hours following administration of tPA through a peripheral vein. Plasma fibrinogen levels in these patients decreased 42 per cent from baseline, and superficial oozing from venipuncture or arterial puncture sites was noted commonly. In addition, two major hemorrhagic complications occurred requiring surgical intervention (pericardial tamponade and hemorrhage from a pelvic tumor). The rate of major bleeding in this study was therefore 5 per cent, noted in conjunction with an 83 per cent moderate or marked improvement in

clinical symptoms and signs within 6 hours. While a precise role for tPA in the treatment of pulmonary embolism has not adequately been defined as of this writing, it is probable that the drug will play a significant role in the future.

REFERENCES

1. Goldhaber, S.Z., Vaughan, D.E., Markis, J.E., Selwyn, A.P., Meyerovitz, M.F., Loscalzo, J., Kim, D.S., Kessler, C.M., Dawley, D.L., Sharma, G.V.R.K., Sasahara, A., Grossbard, E.B., and Braunwald, E.: Acute pulmonary embolism treated with tissue plasminogen activator. Lancet 2:886, 1986.
2. Goldhaber, S.Z., Markis, J.E., Kessler, C.M., Meyerovitz, M.F., Kim, D., Vaughan, D.E., Selwyn, A.P. Loscalzo, J., Dawley, D.L., Sharma, G.V.R.K., Sasahara, A., Grossbard, E.B., and Braunwald, E.: Perspectives on treatment of acute pulmonary embolism with tissue plasminogen activator. Semin. Thromb. Hemost. 13:221, 1987.

396-A (1, 2, and 3 are correct) *(Braunwald, p. 1434)*

Clinical manifestations of heart disease are present in less than 5 per cent of patients with documented pulmonary sarcoidosis, although at autopsy in 20 to 30 per cent of sarcoid cases granulomas were found in the myocardium. The typical pathological feature of sarcoidosis is the presence of noncaseating granulomas which infiltrate the myocardium and eventually become fibrotic scars. The granulomas may involve any region of the heart, although the left ventricular free wall and interventricular septum are the most common sites. The extensive granular scar tissue in the interventricular septum leads to abnormalities in the conduction system. Involvement of cardiac valves is unusual. The murmur of mitral regurgitation is common. However, it appears to be caused by left ventricular dilatation rather than by direct sarcoid involvement of either papillary muscles or the valve.[1]

Sudden death is the most common cause of death in sarcoid heart disease, probably resulting from paroxysmal arrhythmias and AV block. Since the risk of sudden death appears to be greatest in patients with extensive myocardial involvement, it is reasonable to administer glucocorticosteroids in these patients when their disease is active. The diagnosis of sarcoid heart disease may be suspected in appropriate patients with bilateral adenopathy on chest x-ray, in whom there is clinical, echocardiographic, or ECG evidence of myocardial disease. Percutaneous myocardial biopsy may be particularly useful in establishing the diagnosis.

Treatment of myocardial sarcoidosis is difficult, with the arrhythmias being quite refractory to standard therapy. Permanent pacing may be helpful, especially in patients with advanced heart block.

REFERENCE

1. Roberts, W.C., McAllister, H.A., and Ferras, V.J.: Sarcoidosis of the heart. A clinicopathologic study of 35 necropsy patients (Group I) and review of 78 previously described necropsy patients (Group II). Am. J. Cardiol. 63:86, 1977.

397-E   (1, 2, 3, and 4 are correct) (Braunwald, pp. 1517–1519)

Radiation therapy for breast carcinoma and for both Hodgkin's and non-Hodgkin's lymphoma involving the mediastinum may subject the heart to radiation damage. A correlation between the volume of the heart included in the radiation field and the subsequent radiation damage exists. Thus, in patients treated for Hodgkin's disease with mantle therapy radiation in which 60 per cent or more of the cardiac silhouette is included within the treatment beam, the risk of radiation-induced pericarditis is about 5 to 7 per cent with lower doses of radiation, and rises sharply in incidence as higher doses are used.[1] In patients having radiation for breast cancer, in which the volume of the heart included in the field usually is less than 30 per cent, radiation-induced pericarditis occurs in less than 5 per cent; and higher doses of radiation therapy may be used.

While pericardial injury occurs during the course of treatment and is often evident within the first 12 months after completion of therapy, it is clear that radiation pericarditis may become manifested as a chronic pericardial effusion or constrictive process months or years following the original treatments.[2] In this regard, it is important to note that radiation injury may lead to constrictive pericarditis in children, a condition that is otherwise relatively uncommon in this age group.[3] In approximately 50 per cent of patients who have the delayed form of pericardial injury with onset of symptoms between 4 months and up to 20 years following the initial radiation, some degree of cardiac compression is noted. The remaining patients with this disorder will display an asymptomatic pericardial effusion with or without a coexistent pleural effusion on chest roentgenography. Because it is common for patients who undergo a pericardial window drainage for pericardial effusion following radiation therapy to develop late problems with constrictive pericarditis, extensive pericardiectomy is probably the treatment of choice in patients who develop effusive or effusive-constrictive radiation-induced pericarditis.[4]

Five-year survival in patients with postirradiation pericarditis and subsequent pericardiectomy is less than it is in comparable patients who have other causes for their pericarditis. This poor outcome may in part result from underlying myocardial injury as well as a firmly adherent and constricting visceral pericardial layer.

REFERENCES

1. Stewart, J.R., and Fajardo, L.F.: Radiation-induced heart disease: An update. Prog. Cardiovasc. Dis. 27:173, 1984.
2. Applefield, M.M., Slawson, R.G., Hall-Craigs, M., Green, D.C., Singleton, R.T., and Wiernik, P.H.: Delayed pericardial disease after radiotherapy. Am. J. Cardiol. 47:210, 1981.
3. Greenwood, R.D., Rosenthal, A., Cassidy, R., Jaffe, N., and Nadas, A.S.: Constrictive pericarditis in childhood due to mediasternal irradiation. Circulation 50:1033, 1974.
4. Siefert, F.C., Muler, C.D., Oesterle, S.N., Oyer, P.E., Stinson, E.B., and Shumway N.E.: Surgical treatment of constrictive pericarditis: Analysis of outcome and diagnostic error. Circulation 72(Suppl. I):264, 1975.

398-A   (1, 2, and 3 are correct) (Braunwald, pp. 1068–1069)

An ongoing controversy in cardiology is the timing of aortic valve replacement in patients with severe chronic AR. At the center of the issue is the clinical observation that many patients with severe chronic AR lead relatively normal lives for many years, while other patients have a rapid downhill course, sometimes even after valve replacement. From natural history studies carried out prior to modern surgery, the mean survival of patients with AR after the time of diagnosis was 10 years, emphasizing that AR is a long-term illness. In general, current practice dictates that patients who are otherwise healthy and symptom-free despite the presence of severe chronic AR do not require surgical intervention. On the other hand, patients who develop symptoms, and in particular patients who have documented decreases in left ventricular function, are more likely to require surgery.

A variety of tests including exercise tolerance tests, exercise radionuclide examinations, and various echocardiographic studies have been proposed to follow patients with AR and provide information on the appropriate timing of operation. It seems prudent to utilize at least one of these tests to follow a patient's performance and LV function serially.

Patients with severe AR and minimal or no symptoms can be followed provided that the condition is in fact chronic. Patients with infective endocarditis, and AR on that basis, represent a different situation. Patients with endocarditis who experience heart block, congestive heart failure, embolic events, and persistent fever have nearly 100 per cent mortality with medical therapy alone. In general, the earlier an operative procedure is carried out, the better the long-term survival and the lower the mortality.

Results of the early studies of patients with AR demonstrating that an M-mode echocardiographic end-systolic dimension of $\geq$ 5.5 cm predicted poor operative result may no longer be relevant due to recent improvement in operative technique. Thus, patients with dimensions of 6 cm or greater may do well surgically; it is currently not possible to accurately predict the outcome in any given patient based on echocardiographic measurements. Age, overall health, and symptoms are the most important predictors of surgical success in AR.

399-A   (1, 2, and 3 are correct) (Braunwald, pp. 1472–1475)

Primary tumors of the heart are relatively rare, with benign tumors representing approximately 75 per cent of these tumors. The majority of benign cardiac tumors are myxomas, followed in frequency by lipomas, papillary fibroelastomas, rhabdomyomas, fibromas, and other rare tumors. Among the malignant tumors, the most common are sarcomas, and of these the angiosarcoma and rhabdomyosarcoma are the most common forms.

Although it is difficult to differentiate benign from malignant tumors, certain findings may be helpful clinically. The presence of distant metastases, local mediastinal invasion, evidence of rapid growth in tumor size, hemorrhagic pericardial effusion, precordial pain, location of the tumor on the right as opposed to the left side of the heart, and extension into the pulmonary veins are all suggestive of a malignant rather than a benign tumor. Furthermore, infiltration of the myocardium is much more common in malignant than benign tumors. Benign tumors are more likely to occur on the left side of the interatrial septum and to grow slowly. Symptoms produced by benign and malignant tumors are difficult to differentiate since both cause fever, arthralgias, and abnormalities of red and white blood cells. Cardiac symptoms caused by tumors are primarily determined by mechanical interference. Myxomas that are located on the left side are more likely to produce mitral valve symptoms, while malignant tumors more commonly found on the right side of the heart tend to produce signs of right-sided failure such as peripheral edema.

400-B (1 and 3 are correct) *(Braunwald, pp. 1160–1161; 1638–1639)*

Chylomicrons are the largest of the lipoproteins and are composed mostly of triglycerides. They transport dietary triglyceride and cholesterol from the gut to the bloodstream. The chylomicrons are formed from cholesterol and partially digested triglycerides in the intestinal villi. In the cells of the intestinal wall cholesterol is esterified into cholesterol ester, mainly cholesterol oleate, through the enzymatic action of acyl cholesterol acyl transferase (ACAT). The resulting triglyceride particles complex with apolipoproteins and enter the systemic circulation via the lymphatic circulation. In the bloodstream, the chylomicrons bind to lipoprotein lipase, an enzyme on the endothelium that hydrolyzes the triglycerides, releasing free fatty acids. The now protein-enriched chylomicron remnants travel to the liver, where they are taken up by a receptor that recognizes apoprotein E. The presence of chylomicrons in fasting plasma is abnormal and is part of the criteria for the diagnosis of Type I and Type V hypolipoproteinemia. Chylomicronemia per se is not thought to result in premature coronary disease, although the accumulation of remnant particles as a consequence of chylomicron metabolism may be atherogenic.

401-E (1, 2, 3, and 4 are correct) *(Braunwald, pp. 1508–1509)*

Coxsackie virus group B and echovirus type 8 are the viruses most commonly associated with pericarditis in adults.[1] A variety of infections from other viruses may cause acute pericarditis and/or accompanying myocarditis; common entities in this group include mumps, influenza, infectious mononucleosis, poliomyelitis, varicella, and hepatitis B. It should be emphasized that there are no distinctive clinical features of viral pericarditis and that it is probable that many cases of community-acquired idiopathic pericarditis are due to unrecognized viral infection. Spring and fall are the peak seasons for the development of viral or idiopathic pericarditis, coincident with an increased incidence of enterovirus epidemics. Many patients with viral pericarditis report a prodromal syndrome of an upper respiratory tract infection, which they may describe as the "flu," just prior to the onset of chest pain.

In older patients, the diagnosis of viral pericarditis is one of exclusion. Other causes that must be considered include pericarditis due to rheumatoid disorders, recent MI, tuberculosis, and neoplasm.

The illness is usually of short duration and self-limited, although it may follow a dramatic course. In between 15 and 40 per cent of patients a recurrence of pericarditis may follow the acute illness after several weeks, and in a small number of patients such recurrences may continue in the months and years that follow the initial insult.[2] While uncommon, several complications of acute viral or idiopathic pericarditis may occur, including an associated myocarditis, the development of pericardial effusion with or without cardiac tamponade, recurrence, and the late development of constrictive pericarditis.

REFERENCES

1. Sainani, G.S., Dekate, M.P., and Rao, C.P.: Heart disease caused by Coxsackie virus B infection. Br. Heart J. 37:819, 1979.
2. Fowler, N.O., and Harbin, A.D.: Recurrent pericarditis: Follow-up of 31 patients. J. Am. Coll. Cardiol. 7:3000, 1986.

402-A (1, 2, and 3 are correct) *(Braunwald, p. 1161)*

Low-density lipoproteins (LDLs) are the major cholesterol-carrying components of the plasma. LDLs are mainly formed from VLDL breakdown, although they may also be synthesized directly. The major lipid components of LDL are triglyceride and esterified cholesterol. Apo B-100 is the predominant protein present in LDL and comprises approximately 25 per cent of the LDL mass. After LDLs are formed in the liver they are bound by the specific receptors in a variety of tissues, including the liver. In familial hypercholesterolemia there is a decreased number of LDL receptors; however, over 80 per cent of patients with elevated LDL do not have this single-gene disorder but rather have polygenic hypercholesterolemia. Therefore, elevations of LDL due to a primary receptor defect are relatively uncommon. Apo E is the predominant apolipoprotein of high-density lipoproteins (HDLs). It may be "antiatherogenic" because it facilitates the uptake of chylomicron remnants by the liver.

403-B (1 and 3 are correct) *(Braunwald, pp. 1327–1330)*

Nitroglycerin administered sublingually is the drug of choice in the treatment of angina pectoris. The usual sublingual dosage of nitroglycerin is 0.3 to 0.6 mg, and most patients respond within 5 minutes to one or two 0.3 mg tablets. The development of tolerance is rarely a problem with intermittent sublingual usage. Even in patients who have been on chronic nitrates the rapidity of the increase in nitrate levels achieved through buccal absorption usually overwhelms the "tolerant state." However, among the causes for inadequate responses to orally administered nitrates are poor absorption due to dryness of the mouth and a delay in the dissolution of the tablet. This can be remedied by use of either a spray or tablets that contain a moisture gel that can be placed directly on the gum. Nitrates also undergo degradation when left in the open, especially when exposed to light, and it is likely that in the patient described the light on the windowsill caused loss of potency of her pills.

In patients with stable angina, nitrate tolerance appears to develop during four-times-daily therapy with oral isosorbide dinitrate, so that the improvement in exercise tolerance disappears within a matter of a few days. This can be prevented by allowing prolonged drug-free intervals. Thus, one recommendation would be to have the patient take a pill at dinner and not take another until breakfast. This long drug-free interval allows recovery of the response to nitrates. Nitrate tolerance is particularly common with transdermal discs, because they continuously deliver a small dosage and because nitrate levels are maintained constantly.

404-C   (2 and 4 are correct) *(Braunwald, p. 1573)*

The clinical presentation of patients with chronic constrictive pericarditis is determined in part by the degree of elevation of systemic venous and right atrial pressures. In patients with a modest elevation in such pressures, symptoms due to systemic venous congestion may predominate, including edema, ascites, and discomfort due to passive hepatic congestion. When right and left heart filling pressures reach the 15 to 30 mm Hg level, symptoms of pulmonary venous congestion may appear, along with pleural effusions and elevation of the diaphragm due to ascites, all of which contribute to tachypnea and dyspnea. The most important clinical finding in constriction is the elevation of jugular venous pressure, which may be obscured if the patient is examined in the supine position. While elevated jugular venous pressure is a clue to the presence of the disorder, other causes of increased venous pressure must be excluded.

In pure or classic constrictive pericarditis, the presence of pulsus paradoxus is uncommon,[1] although if pericardial fluid is present as well (effusive-constrictive pericarditis), this sign may be observed. Most patients with chronic constrictive pericarditis have an unobtrusive but diffuse precordial movement due to systolic retraction of the apical cardiac impulse.[2] The most distinctive auscultatory finding in constrictive pericarditis is the presence of the *diastolic* pericardial knock, an early diastolic sound that may be heard at the left sternal border and corresponds in timing to the sudden cessation of ventricular filling due to the rigid, constricting pericardium. Pericardial knocks are in general earlier and of higher frequency than the typical S_3 gallop sounds, and may on occasion be confused with the opening snap of mitral stenosis. Most patients with constrictive pericarditis demonstrate hepatomegaly along with prominent hepatic pulsations and other evidence of hepatic dysfunction due to passive liver congestion. Younger patients with competent venous valves may have little or no lower extremity edema. In contrast, older patients with longstanding constrictive pericarditis may have large accumulations of fluid throughout the lower torso and abdominal cavity.

REFERENCES

1. Fowler, N.O.: Constrictive pericarditis: New aspects. Am. J. Cardiol. 50:1014, 1982.

2. Blake, S.: The clinical diagnosis of constrictive pericarditis. Am. Heart J. 106:432, 1983.

405-B   (1 and 3 are correct) *(Braunwald, pp. 1196–1202)*

The normal coronary vascular bed has the ability to reduce its resistance to approximately 20 per cent of basal levels during maximal exercise. The basic principles of fluid mechanics indicate that the pressure drop across a stenosis varies directly with the length of the stenosis and inversely with the fourth power of the radius. Thus changes in the radius are much more important than changes in the length of the stenosis. Furthermore, it can be shown that significant changes in flow do not occur until stenoses are greater than 80 per cent of the original diameter of the vessel. However, the resistance to flow triples as the severity of the stenosis increases from 80 to 90 per cent.[1] As a consequence, even a slight change in the severity of such a stenosis can cause a dramatic alteration in the coronary perfusion pressure distal to the obstruction.

In such a tight stenosis, when flow across the stenosis rises, passive collapse[2] may occur. This is due to substantial energy losses from turbulence (proportional to the square of the flow) which result in an exponential rise in the pressure gradient across the stenosis. Thus at any flow rate, the gradient rises with the degree of stenosis. Therefore, as the transstenotic pressure gradient increases, the distal perfusion pressure will fall significantly, leading to a fall in intraluminal pressure and collapse of the vessel, thereby further augmenting the severity of stenosis.

REFERENCES

1. Klocke, F.J.: Measurements of coronary blood flow and degree of stenosis: Current clinical implications and continuing uncertainties. J. Am. Coll. Cardiol. 1:31, 1983.

2. Epstein, S.E., Cannon, R.O., III, and Talbot, T.L.: Hemodynamic principles in the control of coronary blood flow. Am. J. Cardiol. 56:4E, 1985.

406-E   (1, 2, 3, and 4 are correct) *(Braunwald, pp. 1592–1593)*

The NIH consensus development statement regarding the prevention of venous thrombosis and pulmonary embolism[1] notes that clinically significant pulmonary embolism occurs in approximately 1.6 per cent of the general surgical population. This body therefore recommended prophylaxis in all general surgical patients who meet any of the following criteria: (1) age 40 and over, (2) surgical procedures longer than one hour's duration, (3) obesity, (4) known cancer, or (5) prior pulmonary embolism or DVT. The presence of any of these should dictate the use of 5000 units of heparin subcutaneously every 8 to 12 hours beginning before surgery commences and continuing at least until the patient is ambulatory.

Patients at higher risk should receive a combination of heparin and dihydroergotamine (H-DHE), which has been shown in a variety of clinical trials to be more effective than either drug alone in the prophylaxis of venous thromboembolism.[2] In 1985, the FDA approved one fixed dose of heparin (5000 units) in combination with 0.5 mg of DHE to be administered subcutaneously 2 hours prior to surgery and then every 12 hours for 5 to 7 days. Because of the selective vasoconstrictive effect on veins and venules from the dihydroergotamine preparation, the drug is believed to help counteract venous stasis by accelerating venous return from the legs. However, it should not be used in patients undergoing vascular surgery or in those who have suspected bowel or coronary ischemia.

REFERENCES

1. NIH Consensus Development Statement: Prevention of venous thrombosis and pulmonary embolism. JAMA 256:744, 1986.
2. Gent, M., and Roberts, R.S.: A meta-analysis of the studies of dihydroergotamine plus heparin in the prophylaxis of deep vein thrombosis. Chest 89:3965, 1986.

407-C (2 and 4 are correct) *(Braunwald, pp. 1360–1362)*

The treatment of Prinzmetal's variant angina is similar to that of chronic stable angina in some respects, but several drugs useful in patients with stable angina may provoke paradoxical clinical deterioration in those with Prinzmetal's angina. Patients with both forms of angina are successfully treated with nitrates, which are direct vascular smooth muscle dilators. However, the response in patients with variant angina to beta blockers is variable. In some patients with fixed stenoses beta blockers, by reducing myocardial oxygen demands, will lessen symptoms. In others, however, blockade of beta$_2$ receptors, which are involved in coronary dilation, allows unopposed alpha-adrenoceptor receptor activity leading to coronary vasoconstriction, which may prolong episodes of vasospasm.[1]

In contrast to the beta blockers, the calcium channel antagonists are universally effective in preventing coronary artery spasm associated with variant angina.[2] The three currently available calcium channel antagonists, nifedipine, diltiazem, and verapamil, are all equally effective, although some idiosyncratic responses have been documented. Prazosin, a selective alpha$_1$-adrenoreceptor blocker, has also been found to be of some value. Aspirin, which improves symptoms and decreases infarction in unstable angina, may actually increase the frequency of ischemic episodes in patients with Prinzmetal's angina, because it inhibits synthesis of the naturally occurring vasodilator prostaglandin I$_2$.[3]

REFERENCES

1. Robertson, R.M., Wood, A.J.J., Vaughn, W.K., and Robertson, D.: Exacerbation of vasotonic angina pectoris by propranolol. Circulation 65:281, 1982.
2. Schroeder, J.S., Lamb, I.H., Bristow, M.R., Ginsburg, R., Hung, J., and McAuley, B.J.: Prevention of cardiovascular events in variant angina by long-term diltiazem therapy. J. Am. Coll. Cardiol. 1:1507, 1983.
3. Miwar, K., Kambara, H., and Kawai, C.: Effect of aspirin in large doses on attacks of variant angina. Am. Heart J. 105:351, 1983.

408-A (1, 2, and 3 are correct) *(Braunwald, pp. 1340–1342)*

Several large prospective studies in the 1970's examined the results of surgical as opposed to medical treat-

ment of coronary artery disease. Between 1975 and 1979, the Coronary Artery Surgery Study (CASS) evaluated patients aged 65 or younger with a myocardial infarction or mild angina pectoris. Patients were randomized to medical or surgical therapy if they had significant operable coronary artery disease. In the 7 years of follow-up, cumulative survival in the patients with one-, two-, and three-vessel disease randomized to either the surgical or medical treatment were respectively 92 and 90 per cent for one-vessel disease, 88 per cent in each group for two-vessel disease, and 99 and 83 per cent respectively for patients with three-vessel disease.

An important finding was that certain subgroups were identified who had improved survival with surgical treatment. In particular, a significant advantage favoring surgical treatment was observed in patients with three-vessel disease and an ejection fraction between 35 and 50 per cent. A total of 88 per cent of patients in the surgical group and 65 per cent of those in the medical group were alive after 7 years. Also, in patients with severe angina, surgery improved survival in those with three-vessel disease, regardless of whether ventricular function was normal or depressed.[3] Furthermore, the CASS showed that surgical therapy prolonged survival, particularly in patients with ejection fractions below 26 per cent: 43 per cent five-year survival was found with medical treatment, as compared with 63 per cent with surgical treatment in these patients. These studies suggest that if operative mortality is lower than approximately 7 per cent, surgery is likely to offer an advantage over medical therapy in terms of survival in patients with ischemic myocardium and severely depressed left ventricular function. Surgery also appears to confer an advantage in patients with three-vessel disease and severe angina pectoris.

REFERENCES

1. Passamani, E., Davis, K.B., Gillespie, M.J., Killip, T., and the CASS principal investigators and their associates: A randomized trial of coronary artery bypass surgery. N. Engl. J. Med. 312:1665, 1985.
2. Killip, T., Passamani, E., Davis, K., and the CASS principal investigators and their associates: Coronary artery surgery study (CASS): A randomized trial of coronary bypass surgery. Eight-year follow-up and survival in patients with reduced ejection fraction. Circulation 72(Suppl. V):102, 1985.
3. Kaiser, G.C., Davis, K.B., Fisher, L.D., Myers, W.O., Foster, E.D., Passamani, E.R., and Gillespie, M.J.: Survival following coronary artery bypass grafting in patients with severe angina pectoris (CASS). J. Thorac. Cardiovasc. Surg. 89:513, 1985.

409-A (1, 2, and 3 are correct) *(Braunwald, pp. 1052–1054)*

In the adult with acquired AS, stenosis of a tricuspid aortic valve is usually on a congenital, rheumatic, or degenerative basis. Rheumatic stenosis results from adhesions along the commissures of the cusps leading to retraction and stiffening of the free borders of the cusps with calcific nodules present on both surfaces. Since there is commissural fusion with associated retraction, the rheumatic valve is often regurgitant as well as stenotic. In degenerative or senile calcific AS, the immobility of the aortic valve is due to deposition of calcium at the valve bases rather than at the tips. This now appears to be the most common cause currently of AS in adults in the United States; it is probably due to trauma secondary to normal mechanical stress on the valve. Common associated findings in patients with this form of AS include calcification of the mitral annulus and the coronary arteries, but coexisting AR is uncommon. Both diabetes mellitus and hypercholesterolemia appear to be risk factors for the development of calcific AS.[1] Other causes of AS in adults include rheumatoid involvement of the valve and, very rarely, ochronosis.[2]

REFERENCES

1. Deutscher, S., Rockette, H.E., and Krishanswami, V.: Diabetes and hypercholesterolemia among patients with calcific aortic stenosis. J. Chronic Dis. 37:407, 1984.
2. Ptacin, M., Sebastian, J., and Bamrah, V.S.: Ochronotic cardiovascular disease. Clin. Cardiol. 8:441, 1985.

410-E   (1, 2, 3, and 4 are correct) *(Braunwald, pp. 1023–1026)*

In normal adults the mitral valve orifice is 4–6 cm². When the orifice is reduced to approximately 2 cm², which is consistent with mild MS, blood flow from the LA to the LV occurs only with the development of an abnormal pressure gradient. When the mitral valve opening is reduced further, to approximately 1 cm², critical MS is considered to exist. In this setting, a pressure gradient of approximately 20 mm Hg is recorded, and therefore in the presence of normal LV diastolic pressure, a mean left atrial pressure of approximately 25 to 30 mm Hg is required to maintain normal cardiac output at rest. The severity of mitral valve obstruction is determined by both the transvalvular gradient and the flow rate. The transvalvular flow rate depends directly on the cardiac output and inversely on the heart rate. An increase in heart rate shortens the time for diastole proportionately more than systole and diminishes the time for flow across the mitral valve. Therefore, at any given level of cardiac output (flow rate), tachycardia augments the transmitral valvular pressure gradient.

Hydrodynamic considerations indicate that for any given orifice size the transvalvular gradient is a function of the *square* of the transvalvular flow rate,[1] i.e., a doubling of the flow rate will quadruple the pressure gradient. Thus, a patient with moderate mitral stenosis (e.g., a valve area 2 cm²) at rest would be able to generate a flow of 300 ml per second of diastole with a diastolic pressure gradient of less than 20 mm Hg. However, with exercise and a doubling of the heart rate, the time for diastole will be at least halved. The flow rate would now have to be approximately 600 ml, which would require a much greater diastolic pressure gradient resulting in symptoms of dyspnea and congestive heart failure.

Atrial contraction augments the presystolic transmitral valvular gradient by approximately 30 per cent in patients with MS. A loss of atrial contraction by the development of atrial fibrillation decreases cardiac output by approximately 20 per cent. Furthermore, the rapid ventricular rate common in atrial fibrillation raises the transvalvular pressure gradient. Thus, the importance of sinus rhythm

in patients with MS is determined by both effects on transvalvular flow rate and the ability to raise the presystolic transmitral valve gradient.

REFERENCE

1. Gorlin, R., and Gorlin, S.G.: Hydraulic formula for calculation of the area of stenotic mitral valve, other cardiac valves and central circulatory shunts. Am. Heart J. 41:1, 1951.

411-A   (1, 2, and 3 are correct) *(Braunwald, p. 1164)*

Type IV hyperlipoproteinemia is characterized by increased VLDL, normal or increased cholesterol level, and increased triglycerides. The metabolic defect appears to be an oversynthesis of triglyceride and VLDL by the liver. The genetic disorders that are associated with this disorder include familial hypertriglyceridemia and familial combined hyperlipidemia. Secondary causes of Type IV pattern are common and include excess dietary calories or alcohol, renal failure, diabetes mellitus, hepatocellular disease (glycogen-lipid storage disease), and dysproteinemias. Diabetes is frequently associated with elevated triglycerides; this appears to be due to the elevated insulin levels. Reduced lipoprotein lipase activity occurs in myxedema and renal failure and may account for the elevated triglyceride levels in these conditions. Although neurofibromatosis is associated with an increased incidence of cardiovascular disease, it is not associated with hyperlipoproteinemia.

412-A   (1, 2, and 3 are correct) *(Braunwald, pp. 1316–1319)*

The incidence of coronary artery disease in groups of patients with typical angina, atypical angina, and nonanginal chest pain has been estimated to be about 90, 50, and 10 per cent, respectively. The incidence of coronary artery disease in asymptomatic adults of comparable age is estimated to be about 3 to 4 per cent.[1] In general the clinical manifestations of ischemia are more severe in patients with multivessel than single-vessel disease, but in any individual patient, the nature of the underlying disease cannot be predicted from the severity, nature, duration, or quality of the chest discomfort. This has become particularly evident from studies of patients with advanced coronary artery disease who have so-called "silent ischemia."[2] In general, in patients with the same degree of coronary artery disease, asymptomatic patients have better survival than those with severe angina. When infarction is the first manifestation of ischemic heart disease, it is often associated with single-vessel disease, while initial presentation with angina is more consistent with multivessel disease.[3] Finally, women have angina pectoris at presentation much more frequently than men, in whom fatal and nonfatal myocardial infarctions are relatively more common.[4]

REFERENCES

1. Diamond, G.A., and Forrester, J.S.: Analysis of probability as an aid in the clinical diagnosis of coronary artery disease. N. Engl. J. Med. 300:1350, 1979.

2. Selwyn, A.P., Shea, M., Deanfield, J.E., Wilson, R., Horlock, P., and O'Brien, H.A.: Character of transient ischemia in angina pectoris. Am. J. Cardiol. 58:21B–25B, 1986.
3. Midwall, J., Ambrose, J., Pichard, A., Abedin, A., and Herman, M.V.: Angina pectoris before and after myocardial infarction. Angiographic correlations. Chest 81:681, 1982.
4. Reunanen, A., Suhonen, O., Aromaa, A., Kneckt, P., and Pyorala, K.: Incidence of different manifestations of coronary heart disease in middle-aged Finnish men and women. Acta Med. Scand. 218:19, 1985.

413-B, 414-B, 415-A, 416-C (Braunwald, p. 1167)

Prescribed medications are among the common contributing factors to abnormal serum lipids. Commonly used medications in patients with cardiovascular disease which elevate cholesterol, LDL, triglyceride, and VLDL include thiazide diuretics and beta blockers. Beta blockers have also been shown to lower the HDL fraction of total cholesterol.[1] Although thiazide diuretics have multiple effects, their dominant effects are to increase LDL, VLDL, and triglycerides. Oral contraceptives tend to increase levels of serum cholesterol, but the overall effect on lipids is a function of the relative amounts of estrogen and progesterone in different preparations.[2] Estrogens tend to raise HDL cholesterol and VLDL levels, while progesterone analogs decrease elevated levels of triglycerides and also decrease HDL. Many other drugs including alpha-adrenoreceptor blockers such as prazosin, calcium channel antagonists, angiotensin-converting enzyme inhibitors, and centrally acting antihypertensive drugs such as clonidine and guanabenz have no significant effect on plasma lipoproteins.

REFERENCES

1. Leren, P., Foss, P.O., Helgeland, A., Hjermann, I., Holme, I., and Lund-Larsen, P.G.: Effect of propranolol and prazosin on blood lipids. The Oslo Study. Lancet 2:4, 1980.
2. Wahl, P., Walden, C., Knopp, R., Hoover, J., Wallace, R., Neiss, G., and Rifkind, B.: Effect of estrogen/progestin potency on lipid/lipoprotein cholesterol. N. Engl. J. Med. 308:862, 1983.

417-A, 418-C, 419-B, 420-D (Braunwald, pp. 925–929)

Persistent truncus arteriosus is a rare, serious congenital anomaly in which a single vessel forms the outlet of both ventricles, giving rise to the systemic, pulmonary, and coronary arteries. Persistent truncus arteriosus is always accompanied by a VSD and usually by a right-sided aortic arch. The VSD results from an absence or underdevelopment of the distal portion of the pulmonary infundibulum. This malformation should be distinguished from "pseudotruncus arteriosus," which is the severe form of tetralogy of Fallot with pulmonary atresia, in which the single aorta arises from the heart in the presence of a remnant of pulmonary artery. Differentiation between truncus arteriosus and tetralogy of Fallot by ultrasound may be difficult. The diagnosis may be suspected at cardiac catheterization if the catheter fails to enter the central pulmonary arteries from the RV. Selective angiocardiography and retrograde aortography are necessary to establish the diagnosis and reveal the common trunk arising from the heart, as well as the origin of the pulmonary arteries from this trunk.

Anomalous origin of the coronary artery from the pulmonary artery is a rare malformation which is usually characterized by the *left* coronary artery having its source from the posterior sinus of the pulmonary artery. The most common clinical presentation of this anomaly is the occurrence of MI and subsequent congestive heart failure in an infant. The syndrome usually becomes manifested between 2 and 4 months of age with angina-like symptoms that may be misinterpreted as colic. The diagnosis of anomalous origin of the coronary artery gains support from electrocardiographic demonstration of Q waves in association with ischemic ST-segment alterations and T-wave inversions in lateral chest leads. The diagnosis may be established using retrograde aortography to demonstrate drainage of the left coronary artery into the pulmonary artery. Ventricular arrhythmias may complicate this disorder. Management of infants with anomalous pulmonary origin of the coronary artery depends in part on the degree of left-to-right shunting that is present. The surgical outcome and ultimate prognosis depend on how much myocardial damage the patient has suffered preoperatively.

Coronary arteriovenous fistula also is an unusual anomaly composed of a communication between the coronary system and a cardiac chamber, usually the RV, RA, or coronary sinus. In approximately 55 per cent of cases, the right coronary artery is involved. A majority of these communications lead to a small degree of left-to-right shunting, and patients are most often asymptomatic. Diagnosis thus occurs most commonly because of a loud, superficial continuous cardiac murmur. The ECG and chest x-ray are usually normal in this disorder. Significantly enlarged coronary arteries may be visualized by two-dimensional echocardiography, and occasionally the diagnosis can be made by a combination of this technique and Doppler flow analysis. The usual treatment of this disorder involves closure of the fistula even in asymptomatic patients in order to prevent subsequent symptoms or complications such as infective endocarditis.

Congenital aneurysm of an aortic sinus of Valsalva occurs most frequently in the right coronary sinus and in males, although it is an uncommon anomaly. When such an aneurysm ruptures, the resulting aorticocardiac fistula usually involves a communication with the RV, although when the noncoronary cusp is affected the fistula may drain into the RA. The presence of this disorder may be suspected in a patient with the sudden onset of chest pain, symptoms of decreased cardiac reserve, hyperdynamic pulses, and a loud, continuous, superficial murmur accentuated in diastole. The physical findings may occasionally be difficult to distinguish from those produced by a coronary arteriovenous fistula. ECG may show biventricular hypertrophy and chest x-ray may show generalized cardiac enlargement. Echocardiographic studies may be able to localize the aneurysm, as well as the perturbation in flow produced by the fistula. Diagnosis may be established definitively by retrograde aortography, and cardiac catheterization may reveal a left-to-right shunt at the ventricular level. Preoperative medical management involves treatment of congestive heart failure, arrhythmias, and endocarditis.

Aortic arch obstruction describes a variety of lesions that lead to interruption of a portion of the aortic arch, including localized juxtaductal coarctation, hypoplasia of the aortic isthmus, and frank aortic arch interruption. In contrast to the four lesions mentioned, aortic arch obstruction may exist without accompanying left-to-right shunting.

421-B, 422-C, 423-A, 424-D   *(Braunwald, pp. 1136–1140)*

Each of the cell types listed is involved in the process of atherogenesis, albeit in different ways. *Endothelial cells*, which represent a large and extensive lining of the entire vascular tree, form a highly selective, permeable barrier to the bloodstream and maintain a nonthrombogenic surface. They also actively manufacture and secrete several important vasoactive substances. Endothelial cells have a surface coat of heparan sulfate which helps maintain nonthrombogenicity and are capable of forming prostaglandin derivatives, in particular prostacyclin. The latter is a vasodilator which inhibits platelet aggregation.[1] In addition, endothelial cells secrete tissue plasminogen activator, which may lead ultimately to lysis of fibrin clots and regulation of the local hemostatic milieu, and endothelium-derived relaxing factor (EDRF), which causes vasodilation and also inhibits platelet aggregation. EDRF has recently been identified as nitric oxide and may therefore be considered an endogenous nitrate. Thus, endothelial cells regulate or provide protection against the development of inappropriate thrombus formation through a variety of mechanisms.

The *smooth muscle cell* is orginally derived from the media of the blood vessel and proliferates extensively in the arterial intima to form atherosclerotic plaques. The principal physiological role of this cell in the media of the artery is presumably to maintain arterial wall tone by a capacity to alter contractile state in response to a variety of substances. Thus, prostacyclin may induce relaxation and vasodilation, while numerous vasoactive agents such as epinephrine and angiotensin may cause smooth muscle contraction. Like the macrophage, the smooth muscle cell may become filled with cholesteryl ester and form a "foam cell." In advanced atherosclerotic lesions extensive proliferation of smooth muscle cells in the intima contributes significantly to the development of the mature atherosclerotic lesion.

Macrophages, derived from circulating blood monocytes, are capable of secreting a large number of biologically active substances as they participate in the inflammatory and immune responses. These cells synthesize and secrete a variety of growth factors, which are probably critical in the proliferation of connective tissues which may be involved in development of atherosclerotic lesions. Macrophages become foam cells by extensive accumulation of cholesteryl ester and as such form the principal cells in the fatty streak, the initial lesion of the developing atherosclerotic plaque.

Platelets participate in an important and complex manner with both the endothelium and developing atherosclerotic plaque. Although platelets are capable of little or no protein synthesis, they contain numerous protein substances in their alpha granules which are released upon platelet activation. These include a variety of factors that participate in the coagulation cascade as well as several extremely potent growth factors or mitogens. Growth factors may play an important role in stimulating both vasoconstriction and subsequent proliferation in the injured vessel wall. In addition, the factors released that participate in the coagulation cascade play a role with platelets in the development of thrombi and as such are important clinically in the thrombotic sequelae of atherosclerotic disease.

Each of the cells mentioned plays an important part in the "response-to-injury" hypothesis favored by Ross and colleagues.[2] In this theory, some form of injury occurs to the endothelial cells lining the arterial wall. The subsequent interactions between the underlying portions of the blood vessel, the blood elements, and the various cells mentioned lead to a vascular response to injury and, if unchecked, may ultimately lead to a frank atherosclerotic lesion (see Braunwald, Fig. 35–11, p. 1143).

REFERENCES

1. Moncada, S., Herman, A.G., Higgs, E.A., and Vane, J.R.: Differential formation of prostacyclin (PGX or PGI$_2$) by layers of the arterial wall. An explanation for the antithrombotic properties of vascular endothelium. Thromb. Res. 11:323, 1977.
2. Ross, R.: The pathogenesis of atherosclerosis—An update. N. Engl. J. Med. 314:496, 1986.

425-C, 426-A, 427-A, 428-D, 429-B   *(Braunwald, pp. 1009–1012)*

Cardiac dysfunction in *diphtheria* usually occurs in unimmunized children, especially in the western United States, and appears to be due to abnormal myocardial lipid metabolism due to the diphtheria toxin.[1] Pathologically, extensive fat vacuolization and glycogen depletion is noted in myocytes. Cardiac involvement occurs in approximately 10 per cent of patients with diphtheria and is the most common cause of death from the disease. Heart disease is most easily detected by noting electrocardiographic changes, which may range from ST-segment and T-wave changes to arrhythmias and conduction disturbances, including complete heart block. The appearance of right or left bundle branch block or complete AV block is associated with mortality rates of greater than 50 per cent. In general, treatment for this disorder is not satisfactory. Patients receive diphtheria antitoxin and intravenous penicillin, as well as symptomatic treatment for arrhythmias and congestive failure due to myocardial dysfunction. However, no specific therapy is available. The prognosis is good if the child recovers from the acute episode of diphtheritic cardiomyopathy.

Infection by trypanosomal organisms, especially *Trypanosoma cruzi*, results in Chagas' disease, which occurs most commonly in the Southern United States and which is endemic in Latin America. Trypanosomal myocarditis is an unusual disease in that its most important clinical manifestation is a chronic myocarditis that may not occur until 10 to 30 years after the acute infectious process. There is no satisfactory treatment for the illness. Another trypanosome, *Trypanosoma rhodesiense*, which causes African sleeping sickness, may produce myocardial hemorrhage and a slow degenerative disease resulting in myocardial failure. Cardiac involvement with this parasite is usually mild and is overshadowed by the concomitant encephalitis.

In newborns, Coxsackie B and rubella viruses are the most common causative agents of *infective myocarditis*. Coxsackie B leads to an illness of sudden onset characterized by systemic signs of infection and occasionally cardiac failure. The diagnosis of this viral myocarditis is first suggested by ECG findings that may include atrial or ventricular arrhythmias as well as by marked cardiomegaly and pulmonary vascular congestion on the chest x-ray. When the virus can be isolated from pharyngeal secretions or other body fluids, the diagnosis is strongly suggested. Although general supportive measures are of little benefit in this disorder, the vast majority of children recover from acute episodes of myocarditis with few or no sequelae. After infancy, other agents that may cause such a viral myocarditis include Coxsackie A, influenza, adenovirus, and echovirus. In addition, many of the common viral infectious diseases of childhood, such as mumps and measles, may be associated with a mild myocarditis. Rarely, a child may develop sequelae, such as a permanent conduction defect or a mild cardiac enlargement from viral myocarditis. In some cases, a more severe chronic cardiomyopathy may result. There do not appear to be any predictive criteria to identify which children will ultimately suffer more severe complications.[2]

REFERENCES

1. Challoner, D.R., and Prols, H.G.: Free fatty acid oxidation and carnitine levels in diphtheritic guinea pig myocardium. J. Clin. Invest. 51:2071, 1972.
2. Taliercio, C.P., Seward, J.B., Driscoll, D.J., Fisher, L.D., Gersh, B.J., and Tajik, A.J.: Idiopathic dilated cardiomyopathy in the young: Clinical profile and natural history. J. Am. Coll. Cardiol. 6:1126, 1985.

430-D, 431-B, 432-E, 433-A *(Braunwald, pp. 1052–1056)*

The diagnosis of *aortic stenosis* (AS) by clinical examination rests on several physical findings. Among these are the location and radiation of the murmur and thrill, presence of an aortic ejection sound, characteristics of the aortic component of the second sound, coexisting presence of a regurgitant diastolic murmur, and characteristics of the arterial pulse in both the carotid and peripheral vessels. In the most common form of AS (the acquired nonrheumatic form), the murmur is commonly heard over the second right intercostal space radiating to the neck. An aortic ejection sound is uncommon, and the aortic component of the second heart sound is diminished or absent. A regurgitant diastolic murmur is occasionally heard especially in patients with coexisting hypertension; the carotid pulses are delayed in upstroke and are of diminished volume.

Examination findings in patients with acquired AS due to rheumatic fever are quite similar. One exception is the increased incidence of coexisting aortic regurgitation (AR) due to commissural fusion and retraction of the aortic valve leaflets.

Hypertrophic obstructive cardiomyopathy (HOCM) is

characterized by its prevalence throughout all age groups in contrast to calcific AS, which is observed more frequently in the elderly. In HOCM the systolic murmur is frequently audible along the sternal border and radiates well to the apex. Features characteristic of HOCM are a normal aortic component of the second heart sound, absence of a murmur of AR, and frequent coexistence of mitral regurgitation (MR). It should also be noted that in HOCM the arterial pulse is usually brisk and sometimes bisferiens (classically a spike and dome configuration is noted.)

In *congenital subaortic stenosis* the presence of a fibrous ring below the aortic valve gives rise to a discrete murmur, which is similar to that in valvular AS. Ejection sounds are rare, the aortic component of the second sound is variably present, AR is common, and again the upstrokes are delayed with diminished amplitude.

In *congenital supravalvular* AS the murmur and thrill are most prominent in the first right intercostal space. In this lesion the right carotid and brachial pulses may have normal rates of rise while the left carotid and brachials exhibit slow rates of rise. The peripheral pulses are abnormally strong, and the blood pressure may be higher in the right arm than the left arm. This is thought to be due to the streaming of the aortic outflow jet toward the innominate artery with increased flow to the right side. In this lesion aortic ejection sounds are also rare. The aortic component of the second heart sound is usually normal. AR is uncommon.

In *congenital AS* a common finding is the presence of an aortic ejection sound, which is due to the sudden upward displacement (doming) of the pliant aortic leaflet whose upward motion ceases suddenly, giving rise to a click.

Frequently in aortic outflow tract disease, murmurs are heard at the apex which resemble those produced by MR. In the most common situation a patient with degenerative (senile) calcific AS has a harsh systolic ejection quality murmur in the right second intercostal space which changes in character as the stethoscope is inched toward the apex. This is termed the *Gallavardin phenomenon* and is caused by the selective radiation of high-frequency components of the AS murmur to the apex. This finding is most common in elderly patients because in degenerative calcific AS commissural fusion does not occur and the nonfused cusps may vibrate and produce high-frequency sounds.

REFERENCE

1. Perloff, J.K.: Clinical recognition of aortic stenosis. The physical signs and differential diagnosis of the various forms of obstruction to left ventricular outflow. Prog. Cardiovasc. Dis. 10:323, 1968.

434-B, 435-A, 436-C, 437-E *(Braunwald, pp. 1103–1105)*

Janeway lesions are small macular lesions which are distinguished from Osler nodes by the fact that they are painless and nontender and are most often present in the thenar and hypothenar eminences of the hand and soles of patients with subacute infective endocarditis. They appear much less often on the tips of the fingers or plantar surfaces of the toes. Lesions on the hands and feet blanch with pressure and with elevation of the extremities. In cases of acute valvular infections the lesions tend to be purple and hemorrhagic.

Osler nodes are small raised, nodular, tender lesions present most often in the pulp spaces of the terminal phalanges of the fingers. They may also be present on the backs of the toes, the soles, and the thenar and hypothenar eminences. The most characteristic feature of these lesions is their tenderness. Lesions may be fleeting in some cases, disappearing within a few hours after they have developed; however, they usually persist for 4 to 5 days. Although almost completely restricted to the subacute form of endocarditis, Osler nodes are occasionally present in acute valvular infection. Prevalence of both Osler nodes and Janeway lesions has decreased in recent years, most likely because of early institution of antibiotic therapy and a decrease in both endothelial destruction and frequency of embolic events.

The ocular signs in infective endocarditis include both retinal petechiae and *Roth spots*. These are located in the nerve layer of the retina and look like hemorrhagic exudates. They consist of aggregations of cytoid bodies; histologically they have been shown to be composed of perivascular accumulation of lymphocytes with or without surrounding hemorrhage.

Similarly, embolic events to the myocardium cause a localized inflammatory reaction consisting of collections of lymphocytes and mononuclear cells termed *Bracht-Wächter lesions*. These lesions may eventually replace much of the muscle, contributing to the congestive heart failure seen in chronic endocarditis.

Subungual or splinter hemorrhages are uncommon in patients with infective endocarditis. The characteristic features of the splinter hemorrhage are its linear form and the fact that its distal end does not reach the anterior nail bed; the latter distinguishes this lesion from a true splinter. In some cases, the toes may also be involved but because of the strong association with trauma, splinter hemorrhages are relatively nondiagnostic.

438-C, 439-E, 440-A, 441-D   (Braunwald, pp. 1167–1171)

There are many drugs that have been utilized for treatment of lipid disorders. Part of the explanation for this diversity is the relative lack of effectiveness of any single drug and the fact that several different pathways are responsible for the lipid abnormalities. Although there have been many approaches to treating hyperlipidemia, a national committee has recently provided specific guidelines for elevated cholesterol levels. For example, diet therapy is always recommended initially, but it is usually associated with only a 10 per cent reduction in cholesterol. Patients who have LDL cholesterol levels above 160 mg/dl should be treated with drugs in addition to diet. Patients with total cholesterol above 300 mg/dl often require therapy with more than a single drug.

Nicotinic acid is a B vitamin that is effective in all types of hyperlipoproteinemia except Type I. It decreases LDL by about 25 per cent by blocking hepatic VLDL synthesis. This is associated with numerous side effects,

including cutaneous flushing and gastrointestinal symptoms. Gastrointestinal side effects include gastritis, making it contraindicated in patients with peptic ulcer disease. It also causes abnormalities of liver function, impairment of glucose tolerance, and hyperuricemia, which is usually a significant problem only in patients with preexisting gout or diabetes.

Neomycin sulfate is an aminoglycoside antibiotic that has been shown to decrease LDL by unknown means. It is not well absorbed in the gastrointestinal tract and has both potential nephrotoxic and hepatotoxic effects, so it is not frequently utilized.

Cholestyramine and *colestipol* are quaternary ammonium salts that act as ion exchange resins and bind bile salts in the intestine. This binding results in interruption of the enterohepatic circulation and causes an increased loss of cholesterol in the stool. Cholestyramine and colestipol are particularly effective in Type II hyperlipoproteinemia. They are difficult to administer due to frequent side effects, predominantly involving gastrointestinal distress. They may bind concomitantly administered medications such as digitalis, phenobarbital, thiazides, warfarin, and tetracycline, and therefore may be associated with a decrease in the prothrombin time in patients taking warfarin.

Probucol is another drug that lowers LDL but also has the side effect of lowering HDL. Its mechanism of action is unknown at this time, but it is thought to increase clearance of LDL via the scavenger or macrophage pathways. It is most frequently used in conjunction with other agents such as the bile acid sequestrants.

Gemfibrozil is a fibric acid derivative that is effective in lowering VLDL, LDL, and triglycerides. Although the exact mechanism of action is unknown, it does appear to increase lipoprotein lipase activity. The most common side effects are nausea and gastrointestinal discomfort, although impaired glucose intolerance has also been noted. All fibric acid derivatives may potentiate the effects of coumarin anticoagulants so that patients on warfarin will have an increased prothrombin time.

REFERENCE

1. Report of the National Cholesterol Education Program expert panel on detection, evaluation and treatment of high blood cholesterol in adults. Arch. Intern. Med. *148:*36, 1988.

442-C, 443-A, 444-B   (Braunwald, p. 1332)

The physician should be aware that many drugs can affect the uptake and metabolism of beta blockers. Cimetidine reduces the hepatic metabolism of beta blockers, resulting in prolongation of the serum half-life and increased plasma levels. This is particularly true for the lipophilic beta blockers such as propranolol and metoprolol, in contrast to the hydrophilic blockers such as atenolol and nadolol, which are not as extensively metabolized. The barbiturates induce hepatic microsomal enzymes, and therefore enhance metabolism of beta blockers and reduce their plasma levels. Although lidocaine has no effect on beta blockers, propranolol reduces the hepatic clearance of lidocaine and may result in increased lidocaine levels.

Aluminum hydroxide gel, a common form of antacid, can delay or reduce gastrointestinal absorption of beta blockers, causing diminished plasma levels. This is particularly important with respect to hydrophilic beta blockers such as atenolol and nadolol, which normally are not as readily absorbed from the gastrointestinal tract and whose action is more affected by concomitant administration of these antacids. Calcium carbonate antacids do *not* alter absorption.

There are a number of interactions of the beta blockers with commonly administered drugs. The hypotension, bradycardia, and negative inotropy associated with verapamil may be additive with beta blockers, and concomitant usage requires careful patient monitoring. Aminophylline, which increases cyclic AMP by inhibiting phosphodiesterase, is antagonized by concurrent use of beta blockers. This effect may contribute to the bronchoconstriction observed in patients with asthma. Propranolol may also induce hypoglycemia and exacerbate the effects of antidiabetic agents, particularly long-acting drugs. Finally, the withdrawal syndrome observed in patients on clonidine, resulting in increased epinephrine release, may be exacerbated by beta blockade due to resulting unopposed alpha-adrenoceptor tone.

445-B, 446-C, 447-D, 448-A (Braunwald, pp. 1078–1080)

The development of artificial cardiac valves has dramatically improved the surgical outcome for all patients with valvular heart disease. The valves can be classified into mechanical prostheses and bioprosthetic tissue valves as well as into the various subtypes of discs, balls, and cages that are utilized to approximate normal valve function.

Mechanical prosthetic valves are classified into two groups: caged ball and tilting disc valves. The Starr-Edwards caged ball valve was one of the earliest valves and has a long record of predictable performance. However, its major disadvantage is the bulky cage design, which makes it unsuitable for patients with a small LV cavity or a small aortic annulus. Furthermore, the flow characteristics and action of the ball in the cage result in low-level hemolysis and elevation of lactate dehydrogenase. Tilting disc valves have become more widely employed, primarily because they are less bulky and have a lower profile than the caged ball valve. The Björk-Shiley valve has a suspended tilting disc occluder. Certain models of this valve have been characterized by two problems: sudden thrombosis with acute obstruction and strut fracture. The valves associated with strut fracture are no longer being produced. The Lillehei-Kaster valve is another pivoting disc valve which has a relatively high incidence of thrombosis, precluding its use in the mitral position. The St. Jude valve has two semicircular discs that pivot between open and closed positions without need for supporting struts. It has a lower transvalvular gradient than other caged ball or tilting disc types and appears to have particularly favorable hemodynamic characteristics in the smaller sizes, making it especially useful in children.

All of the mechanical prosthetic valves are extremely durable, lasting up to 20 years, but they are associated with a high incidence of thromboembolism, greatest in the first postoperative year. Without anticoagulation the incidence of thromboembolism is three- to sixfold higher than in properly anticoagulated patients.[1] Despite treatment with anticoagulants, the incidence of thromboembolic complications with the best mechanical prosthesis is still one to two nonfatal events per 100 patient years. The incidence is significantly higher for prostheses in the mitral than in the aortic position. Thrombosis of mechanical prostheses in the tricuspid position is extremely high, most likely due to the lower transvalvular pressure gradients, and for this reason bioprostheses are preferred at this site. Furthermore, it should be noted that administration of warfarin carries its own mortality and morbidity, estimated at 0.2 and 2.2 per 100 patient years, respectively.

Because of the high risk of thromboembolism inherent in the mechanical prosthetic valves, tissue valves have been developed. Among the tissue valves that are currently available, the Hancock valve is a porcine heterograft valve, as is the Carpentier-Edwards. There also is an Ionescu-Shiley pericardial xenograft consisting of bovine pericardium. This valve appears to have a relatively high primary failure rate due to calcification and tearing at the attachments to the struts. Recently, human homograft valves have been utilized with increasing success.

The porcine heterografts require anticoagulation during the first 3 months while the sewing ring becomes endothelialized. Thereafter, anticoagulants are not required for porcine valves in the aortic position and the thromboembolic rate is approximately 1 to 2 per 100 patient years without these drugs.[2] Patients with these valves in the mitral valve position who are in sinus rhythm generally do not require anticoagulant treatment. However, in patients in atrial fibrillation these valves are associated with an increased incidence of thromboembolism most likely due to LA thrombi. Anticoagulation is in general advocated.

In terms of selecting artificial valves, the relative risks and benefits of durability, endocarditis, hemodynamics, high versus low profile, and thromboembolism must be evaluated. In general, tissue valves are preferred over mechanical prostheses in patients in whom anticoagulation is difficult or in whom it is especially hazardous because they are prone to hemorrhage or are noncompliant. The common recommendation is to employ mechanical prosthetic valves in patients under the age of 65 to 70 who have no contraindications to anticoagulants. Bioprostheses are recommended for patients with coexisting disease that is likely to make them prone to hemorrhage, those who are noncompliant, those unable to take anticoagulants for other reasons, women who may become pregnant, and those of an age at which the durability is of lesser importance.

REFERENCES

1. Harker, L.A.: Antithrombotic therapy following mitral valve replacement. In Duran, C., et al. (eds.): Recent Progress in Mitral Valve Disease. London, Butterworths, 1984, pp. 340–348.

2. Zussa, C., Ottino, G., diSumma, M., Poletti, G.A., Zattera, G.F., Pansini, S., and Morea, M.: Porcine cardiac bioprostheses: Evaluation of long-term results in 990 patients. Ann. Thorac. Surg. 39:243, 1985.

449-A, 450-A, 451-D, 452-C *(Braunwald, pp. 1116–1125)*

Although the choice of specific antimicrobial therapy for infective endocarditis depends on the nature of the organism in the blood and the susceptibility to various drugs, there are standard treatment regimens suggested for initial therapy before results of sensitivity testing become available. For many relatively nonvirulent organisms, patients have frequently been ill for several weeks so that a delay of 2 to 3 days in treatment to establish a definitive diagnosis and antibiotic susceptibility is not contraindicated. However, for some of the more aggressive organisms such as those listed here, including staphylococci and Pseudomonas, rapid initiation of therapy is necessary to prevent destruction of valve leaflets, papillary muscles, and chordae tendineae. Although it is not always clear what the ideal dosages are for treatment, bolus injections of high doses of antibiotics are associated with a higher cure rate.

The duration of therapy again is empirical. Although many physicians treat for only 4 weeks, for complicated infections therapy may be extended for 6 weeks. Staphylococci are difficult to eradicate, and resistance to methicillin has been increasingly documented. About 15 per cent of infections caused by *Staph. aureus* that occur outside a hospital, and more than 90 per cent that develop during hospitalization, are caused by penicillin-resistant strains. Thus, in the case of hospital-acquired *Staph. aureus* it is appropriate to commence therapy with vancomycin, 500 mg intravenously every 6 hours. If the patient fails to respond to this regimen an aminoglycoside may be added, although the data on its value are controversial. Oral rifampin has also been suggested to be a useful addition. The Working Party of the British Society for Antimicrobial Chemotherapy[1] recommended for the initial treatment of staphylococcal endocarditis flucloxacillin 2 gm IV every 4 hours plus lucitic acid 500 mg orally every 8 hours plus gentamicin 120 mg for the first dose followed by 80 mg IV every 8 hours.

Staphylococcus epidermidis infections are almost always methicillin resistant and are among the most common forms of prosthetic valve endocarditis. In native valve endocarditis with this organism, vancomycin alone is effective. However, in prosthetic valve endocarditis, it is recommended that therapy be begun with both vancomycin and gentamicin, with rifampin added as needed.

Pseudomonas aeruginosa infection causes rapid valve destruction. Therefore, it is recommended that two drugs be used to treat the infection, an aminoglycoside and a synthetic penicillin. Recent success has been achieved with pipericillin as well as ticarcillin as the synthetic penicillin portion of this regimen.

Escherichia coli acquired in the community is quite susceptible to standard therapy with a single agent such as ampicillin, although the drug must be given in relatively high amounts (12 gm/day). However, in hospitalized patients *E. coli* frequently carries multiple resistances so that initial therapy should be begun with an aminoglycoside and either ticarcillin or pipericillin. Therapy for the other enterobacteriaceae (Klebsiella, Proteus) is similar to that for *E. coli*.[2]

REFERENCES

1. Working Party of the British Society for Antimicrobial Chemotherapy: Antibiotic treatment of streptococcal and staphylococcal endocarditis. Lancet 2:815, 1985.
2. Wilson, W.R., and Geraci, J.E.: Antibiotic treatment of infective endocarditis. Annu. Rev. Med. 34:413, 1983.

453-C, 454-B, 455-A, 456-A *(Braunwald, pp. 1505–1507)*

Clinical distinction between patients with constrictive pericarditis and those with restrictive physiology due to such diseases as amyloidosis, hemochromatosis, and the hypereosinophilic syndrome may be very difficult. Both restrictive cardiomyopathy and constrictive pericarditis may show the electrocardiographic changes of atrial fibrillation, left atrial abnormality, diffuse low voltage, and T-wave flattening. The presence of atrioventricular block and conduction disturbances may favor the diagnosis of restrictive cardiomyopathy. While findings at cardiac catheterization may be of some help in differentiating these two conditions, some patients will defy all analyses and a final diagnosis of one entity or the other will not be possible. In both conditions, RV and LV diastolic pressures are elevated, stroke volume and cardiac output are decreased, and LV end-diastolic volume is normal or decreased, with impaired diastolic filling. A frame-by-frame analysis of LV filling in one study has been used as a method to differentiate between constrictive pericarditis and restrictive cardiomyopathy,[1] demonstrating that early diastolic filling tends to be excessively rapid (80 per cent in the first half of diastole) in constrictive pericarditis in contrast with that seen in restrictive cardiomyopathy.

A diagnosis of restrictive cardiomyopathy is more likely when marked RV systolic hypertension is present (pressure greater than 60 mm Hg) and is also suggested when LV and RV diastolic pressures at rest or during exercise differ by more than 5 mm Hg.[2] It should be noted, however, that some patients with restrictive cardiomyopathy may have hemodynamics at rest and during exercise which are indistinguishable from constrictive pericarditis, including sustained and complete equilibration of RV and LV pressures as well as the presence of a dip-and-plateau pattern in the ventricular wave form.[3] Angiography in these conditions reveals a straightening of the right heart border in both cases, as well as thickening of the heart border due to either pericardial or myocardial thickening. However, while a decreased motion of the RV free wall is seen in both conditions, normal motion of the crista supraventricularis is usually present in constrictive pericarditis but not in restrictive cardiomyopathy.[4] Echocardiographic examination in some patients with restrictive cardiomyopathy may reveal abnormal ventricular myocardial thickening with a peculiar "sparkling" appearance if amyloidosis is present. However, in general, echocardiography is not capable of distinguishing between these two entities in a definitive manner. Endomyocardial biopsy may prove useful in the diagnosis of amyloidosis or hemochromatosis[5] but does not usually provide an adequate method for distinguishing between constriction and restriction on a consistent basis.

REFERENCES

1. Tyberg, T.I., Goodyer, A.V.N., Hurst, V.W., Alexander, J., and Langon, R.A.: Left ventricular filling in differentiating restrictive amyloid cardiomyopathy and constrictive pericarditis. Am. J. Cardiol. 47:791, 1981.
2. Meaney, E., Shebatai, R., and Bhargava, V.: Cardiac amyloidosis, constrictive pericarditis and restrictive cardiomyopathy. Am. J. Cardiol. 38:547, 1976.
3. Lorell, B.H., and Grossman, W.: Profiles in constrictive pericarditis, restrictive cardiomyopathy and cardiac tamponade. In Grossman, W. (ed.): Cardiac Catheterization and Angiography. 3rd ed. Philadelphia, Lea and Febiger, 1986, pp. 427–445.
4. Chang, L.W., and Grollman, J.H., Jr.: Angiographic differentiation of constrictive pericarditis and restrictive cardiomyopathy due to amyloidosis. Am. J. Radiol. 130:451, 1978.
5. Eagle, K.A., and Southern, J.F.: A 62-year-old woman with right-sided congestive heart failure. N. Engl. J. Med. 319:932, 1988.

457-D, 458-C, 459-B, 460-A, 461-C (Braunwald, pp. 1163–1171)

While treatment for the specific hyperlipoproteinemias must be tailored for individual patients, and secondary causes of various phenotypic patterns must first be excluded, some general comments may be made regarding therapeutic approaches to these disorders. Dysbetalipoproteinemia, or Type III hyperlipoproteinemia, is an uncommon disorder marked by cholesterol levels in the 300 to 1000 mg/dl range and elevated triglyceride levels as well, which are derived from incomplete metabolism of chylomicrons and VLDL. The use of clofibrate, which decreases both LDL and VLDL cholesterol, has proven useful in this disorder.[1] Nicotinic acid may also be effective. Clofibrate exerts its action by increasing lipoprotein lipase activity and the biliary excretion of sterols, with a decrease in triglyceride levels of approximately 40 per cent. Whereas the drug effects only a modest decrease in cholesterol in patients with elevations of LDL, in patients with intermediate-density lipoprotein elevations (such as those with Type III hyperlipoproteinemia), the drug is a mainstay of therapy.

The majority of patients with the phenotype Type II hyperlipoproteinemia have polygenic hypercholesterolemia that may be first treated with diet alone. In this hyperlipoproteinemia, elevated total plasma cholesterol is noted, primarily due to an increase in LDL cholesterol. This disorder may account for up to 85 per cent of individuals detected to have elevated cholesterol by routine screening. Dietary treatment alone in these patients usually leads to a substantial reduction in hypercholesterolemia. In some individuals in whom dietary therapy is not effective or in whom compliance is a problem, drug therapy may be necessary and is often begun with either the bile acid sequestrant cholestyramine or nicotinic acid.

Heterozygous familial hypercholesterolemia, another Type II hyperlipoproteinemia phenotype, requires a different therapeutic approach. The gene frequency for this autosomal dominant disorder is approximately 1 in 500 for the heterozygote, and carries a strong association with premature atherosclerosis. Levels of LDL are elevated in this disorder, and those of HDL may be reduced, with a deficiency of the cell-surface receptor for LDL being the biochemical characteristic of the disorder. Treatment of the disorder may be approached in a variety of ways. The recent approval by the FDA of the HMG CoA reductase inhibitor lovastatin provides one proven alternative for the treatment of this disorder. This agent, alone or in conjunction with bile acid sequestrants, is capable of dramatically lowering circulating plasma cholesterol levels. It works by leading to a decrease in cholesterol synthesis in hepatic and other cells, and a concomitant increase in the level of LDL receptors on the cell surface, resulting in an increased rate of clearance of LDL from the plasma. Patients receiving this agent should be monitored for the development of liver function abnormalities and the development of myositis, which are occasionally associated with the drug.

Lipoprotein lipase deficiency is a primary genetic disorder with the phenotype of Type I hyperlipoproteinemia. While the disorder is not associated with premature atherosclerosis, abdominal pain and pancreatitis are frequent complications. This primary familial form of Type I hyperlipoproteinemia may occur due to the lack of apo protein C-II, the activator of lipoprotein lipase. The phenotype may also be seen in association with poorly controlled diabetes mellitus, pancreatitis, or dysglobulinemia. The disorder is generally diagnosed at an early age, and treatment is quite difficult. Drug therapy is not effective for lipoprotein lipase–deficient patients; therefore, the cornerstone of therapy is a fat-restricted diet, which is designed to lower triglyceride levels to less than 1000 mg/dl. In addition, dietary fat is limited to 10 to 25 gm/day, and medium-chain triglycerides may be used to enhance dietary compliance and provide needed calories.

Type IV hyperlipoproteinemia either may be due to a genetic disorder or may be secondary to another disease. It is caused by the accumulation of VLDL and triglycerides in the plasma, leading to elevated triglyceride levels in the 200 to 500 mg/dl range with or without accompanying hypercholesterolemia. The treatment of Type IV hyperlipoproteinemia primarily involves weight control and aggressive dietary management. Alcohol consumption is restricted and aggressive therapy of any underlying diabetes is implemented. In unusual circumstances, drug therapy may be necessary for patients at risk for pancreatitis. In these instances, the choice of drugs must be individualized according to the etiology of the elevated LDL fraction. In general, however, dietary therapy suffices. The risk for patients with familial hypertriglyceridemia is not as well defined with respect to atherosclerosis, since the concentrations of LDL and total cholesterol in these patients are frequently normal.[2]

REFERENCES

1. Schaefer, E.J.: Dietary and Drug Treatment. In Brewer, H.B. (moderator): Type III hyperlipoproteinemia: Diagnosis, molecular effects, pathology, and treatment. Ann. Intern. Med. 98:623, 1983.

2. Sniderman, A.D., Wolfson, C., Teng, B., Franklin, F.A., Bachorik, P.S., and Kwiterovich, P.O.J.: Association of hyperapobetalipoproteinemia with endogenous hypertriglyceridemia and atherosclerosis. Ann. Intern. Med. 97:833, 1982.

462-C, 463-A, 464-B, 465-D *(Braunwald, pp. 1248–1249; Forrester, J.S., Diamond, G., Chatterjee, K., and Swan, H.J.C.: Medical therapy of acute myocardial infarction by application of hemodynamic subsets. N. Engl. J. Med. 295:1356, 1404, 1976.)*

The use of hemodynamic monitoring in acute myocardial infarction was pioneered by Forrester and colleagues and marked a major advance in our ability to diagnose and treat patients with this condition. The hemodynamic data provided by these investigators describe four types of patients. Patient A has both a normal cardiac index and pulmonary capillary wedge pressure. Patients with AMI with normal perfusion and without pulmonary congestion have an excellent prognosis with a mortality of approximately 2 per cent. These patients in general require little in the way of pharmacological intervention but may benefit from the use of beta blockade to decrease long-term mortality.[1] One important piece of data first provided by the study of Forrester and colleagues is that approximately 25 per cent of patients with cardiac indices less than 2.2 liters/M/m^2 and 15 per cent of patients with abnormally elevated PCW pressures are not recognized clinically to have evidence of either of these abnormalities. Thus the truly "normal" hemodynamics illustrated in patient A may be found in fewer patients than those judged to belong to this group solely on the basis of a clinical impression.

Patient B has a moderate reduction in cardiac index and a markedly elevated pulmonary capillary wedge pressure. This patient thus displays moderate left ventricular failure and is most appropriately treated first with diuretic therapy to relieve associated dyspnea, hypoxemia, and pulmonary vascular congestion. In the series of patients defined by Forrester and colleagues, this group had a mortality of approximately 10 per cent. It should be noted that the *degree* to which the pulmonary capillary wedge and CI are abnormal has a marked influence upon mortality. For example, Rackley and colleagues reported that in patients with a PCW of > 15 mm Hg and a cardiac index < 2.0 liters/M/m^2 a mortality of 93 per cent was present, while in patients with a PCW < 15 mm Hg and a cardiac index < 2.0 the mortality was 63 per cent.[2]

The patient in example C has a moderately depressed cardiac index and an unusually low PCW for the AMI setting. This patient probably has hypovolemic hypotension and should be treated first with a challenge with intravenous saline in an attempt to increase both filling pressures and cardiac index. Exclusion of hypovolemia as the cause of hypotension in this patient would require documentation of a persistently reduced cardiac output despite PCW pressures exceeding 14 to 18 mm Hg. (It should be noted that documentation of such persistent hypotension with elevated PCW would lead to reclassification of the patient in hemodynamic terms.) In addition, patients with hypotension due to right ventricular infarction may be confused with that caused by hypovolemia because of the associated normal or minimally elevated left ventricular filling pressure noted in this condition. Diagnosis of right ventricular infarction requires a knowledge of the clinical presentation of this lesion and hemodynamic alterations that frequently accompany it (see Braunwald, pp. 122, 1242). Fortunately, both hypovolemia and right ventricular infarction with hypotension are initially treated with intravenous saline.

The hemodynamic data in example D illustrate a markedly depressed cardiac index together with a markedly elevated pulmonary capillary wedge pressure. This combination of pulmonary congestion and hypoperfusion defines cardiogenic hypotension or shock and carries a mortality well in excess of 50 per cent in most series. Patients with cardiogenic shock usually have at least 40 per cent of the left ventricle damaged, assuming that no underlying mechanical complications are contributing to the hemodynamic profile. Evaluation of cardiogenic shock must begin with immediate hemodynamic monitoring in an attempt to exclude mechanical defects that might initiate circulatory collapse, such as mitral regurgitation, ventricular septal defect, and ventricular aneurysm or pseudoaneurysm. In the absence of such defects, global impairment of left ventricular function is the underlying cause of circulatory collapse. Stabilization of patients with this syndrome using dopamine, dobutamine, and/or intraaortic balloon counterpulsation is often possible. In general, however, improvement in this population is only temporary, and "balloon dependence" is common.[3]

REFERENCES

1. Yusuf, S., Peto, R., Lewis, J., Collins, R., and Sleight, P.: Beta blockade during and after myocardial infarction: An overview of the randomized trials. Prog. Cardiovasc. Dis. 27:335, 1985.
2. Rackley, C.E., Satler, L.F., Pearle, D.L., Del Negro, A.A., Pallas, R.S., and Kent, K.E.: Use of hemodynamic measurements for management of acute myocardial infarction. *In* Rackley, C.E. (ed.): Advances in Critical Care Cardiology. Philadelphia, F.A. Davis Co., 1986, pp. 3–16.
3. Corral, C.H., and Vaughn, C.C.: Intra-aortic balloon counterpulsation: An eleven year review and analysis of determinants of survival. Texas Heart Inst. J. 13:39, 1986.

466-D, 467-B, 468-C, 469-A *(Braunwald, pp. 1717–1718; 1725–1727; and Table 33–14, p. 1062)*

Aortic regurgitation (AR) is frequently the initial cardiac manifestation of both Marfan syndrome and ankylosing spondylitis. It may be caused by primary disease of the aortic valve leaflets, by disease of the wall of the aortic root, or both. Rheumatic fever is a common cause of primary disease of the aortic valve leading to regurgitation. The cusps become infiltrated with fibrous tissues and retract, preventing cusp apposition during diastole and leading to regurgitation through a defect in the center of the valve. AR is more common in association with rheumatic aortic stenosis than with senile calcific aortic stenosis. Other primary valvular causes of AR include infective endocarditis, trauma, rheumatoid disease, and less commonly systemic lupus erythematosus and Whipple's disease.

Recently, disease of the aortic root has become an increasingly common cause of AR, accounting for the condition in approximately one-third of all patients.[1] Among the diseases which produce AR by causing dilatation of the ascending aorta are annuloaortic ectasia, cystic medial necrosis of the aorta, syphilitic aortitis, ankylosing spondylitis, Behçet's syndrome, relapsing polychondritis, systemic hypertension, and osteogenesis imperfecta.

Syphilitic aortitis has become rare during the last several decades, but as general medical therapy of patients with Marfan syndrome and ankylosing spondylitis has improved, more of these patients are now living to an age at which aortic disease becomes an important part of their illnesses. In ankylosing spondylitis, a high incidence of AV conduction disturbances is present. The aorta is markedly abnormal with a thickening of adventitia, degeneration of the media, intimal proliferation, and abnormal vasa vasorum consistent with autoimmune disease. The basal portion of the aortic valve cusps are thickened and shortened and commissures are normal.

Marfan syndrome tends to be a disease of younger patients. Both aortic and mitral regurgitation are common in Marfan syndrome; however, conduction disturbances are rare. The abnormalities in the aorta are essentially confined to the media, where cystic medial necrosis develops. Because of the more extensive destruction of the supporting media, aneurysms of the aorta are more common in Marfan syndrome than in ankylosing spondylitis.

REFERENCE

1. Olson, L.J., Subramanian, R., and Edwards, W.D.: Surgical pathology of pure aortic insufficiency: A study of 225 cases. Mayo Clin. Proc. 59:835, 1984.

470-A, 471-A, 472-D, 473-B, 474-B (Braunwald, pp. 936–938)

Discrete subaortic stenosis accounts for between 8 and 10 per cent of all cases of congenital aortic stenosis (AS) and is seen more commonly in males than in females. The disorder is characterized by a membranous diaphragm that encircles the left ventricular outflow tract beneath the base of the aortic valve. While the diastolic murmur of aortic regurgitation is heard more commonly in this disorder and an ejection sound is rarely appreciated, distinction of subvalvular from valvular AS is difficult by clinical means alone. Dilatation of the ascending aorta is common in this condition, but calcification of the valve itself is not observed. Echocardiography has proven extremely useful in the diagnosis of this disorder and in identifying the coexistence of hypertrophic subaortic stenosis or in differentiating between these two disorders. The definitive diagnosis, however, is provided by recording pressure tracings as a catheter is withdrawn across the outflow tract or by direct visualization of the site of obstruction with LV angiography (see Braunwald, Fig. 30–34, p. 935). The mild aortic regurgitation that is commonly appreciated in patients with discrete subaortic stenosis appears to be a result of thickening of the valve and decreased mobility of valve cusps due to trauma

created by a high-velocity stream of blood flowing through the subaortic diaphragm. Discrete subaortic stenosis of any degree merits consideration for elective repair. Operative repair is frequently curative.[1]

Supravalvular AS is a congenital narrowing of the ascending aorta, which originates at the superior margin of the sinuses of Valsalva above the level of the coronary arteries. Three anatomical types of supravalvular AS are recognized, the most common of which is the hourglass type in which thickening and disorganization of the aortic media leads to a constriction or annular ridge at the superior margin of the sinuses of Valsalva. Less commonly a membrane is noted, with a small central opening stretched across the lumen of the aorta. A third form occurs in which uniform hypoplasia of the ascending aorta is also noted. What makes the clinical picture of supravalvular obstruction unique is its association with idiopathic infantile hypercalcemia, a disease that may be related to abnormal vitamin D metabolism.[2] "Williams syndrome" is a term applied to the constellation of clinical findings that include the cardiac abnormalities of supravalvular aortic stenosis and a multisystem disorder. The disorder includes a peculiar elfin facies (see Braunwald, Fig. 30–37, p. 937), mental retardation, auditory hyperacusis, narrowing of peripheral, systemic, and pulmonary arteries, inguinal hernia, strabismus, and abnormalities of dental development. Some patients may show an association of valvular pulmonary stenosis or peripheral pulmonary artery stenosis, and rarely mitral valve abnormalities may occur. However, tricuspid stenosis is not a part of this syndrome or of the disease discrete subaortic stenosis. While the physical findings in supravalvular AS resemble those in valvular AS for the most part, the presence of an especially prominent transmission of a thrill or murmur into the jugular notch, a late systolic or continuous murmur due to peripheral pulmonary artery stenoses, or a significant difference between the arterial pressures recorded in the upper extremities may suggest the diagnosis of supravalvular AS. This last finding occurs due to selective streaming of blood into the innominate artery from the constricting lesion.[3]

Echocardiography is extremely valuable in localizing the site of obstruction of supravalvular AS, and retrograde aortic catheterization may be used to quantitate precisely the degree of hemodynamic abnormality present. Operative repair of this disorder is most successful when little or no hypoplasia of the ascending aorta and arch is present and when the obstruction is discrete and significant. In these instances, the aortic lumen may be widened by the insertion of a fabric patch. In patients with a markedly hypoplastic ascending aorta, however, operative repair usually succeeds only in displacing the pressure gradient distally and is therefore not advised.

REFERENCES

1. Newfeld, E.A., Muster, A.J., Paul, M.H., Idress, F.S., and Riker, W.L.: Discrete subvalvular aortic stenosis in childhood. Am. J. Cardiol. 38:53, 1976.
2. Taylor, A.B., Stern, R.H., and Bell, N.H.: Abnormal regulation of circulating 25-hydroxy vitamin D in the Williams syndrome. N. Engl. J. Med. 306:972, 1982.
3. Goldstein, R.E., and Epstein, S.E.: Mechanism of elevated innominate artery pressures in supravalvular aortic stenosis. Circulation 42:23, 1970.

475-A, 476-C, 477-B, 478-A, 479-D   *(Braunwald, pp. 1587–1588)*

Since a controlled trial demonstrated a decrease in mortality rate for PE patients treated with heparin,[1] intravenous heparin therapy has been a cornerstone of the therapeutic approach to the patient with pulmonary embolism. Most studies which have compared continuous and intermittent infusion of heparin have found that the frequency of major hemorrhage was greater with intermittent transfusions.[2] In addition, intermittent therapy leads to wide fluctuations in the partial thromboplastin time (PTT). Therefore, it is recommended that heparin be administered by continuous intravenous infusion after an initial bolus in patients with suspected acute pulmonary embolism. The actual heparinization process is empirical; in most cases, an initial loading bolus of approximately 5000 units is administered and is followed by a continuous intravenous infusion of approximately 1000 units per hour. Subsequently the PTT is checked every 4 to 6 hours until the desired clinical range is attained. The PTT should in general be maintained at 1.5 to 2 times normal values, with an effort made to assure at least twice the normal value in patients with proven pulmonary embolism.

Hemorrhage is the single most important adverse effect of heparin therapy. Complications of heparin therapy include a mild thrombocytopenia that is thought to be a direct and nonimmune-mediated effect of the drug, as well as true "heparin-associated thrombocytopenia," which occurs more frequently with beef lung heparin than with pork gut heparin and which may be accompanied by dramatic thrombocytopenia as well as associated thrombosis due to an immune-mediated mechanism. While rarer, heparin-associated thrombocytopenia may be life-threatening, and may be acompanied by unusual thrombotic events involving the skin or major arteries.[3]

Streptokinase and urokinase are proteins capable of activating endogenous plasminogens to form plasmin, which may actually lyse clots that have recently formed. This is unlike heparin, which acts primarily to prevent thrombus extension but does not promote frank dissolution of recently formed clots. Although single-bolus therapy with urokinase has been proposed, no comparison between continuous intravenous therapy and intermittent dosing has yet been performed. Laboratory confirmation of the achievement of a lytic state may be carried out with a variety of tests, the most sensitive of which is the thrombin time (see Braunwald, Table 47–6, p. 1587). Increases in fibrin degradation products, thrombin time, whole blood euglobulin lysis time, PT, or PTT all may be noted following the administration of first-generation thrombolytic agents. The risk of bleeding from streptokinase or urokinase has not been shown to correlate directly with a specific laboratory abnormality or with the dose of the lytic agent administered. Randomized trials comparing streptokinase or urokinase administration with heparin therapy for pulmonary embolism have demonstrated more rapid clot lysis with the former agents but have *not* demonstrated any reduction in mortality. Therefore, the decision to employ thrombolytic therapy in patients with pulmonary embolism must rely in part upon the particular clinical situation. Particular attention must be paid to any contraindications to thrombolytic therapy that may exist (see Braunwald, Table 47–7, p. 1588), and simultaneous administration of antiplatelet agents should be *avoided* whenever possible. Bleeding or hemorrhagic complications are the most important adverse effect of therapy with streptokinase or urokinase. In the urokinase pulmonary embolism trial (UPET), bleeding episodes requiring a transfusion of more than two units of blood or leading to a decrease in hematocrit of more than 10 points occurred in 27 per cent of treated patients in the study. The most serious of such episodes is intracranial bleeding, which occurs in one or two out of every 1000 patients treated with urokinase or streptokinase. Severe bleeding complications may require administration of fresh frozen plasma or cryoprecipitate.

REFERENCES

1. Barritt, D.W., and Jordan, S.C.: Anticoagulant drugs in the treatment of pulmonary embolism. A controlled trial. Lancet 1:1309, 1960.
2. Kelton, J.G., and Hirsch, J.: Bleeding associated with antithrombotic therapy. Semin. Hematol. 17:259, 1980.
3. Powers, P.J., Kelton, J.G., and Carter, C.J.: Studies on the frequency of heparin-associated thrombocytopenia. Thromb. Res. 33:439, 1984.
4. Urokinase Pulmonary Embolism Trial: A National Cooperative Study. Circulation 47 and 48 (Suppl. II): 1, 1973.

480-D, 481-C, 482-B, 483-B, 484-A   *(Braunwald, pp. 1013–1016)*

Type II glycogen storage disease (Pompe's disease) is an autosomal recessive disorder that results from a deficiency of a lysosomal enzyme that hydrolyzes glycogen into glucose. This results in deposition of excessive amounts of glycogen in a generalized fashion, but especially in the heart, the skeletal muscles, and the liver. The clinical consequences include cardiomegaly—often of a marked degree—and the subsequent development of congestive heart failure. The disease usually is detected in the early neonatal period and is marked by a failure to thrive, progressive hypotonia, lethargy, and a weak cry.[1] The ECG may demonstrate extremely tall and broad QRS complexes, with a P-R interval that is commonly less than 0.09 second (see Braunwald, Fig. 32–3, p. 1013). This shortening of the P-R interval may be caused by facilitated atrioventricular conduction as a consequence of the glycogen deposition. The differential diagnosis includes other causes of cardiac failure in the early months of life, including endocardial fibroelastosis, anomalous pulmonary origin of the left coronary artery, the variety of fixed and dynamic forms of LV outflow tract obstruction, coarctation of the aorta, and myocarditis. The presence of skeletal muscular *hypotonia* and short P-R interval helps to suggest the diagnosis of glycogen storage disease type II. The disease is uniformly fatal, and patients usually die within the first year of life.

The mucocutaneous lymph node syndrome (Kawasaki's disease) was first described in Japan in 1967 and has subsequently been reported both in the Orient and throughout Europe and North America. The disease usually occurs in children between the ages of 2 and 10 years and is commonly associated with a fever lasting 5 days or longer that is unresponsive to antibiotics, as well as bilateral congestion of the ocular conjunctivae and fissuring of the lips, injected oropharangeal mucosa, and strawberry tongue. These manifestations may then be followed by a rash and edema of the hands and feet, accompanied by palmar and plantar erythema. The disease progresses to a phase of cutaneous desquamation within approximately 2 weeks. Other noncardiovascular complications of the illness may include arthritis, pulmonary infiltrates, and hydrops of the gallbladder. In addition, cervical adenopathy, diarrhea, and a variety of laboratory abnormalities may become apparent.

The etiology of Kawasaki's disease continues to be obscure, although some evidence for a viral cause has been accumulated. Cardiovascular involvement in the disorder may include myocarditis and pericarditis resulting in congestive heart failure and/or arrhythmias. Coronary angiitis, which may include the development of coronary artery aneurysms, is also noted. These cardiac complications are primarily responsible for the associated acute mortality of 1 to 3 per cent in the disease. Approximately half of the children who develop coronary artery aneurysms during the acute phase of Kawasaki's disease have normal-appearing vessels by angiography 1 to 2 years following the illness.[2] No treatment has proven effective in the prevention of coronary artery aneurysms, although a variety of agents have been utilized. Apparently, corticosterid therapy during the acute phase of the illness is detrimental, while high-dose salicylate treatment is advised in all patients. Recently, investigators have had success using gamma globulin during the acute phase, with substantial reduction in the formation of coronary arterial aneurysms.[3] In general, coronary angiography is recommended in patients with symptoms of cardiovascular involvement and/or signs of such involvement by physical examination or laboratory evaluation.

REFERENCES

1. Hwang, G., Meng, C.C., Lin, C.Y., and Hsu, H.C.: Clinical analysis of five infants with glycogen storage disease of the heart—Pompe's disease. Jpn. Heart J. 27:25, 1986.
2. Kato, H., Ichinose, E., Matsunaga, S., Suzuki, K., and Rikatake, N.: Fate of coronary aneurysms in Kawasaki disease: Serial coronary angiography and long-term follow-up study. Am. J. Cardiol. 49:1758, 1982.
3. Newburger, J.W., Takahasi, M., Burns, J.C., Beiser, A.S., Chung, K.J., Duffy, C.E., Glode, M.P., Mason, W.H., Reddy, V., Sanders, S.P., Shulman, S.T., Wiggins, J.W., Hicks, R.V., Fulton, D.R., Lewis, A.B., Leung, D.Y.M., Colton, T., Rosen, F.S., and Melish, M.E.: The treatment of Kawasaki syndrome with intravenous gamma globulin. N. Engl. J. Med. 315:341, 1986.

485-A, 486-C, 487-A, 488-D, 489-B (Braunwald, pp. 1140–1143)

The fatty streak is the earliest lesion of atherosclerosis and can usually be found in the aorta of young children. On gross inspection, a fatty streak has a yellow discoloration due to the large amount of lipid deposited in the foam cells that comprise the lesion. These foam cells are principally lipid-laden macrophages, together with a small number of lipid-filled smooth muscle cells that accumulate beneath the macrophage layer as the lesions enlarge.

The lipid that is present is in the form of cholesteryl ester or cholesterol. Analyses of the distribution of fatty streaks in coronary arteries of children and young adults reveal that they occupy the same anatomical sites as the more advanced lesions (fibrous plaques) of atherosclerosis. Over time, fatty streaks enlarge to occupy an increasing surface area of the coronary arteries, and these sites often precede the formation of advanced lesions.[1] Data such as these lend support to the notion that the fatty streak is in many instances—if not in most—the precursor to the advanced occlusive form of atherosclerosis. Using monoclonal antibodies directed against cell-specific markers, the fatty streak has been demonstrated to consist principally of lipid-laden macrophages, regardless of its site of origin (see Braunwald, Fig. 35–9, p. 1141).

The more advanced lesion of atherosclerosis is usually termed the "fibrous plaque." Fibrous plaques appear grossly white, and often protrude into the lumen of the artery. Therefore, they are more likely to become involved in thrombosis, hemorrhage, and/or calcification. Fibrous plaques consist of a variety of cells, especially large numbers of intimal smooth muscle cells, along with macrophages. Lipid deposition in both of these cell types occurs in the fibrous plaque. In addition, fibrous plaques seem to be covered consistently by a fibrous tissue cap. The fibrous plaque lesion appears to be composed of several layers. The fibrous cap of each lesion involves a smooth muscle cell and connective tissue matrix, which is exceedingly dense. Beneath this may be found a mixture of smooth muscle cells, macrophages, and lymphocytes. Large amounts of connective tissue are also found in this cellular sublayer. Still deeper in the fibrous plaque, there is frequently a zone of necrotic tissue, which may contain areas of cholesterol and calcification, as well as enlarged foam cells. Interestingly, the material that constitutes a fibrous plaque varies, depending upon the individual risk factors present in a given patient. For example, it is common that fibrous plaques observed in the femoral arteries of heavy cigarette smokers are extremely fibrous, with relatively little lipid, while those from individuals with hypercholesterolemia often have large areas of lipid deposition within the plaque.[2]

The general pattern of distribution of advanced atherosclerotic lesions in humans shows a predilection for the abdominal aorta, with lesions most prominent near the ostia of major branches. The renal arteries appear to be spared from atherosclerosis except at their ostia.[3] Coronary arteries generally demonstrate a more intense involvement with atherosclerosis, and lesions are often located within their first 6 cm. Understanding the cell types and patterns that constitute both the developing and mature lesions of atherosclerosis is important to formulating hypotheses of both atherogenesis and of the conversion of a plaque from the quiescent to the clinically active state.

REFERENCES

1. McGill, H.C., Jr.: Persistent problems in the pathogenesis of atherosclerosis. Arteriosclerosis 4:443, 1984.
2. Ross, R., Wight, T.N., Strandness, E., and Thiele, B.: Human atherosclerosis: I. Cell constitution and characteristics of advanced lesions of the superficial femoral artery. Am. J. Pathol. 114:79, 1984.

3. Glagov, S., and Oxoa, A.: Significance of the relatively low incidence of atherosclerosis in the pulmonary, renal and mesenteric arteries. Ann. NY Acad. Sci. 149:940, 1968.

490-A, 491-C, 492-B, 493-A, 494-B (Braunwald, pp. 991–992; 1069–1076; 1439–1440)

Tricuspid stenosis (TS) is most commonly rheumatic in origin and almost never occurs as an isolated lesion but rather usually accompanies mitral valve disease, with involvement of the aortic valve frequently noted as well. The pathophysiology of the lesion is quite similar to that of mitral stenosis (MS). The lesion results in a characteristic low-cardiac output state which presents as fatigue and right-sided heart failure, including uncomfortable hepatomegaly, abdominal swelling due to ascites, and anasarca. While MS is usually present with TS, the characteristic symptoms associated with that lesion are usually absent. Thus the absence of symptoms of pulmonary congestion in a patient with tight MS should suggest the possibility of TS. The physical findings are subtle and are notable for signs of right-sided heart failure in the presence of clear lung fields. Auscultation usually reveals signs of MS, and these often overshadow the more subtle findings of TS. The diastolic murmur of TS is commonly heard best along the lower left sternal border in the fourth intercostal space and is usually softer, higher pitched, and shorter in duration than the murmur of MS. The management of severe TS is surgical and requires mitral valvulotomy or valve replacement in patients in whom tricuspid orifice areas are less than approximately 2.0 cm². In general, tissue valves are used preferentially in the tricuspid position because of the risk of thrombosis of mechanical prostheses.

The most common form of pulmonic stenosis (PS) is congenital. A much rarer form of PS results from carcinoid plaques, present in the outflow tract of the right ventricle in patients with malignant carcinoid. These can cause constriction of the pulmonic valve ring, retraction and fusion of the cusps, and PS with or without accompanying pulmonic regurgitation. Carcinoid heart disease also involves the tricuspid valve and most commonly leads to tricuspid regurgitation. However, some degree of TS is sometimes noted with carcinoid involvement of the tricuspid valve.[1]

Most adults with mild to moderate PS are asymptomatic, and it is only in the more severe forms of the disease that symptoms of dyspnea and fatigue secondary to an inadequate cardiac output response to exercise are noted. Patients with severe grades of PS may develop tricuspid regurgitation and frank RV failure. The severity of PS is grouped according to the peak systolic pressure gradient between the RV and the pulmonary artery. Gradients of 50 to 79 mm Hg are considered moderate, while those greater than 80 mm are severe. In most patients, valvular PS is a relatively stable or at most slowly progressive disease. The physical examination in patients with PS is notable for a systolic thrill present along the left upper sternal border of the chest, a prominent systolic ejection murmur heard most clearly in the location of the thrill, and often an associated ejection click. In contrast to the inspiratory increase in most right-sided cardiac sounds, the intensity of the pulmonic click in PS *decreases* with inspiration.[2] Increasing degrees of severity of PS lead to increases in both the length and the intensity of the murmur, with peaking of the murmur occurring later in systole in the more severe forms of the lesion. A normal pulmonic component of the second heart sound and a murmur that is less than grade 4 out of 6 in intensity suggests a gradient that is less than 80 mm Hg and hence at most moderate PS. Echocardiography can usually define the lesion, and Doppler echocardiography allows accurate estimation of the gradient across the pulmonary valve in many cases. In adults the use of percutaneous balloon valvuloplasty for typical valvular PS is both safe and effective and is now considered by many cardiologists to be the treatment of choice for this lesion.[3] Interestingly, studies have shown no significant restenosis in follow-up catheterizations of patients initially treated with balloon valvuloplasty.

REFERENCES

1. Ross, E.M., and Roberts, W.C.: The carcinoid syndrome. Comparison of 21 necropsy subjects with carcinoid heart disease. Am. J. Med. 79:339, 1985.
2. Feldman, T., and Borow, K.M.: Adults with pulmonic stenosis: Management. Cardiovasc. Med. 9:711, 1984.
3. Kan, J.S., White, R.I., Mitchell, S.E., Anderson, J.H., and Gardner, T.J.: Percutaneous transluminal balloon valvuloplasty for pulmonary valve stenosis. Circulation 69:554, 1984.

495-B, 496-B, 497-A, 498-B (Braunwald, p. 1606)

Cor pulmonale is most commonly caused by chronic obstructive pulmonary disease (COPD). This disease consists of chronic bronchitis, emphysema, and bronchial asthma. However, atopic asthma does *not* produce chronic cor pulmonale. In most patients with COPD, chronic bronchitis and emphysema coexist, but cor pulmonale is restricted to those with functionally significant airway disease, i.e., bronchitis, with or without emphysema.[1]

A common classification scheme places chronic bronchitis at one extreme and emphysema at the other in the continuum of COPD. Classically, patients with chronic bronchitis are termed "blue bloaters" and have chronic cough and sputum production, recurring respiratory infections, secondary erythrocytosis, and repeated bouts of right heart failure. Physiologically, these patients have hypoxemia and hypercapnea at rest, normal diffusion capacity, elevated residual volumes, and functional residual capacity, with relatively normal values for total lung capacity and pulmonary compliance. On chest x-ray, these patients usually have moderately hyperinflated lungs, increased bronchovascular markings, and rather commonly, cardiomegaly.

In contrast, patients with predominant emphysema, classically described as "pink puffers," present with dyspnea, while cough and sputum production are considerably less prominent. Erythrocytosis is uncommon, and right heart failure tends to occur only as a terminal event. Because these patients hyperventilate, the alveolar-arterial gradient for oxygen is abnormally elevated, but arterial oxygen tension is usually normal or slightly depressed and hypercapnea is rare. Standard spirometric indices are usually similar to those observed in chronic bronchitis, but the pink puffer has abnormally low diffusing capacity and greatly increased lung volumes and pulmonary compliance. Because of this, the cardiac silhouette frequently appears smaller than normal. Because the primary pathological defect in this illness is destruction of the alveolar septa, these patients initially have normal or near-normal pulmonary artery pressures at rest, and it is only with severe loss of lung parenchyma that secondary changes occur in the vasculature and resting pulmonary artery hypertension and cor pulmonale develop. In contrast, patients with chronic bronchitis become hypoxic early in the course of their illness and therefore have elevated pulmonary pressures at rest.

REFERENCE

1. Thurlbeck, W.M., Henderson, J.A., Fraser, R.G., and Bates, D.V.: Chronic obstructive lung disease. A comparison between clinical, roentgenologic, functional and morphologic criteria in chronic bronchitis, emphysema, asthma, and bronchiectasis. Medicine 48:51, 1970.

499-A, 500-C, 501-D, 502-A, 503-B *(Braunwald, pp. 113–114; 978–982; 1052–1060; 1717–1718)*

A illustrates a parasternal short-axis two-dimensional echocardiographic image at the level of the aortic valve in which a bicuspid (but otherwise normal) aortic valve is present. *B* illustrates a parasternal two-dimensional echocardiographic image of valvular aortic stenosis with thickening of the aortic valve leaflets and a decrease in aortic valve leaflet separation, or "doming."

A bicuspid aortic valve is probably the most common congenital cardiac anomaly. Most frequently, the bicuspid valve is functionally normal early in life but may become thickened, fibrotic, calcified, and stenotic during adulthood. By the age of 45, approximately half of all bicuspid valves show some degree of stenosis.[1] The bicuspid valve is also a common cause of congenital valvular aortic stenosis (AS), a lesion that may be associated with coarctation of the aorta and, less frequently, atrial septal defect or isolated pulmonic stenosis. Thus in young or middle-aged adults, the presence of isolated valvular AS is usually congenital in origin rather than due to rheumatic disease. Interestingly, aortic valve prolapse may be noted in association with a bicuspid aortic valve,[2] and may occasionally lead to aortic regurgitation that requires valve replacement. Two-dimensional echocardiography is quite useful in making the diagnosis of bicuspid aortic valve, although the diagnosis can occasionally be confusing due to the presence on echocardiography of a fused commissure resembling a third leaflet.[3] All patients with known bicuspid aortic valve require antibiotic prophylaxis against infective endocarditis.

The changes causing AS that occur in a bicuspid valve resemble those occurring in senile degenerative calcific stenosis of a tricuspid aortic valve, which is illustrated in *B*. Senile calcific AS has a pathophysiology similar to stenosis occurring upon a bicuspid valve but presents several decades later. The natural history of this form of AS includes a long latent period during which a gradual

increase in LV outflow tract obstruction occurs, leading to a similarly gradual increase in the pressure load on the LV while the patient remains asymptomatic.

In untreated patients, the appearance of any of the cardinal symptoms of AS heralds a poor prognosis. Thus, survival curves show that the interval from the onset of symptoms to the time of death is approximately 5 years in patients with angina, 3 years in patients with syncope, and 2 years in patients with congestive heart failure (see Braunwald, Fig. 33–28, p. 1058).[4] Approximately two-thirds of patients with critical AS have angina, which usually is similar clinically to angina which is observed in patients with coronary artery disease. It occurs because of the increased oxygen needs of the hypertrophied myocardium and/or reduction of oxygen delivery due to excessive compression of coronary vessels.[5]

Medical management of AS includes careful counseling of patients regarding the hazards of endocarditis and the need for endocarditis prophylaxis prior to both dental and invasive procedures, as well as discussions regarding the potential symptoms that may arise in the asymptomatic patient. It is crucial that patients understand that the earliest appearance of symptoms should be reported to their physician. In addition, noninvasive assessment of the severity of obstruction by Doppler echocardiography should be performed at regular intervals. In most adults with AS, aortic valve replacement should be recommended when symptoms appear and documented hemodynamic evidence of critical obstruction is present.

Ankylosing spondylitis leads to a dilatation of the aortic valve ring with fibrous thickening and scarring, as well as focal inflammatory lesions involving the aortic valve cusps. Dilatation of the sinuses of Valsalva and focal degenerative changes in the ascending aorta may also be involved. Aortic regurgitation may result from shortening and thickening of the valve cusps and their displacement by aortic root dilatation (see Braunwald, Fig. 54–9, p. 1717).

REFERENCES

1. Fenoglio, J.J., McAllister, H.A., DeCastro, C.M., Davia, J.E., and Cheitlin, M.D.: Congenital bicuspid aortic valve after age 20. Am. J. Cardiol. 39:164, 1977.
2. Shapiro, L., Thwaites, B., Westgate, C., and Donaldson, R.: Prevalence and clinical significance of aortic valve prolapse. Br. Heart J. 54:179, 1985.
3. Brandenburg, R.O., Tajik, A.J., Edwards, W.D., Reeder, G.S., Shub, C., and Seward, J.B.: Accuracy of two-dimensional echocardiographic diagnosis of congenitally bicuspid aortic valve—echocardiographic-anatomic correlation in 115 patients. Am. J. Cardiol. 51:1469, 1983.
4. Ross, J., Jr., and Braunwald, E.: The influence of corrective operations on the natural history of aortic stenosis. Circulation 37(Suppl. V):61, 1968.
5. Lombard, J.T., and Selzer, A.: Valvular aortic stenosis: A clinical and hemodynamic profile of patients. Ann. Intern. Med. 106:292, 1987.

504-C, 505-C, 506-D, 507-A *(Braunwald, pp. 1283–1284)*

Rupture of the interventricular septum in the presence of AMI usually occurs secondary to anterior infarction and in patients with multivessel coronary artery disease.[1]

Patients with an anterior infarction that leads to rupture tend to have a septal defect that is apical in location, whereas inferior infarctions are associated with perforation of the basal septum. Partial or total rupture of a papillary muscle in the setting of AMI usually is due to damage to the posteromedial papillary muscle due to inferior wall infarction. Such a papillary muscle rupture occurs with relatively small infarctions in approximately half of the cases, in contrast to rupture of the ventricular septum, which almost always occurs with larger infarcts.[2]

Clinically, patients with both lesions develop a new murmur, which is usually holosystolic. The murmur associated with rupture of the interventricular septum is often more obvious, but clinical distinction between the two entities in question may be difficult. In both lesions, the murmur may decrease or disappear as arterial blood pressure falls with the progressive hemodynamic compromise that invariably ensues. The use of echocardiography to identify partial or complete rupture of a papillary muscle and ventricular septal defect is often helpful.[3] However, the definitive diagnosis and distinction between acute ventricular septal rupture and mitral regurgitation is accomplished by insertion of a pulmonary artery balloon catheter, which allows the detection of a "step-up" in oxygen saturation in blood samples from the right ventricle and pulmonary artery in patients who have developed an acute ventricular septal rupture.[4] Patients with both lesions may develop tall v waves in the pulmonary papillary wedge tracing; therefore, this finding is not useful in distinguishing between the two lesions. Hemodynamic monitoring of right and left ventricular filling pressures, as well as measurement of cardiac output and systemic vascular resistance, are helpful guides during vasodilator therapy. The latter may allow stabilization of a patient's condition prior to diagnostic catheterization and subsequent surgical repair.

REFERENCES

1. Radford, M.J., Johnson, R.A., Daggett, W.M., Fallon, J.T., Buckley, M.J., Gold, H.K., and Leinbach, R.C.: Ventricular septal rupture: A review of clinical and physiologic features and an analysis of survival. Circulation 64:545, 1981.
2. Nishimura, R.A., Schaff, H.V., Shub, C., Gersh, B.J., Edwards, W.D., and Tajik, A.: Papillary muscle rupture complicating acute myocardial infarction: Analysis of 17 patients. Am. J. Cardiol. 51:373, 1983.
3. Come, P.C., Riley, M.F., Weintraub, R., Morgan, J.P., and Nakao, S.: Echocardiographic detection of complete and partial papillary muscle rupture during acute myocardial infarction. Am. J. Cardiol. 56:787, 1985.
4. Meister, S.G., and Helfant, R.H.: Rapid bedside differentiation of ruptured interventricular septum from acute mitral insufficiency. N. Engl. J. Med. 287:1024, 1972.

508-C, 509-B, 510-A, 511-B   (Braunwald, pp. 1430–1434; 1501–1507)

The clinical and hemodynamic features of restrictive heart disease such as that which may be caused by cardiac amyloidosis are very similar to those of chronic constrictive pericarditis. Endomyocardial biopsy, CT scanning, and magnetic resonance imaging may be useful in differentiating the two diseases. The typical hemodynamic feature present in both conditions is the deep and rapid early decline in ventricular pressure at the onset of diastole, with a rapid rise to a plateau in early diastole, termed the "square root" sign. In the atrial tracings, the dip and plateau is manifested as a prominent "y descent" followed by a rapid rise in pressure. The x descent may also be prominent, and the combination results in a characteristic M or W wave form in the atrial pressure tracing. Both systemic and pulmonary venous pressures are usually elevated. In general, patients with restrictive heart disease have left ventricular filling pressures that exceed right ventricular filling pressures by more than 5 mm Hg, and this difference can be accentuated by exercise. This is because in restrictive disease, as opposed to constrictive disease, the "encasement" of the heart is relative. Furthermore, the pulmonary artery systolic pressure is often greater than 45 mm Hg in patients with restrictive cardiomyopathy but is usually lower in constrictive pericarditis.[1] Finally, the plateau of the right ventricular diastolic pressure is usually at least one-third of the peak right ventricular systolic pressure in patients with constrictive pericarditis, while it is frequently less than one-third in patients with restrictive cardiomyopathy.

REFERENCE

1. Shabetai, R.: Profiles in constrictive pericarditis, cardiac tamponade and restrictive cardiomyopathy. In Grossman, W. (ed.): Cardiac Catheterization and Angiography. Philadelphia, Lea and Febiger, 1974, p. 304.

512-C, 513-A, 514-B, 515-B, 516-C   (Braunwald, pp. 1563–1566)

Takayasu's arteritis, which is also referred to as "aortic arch syndrome," "pulseless disease," "reversed coarctation," "young female arteritis," and "occlusive thromboaortopathy," is a disease of unknown etiology characterized by marked fibrous and degenerative scarring of the elastic fibers of the vascular media. The disease may be subclassified depending upon sites of involvement and commonly involves the aorta and carotid arteries. The disease is much more common in women than it is in men, and in most patients the disease has its onset during the teenage years.[1] Patients not uncommonly present initially with a systemic illness characterized by fever, malaise, weight loss, night sweats, arthralgias, pleuritic pain, anorexia, and fatigue. Regardless of whether or not a patient goes through this initial phase, after a latent period, symptoms and signs referable to the obliterative and inflammatory changes in affected blood vessels begin to appear. These often include diminished or absent pulses, narrowing of affected arteries, hypertension, and in approximately one-fourth to one-third of patients, heart failure, which is usually seen in very young patients as a consequence of systemic hypertension.

A minority of patients have involvement primarily of the abdominal aorta and may therefore have abdominal angina, lower extremity claudication, and hypertension due to renal arterial involvement. More commonly, patients manifest symptoms and signs due to upper extremity arterial involvement. Common laboratory abnormalities include elevated sedimentation rate, low-grade leukocytosis, and mild normocytic anemia. A typical pattern is often seen on arteriography and may include a "rat-tail" appearance of the thoracic aorta (see Braunwald, Figs. 46–19 and 46–20, pp. 1564–1565).

Therapy of this disorder includes treatment with steroids of patients with documented systemic symptoms and/or clinical progression of the disease. In patients who remain unresponsive, cyclophosphamide may be added. In addition, platelet-inhibitory agents such as aspirin and dipyridamole are often used to treat the symptoms of transient ischemia as well as to prevent progression of the disease, although clinical trials of efficacy of these agents have not yet been performed. Survival in general depends on the degree and number of complications that develop during the course of the illness. The use of corticosteroid therapy, cytotoxic agents, and appropriate surgery has lead to excellent 5-year survival rates.[2]

Giant cell arteritis is a disease of unknown etiology characterized by granulomatous inflammation of the media of small- to medium-caliber arteries with a special predilection for vessels of the head and neck. The disease is also known as "granulomatus arteritis" and "temporal arteritis" and is seen primarily in elderly people. Clinically, the classic triad of severe headache, fever, and marked malaise characterize the illness. The headaches are often extremely severe and are typically localized over the involved temporal arteries. Claudication of the jaw muscles during chewing is present in up to two-thirds of patients and is considered to be very suggestive of the illness.[3] Involvement of the ophthalmic artery leads to visual symptoms in between 25 and 50 per cent of patients and may result in irreversible blindness. The syndrome of polymyalgia rheumatica, consisting of diffuse muscular aching and stiffness, occurs in close to 40 per cent of patients with giant cell arteritis.[4] In a minority of cases, involvement of the aorta or its major branches may lead to symptoms and signs similar to those of Takayasu's arteritis, although interestingly, renal artery involvement is almost never seen in this disorder.

Patients with giant cell arteritis appear ill and almost always have fever. Affected vessels feel abnormal to palpation and are tender, allowing experienced examiners to make the diagnosis of temporal arteritis at the bedside by identifying an indurated, beaded, tender, temporal artery. Laboratory tests often reveal a very high sedimentation rate, normochromic normocytic anemia, and elevated acute phase reactants. Biopsy of an involved temporal artery allows confirmation of the diagnosis.

Management of granulomous arteritis includes early intervention with high-dose steroid therapy (60 to 80 mg of prednisone per day). Steroids may be titrated against the sedimentation rate and clinical symptoms and gradually tapered to a maintenance dose, which is typically continued for 1 to 2 years. Early administration of steroid therapy is crucial to the prevention of involvement of the ophthalmic arteries and possible blindness.

REFERENCES

1. Lupi-Herrera, E., Sanchez-Torres, G., Marcushamer, J., Mispirela, J., Horowitz, S., and Espino Vela, J.: Takayasu's arteritis. Clinical study of 107 cases. Am. Heart J. 93:94, 1977.

2. Shellbamer, J.H., Volkman, D.J., Parillo, J.E., Lawley, T.J., Johnston, M.R., and Fauci, A.S.: Takayasu's arteritis and its therapy. Ann. Intern. Med. 103:121, 1985.

3. Huston, K.A., and Hunder, G.G.: Giant cell (cranial) arteritis: A clinical review. Am. Heart J. 100:99, 1980.

4. Chuang, T., Hunder, G.G., Ilstrup, D.M., and Kurland, L.T.: Polymyalgia rheumatica. Ann. Intern. Med. 97:672, 1982.

517-C, 518-A, 519-A, 520-B *(Braunwald, pp. 1028, 1039, 1055)*

The systolic murmur is the most prominent auscultatory finding in mitral regurgitation (MR), but it must be differentiated from the systolic murmur heard in aortic stenosis (AS), tricuspid regurgitation, and ventricular septal defect. In most cases the systolic murmur of MR commences immediately after a soft S_1 and extends to S_2. The murmur may persist beyond S_2, obscuring A_2 in some instances because of a persistent pressure difference between the left ventricle and the left atrium. The holosystolic murmur in chronic MR is usually constant in intensity, blowing, high-pitched, and loudest at the apex. The murmur of AS, on the other hand has a crescendo-decrescendo pattern, is usually much less musical than the murmur of MR, and is followed by a single S_2. However, these murmurs can frequently be confused with each other; several dynamic maneuvers are helpful in their differentiation.

The dynamic maneuvers can be conceptualized as altering either preload (the left ventricular end-diastolic pressure or volume) or afterload (left ventricular systolic pressure). In general, the intensity of regurgitant murmurs is reduced while that of stenotic murmurs is increased by a fall in afterload. Regurgitant murmurs are minimally affected by alterations in preload while stenotic murmurs are significantly affected by changes in preload. Thus, handgrip, which increases the peripheral resistance, tends to have little effect on the murmur of AS but will increase the murmur of MR. Amyl nitrite, which causes an immediate and marked drop in blood pressure, will make an MR murmur softer while an AS murmur will become louder due to the increased velocity of LV ejection following the reflex increase in cardiac output. During slow atrial fibrillation, with significant beat-to-beat variation in left ventricular stroke volume, there will be marked beat-to-beat changes in the intensity of the murmur of AS but little change in the murmur of MR; similar findings occur with ventricular premature beats. The murmurs of AS and MR are both usually diminished during the strain phase of the Valsalva maneuver due to a decrease in the preload with resulting decrease in total cardiac output and blood flow.[1]

REFERENCE

1. Dalen, J.E., and Alpert, J.S.: Valvular Heart Disease. 2nd ed. Boston, Little, Brown and Company, 1987.

521-C, 522-C, 523-C, 524-C, 525-C *(Braunwald, pp. 953–957; 961–963)*

In complete transposition of the great arteries, the aorta arises from the right ventricle while the pulmonary artery arises from the left ventricle. Because the origin of the aorta is to the right and anterior to the main pulmonary artery, this disorder is often termed dextro or D-transposition. Complete transposition is a common and potentially lethal form of congenital heart disease. The resulting anatomical disarrangement results in two separate and parallel circulations that usually communicate through an atrial septal defect. In addition, two-thirds of the patients have a patent ductus arteriosus and about one-third have an associated ventricular septal defect. Infants with complete transposition are particularly susceptible to the early development of pulmonary vascular obstructive disease.[1] They usually present at birth with dyspnea and cyanosis as well as progressive hypoxemia and congestive heart failure. Cardiac murmurs are of little diagnostic significance and are actually absent in up to one-half of infants with complete transposition.

Electrocardiographic findings include right axis deviation, right atrial enlargement, and right ventricular hypertrophy. Echocardiography may be extremely useful in making the diagnosis of complete transposition. Cardiac catheterization with angiography allows confirmation of the anatomical arrangement of the great arteries and establishes the presence of associated lesions. Palliative balloon atrial septostomy at the time of catheterization in the newborn serves to enlarge the interatrial communication and improves oxygenation. While medical management of this disorder is often of limited value and is primarily symptomatic, the development of corrective surgical operation for infants born with transposition has greatly improved their prognosis.[2] Operative repair using the Mustard technique or the Senning procedure allows atrial rerouting of blood flow with clinical improvement that is usually quite dramatic. While the procedures are usually well tolerated, there appears to be a high incidence of early and late postoperative dysrhythmias in these repairs.

Total anomalous pulmonary venous connection is the result of persistent communication of all of the pulmonary veins either to the right atrium directly or to the systemic veins and their tributaries. Because all pulmonary venous blood therefore returns to the right atrium, an interatrial communication is an integral part of this malformation in viable infants. The anatomical varieties of total anomalous pulmonary venous connection are subdivided based on the level of abnormal drainage (see Braunwald, Fig. 30–71 and Table 30–10, p. 962). The physiological consequences and subsequent clinical manifestations of this disorder depend upon the size of the interatrial communication that is present as well as upon the height of the pulmonary vascular resistance.[3] Most patients with total anomalous pulmonary venous connection develop symptoms during the first year of life and 80 per cent die before age 1 if left untreated.

Infants with this disorder have early onset of severe dyspnea, pulmonary edema, right heart failure, and cyanosis. Cardiac murmurs are usually not a prominent finding. Multiple heart sounds are often heard, including a prominent S_1 followed by an ejection sound and a fixed and widely split S_2, as well as an S_3 and S_4. The ECG usually shows right-axis deviation and right atrial and ventricular hypertrophy. In some instances, echocardiographic identification of anomalous pulmonary venous

connection to the systemic veins, coronary sinus, or right atrium may be made. Analysis of oxygen saturations at cardiac catheterization as well as selective pulmonary arteriography will establish the diagnosis. Balloon atrial septotomy may provide dramatic palliation for infants with this disorder.[4] Unless pulmonary vascular disease has developed prior to correction, the results of operation for total anomalous pulmonary venous connection in patients beyond infancy are generally favorable.[5] Surgical correction usually involves anastomosis between the pulmonary venous channels and left atrium as well as closure of the atrial septal defect.

REFERENCES

1. Lakier, J.B., Stanger, P., Heyman, M.A., Hoffman, J.I.E., and Rudolph, A.M.: Early onset of pulmonary vascular obstruction in patients with aortopulmonary transposition and intact ventricular septum. Circulation 51:875, 1975.
2. Castaneda, A.R., Norwood, W.I., Jonas, R.A., Colon, S.D., Sanders, S.P., and Lang, P.: Transposition of the great arteries and intact ventricular septum: Anatomical repair in the neonate. Ann. Thorac. Surg. 38:438, 1984.
3. Gathman, G.E., and Nadas, A.S.: Total anomalous pulmonary venous connection: Clinical and physiologic observations in 75 pediatric patients. Circulation 42:143, 1970.
4. Ward, K.E., Mullins, C.E., Huhta, J.C., Nihill, M.R., McNamara, D.G., and Cooley, D.A.: Restrictive interatrial communication in total anomalous pulmonary venous connection. Am. J. Cardiol. 57:1131, 1986.
5. Reardon, M.J., Cooley, D.A., Kubrusly, L., Ott, D.A., Johnson, W., Kay, G.L., and Sweeney, M.S.: Total anomalous pulmonary venous return: Report of 201 patients treated surgically. Texas Heart Inst. J. 12:131, 1985.

526-A, 527-B, 528-D, 529-B *(Braunwald, p. 1127)*

There is considerable dispute concerning the selection of appropriate prophylactic antibiotics to prevent infective endocarditis in patients with cardiac disease. However, a few rules have been agreed upon. First, the procedures for which chemoprophylaxis is necessary include those that may cause substantial bacteremia, such as dental and oral surgical procedures, open-heart surgery, tonsillectomy, gastrointestinal and genitourinary operations, instrumentation or biopsies, nasal intubation, rigid bronchoscopy, and incision and drainage of abscesses. Patients at particularly high risk for endocarditis (such as those with surgically created shunts, prosthetic valves, conduits, and patches) should also receive prophylaxis for percutaneous liver biopsy, gastrointestinal endoscopy, barium enema, complicated vaginal delivery, bladder catheterization, and diagnostic cardiac catheterization.

Second, the specific prophylactic program should be directed at the organisms most likely to be involved in transient bacteremia. Thus, the bacterium present in blood following dental manipulation and operations of the upper respiratory tract is predominantly *Streptococcus viridans*, although some staphylococci may also circulate. Transient bacteremia associated with procedures involving the urinary, gastrointestinal, and genital tracts usually includes gram-negative bacteria and occasionally staphylococci.

Based on these general recommendations, guidelines for prophylaxis have been established by the American

Heart Association[1] and by the British Society for Anti-microbial Chemotherapy.[2] Patient No. 1 (who is not at high risk) undergoes a simple dental extraction and would be adequately covered by oral amoxicillin given immediately before the procedure. Patient No. 2, who is to undergo dental extraction, is at higher risk for endocarditis by virtue of having an aortic valve prosthesis. This patient should receive intravenous amoxicillin and gentamicin both before and after the procedure. Similarly, patient No. 4, who will undergo genitourinary surgery, should also receive aminoglycoside prophylaxis because of the nature of the organisms likely to cause bacteremia. Patient No. 3, undergoing general anesthesia in a relatively uncomplicated procedure, would be most appropriately covered with an intravenous antibiotic regimen different from any of those listed, such as amoxicillin 1 gm IM or IV followed by 0.5 gm orally or IM 6 hours later.

Patients at high risk who are allergic to penicillin may be treated with vancomycin 1 gm IV plus gentamicin 120 mg IM or IV for procedures associated with significant bacteremia. For patients allergic to penicillin who are undergoing simple procedures involving local anesthesia, erythromycin 1.5 gm orally 1 hour before and 0.5 gm 6 hours later is a reasonable treatment.

REFERENCES

1. Shulman, S.T., Amren, D.P., Bisno, A.L., et al: Prevention of bacterial endocarditis: A statement for health professionals by the committee on rheumatic fever and infective endocarditis of the council on cardiovascular disease in the young. Circulation 70:1123A, 1984.
2. Working Party of the British Society for Antimicrobial Chemotherapy. Lancet 2:1323, 1982.

530-A, 531-B, 532-A, 533-A (Braunwald, pp. 1325–1335)

There is currently significant controversy about whether calcium antagonists or beta blockers should be employed first in the treatment of chronic stable angina in patients in whom sublingual nitroglycerin alone is insufficient. It appears that both classes of drugs are equally effective and both have minor but frequent side effects. Thus, the associated conditions and unique attributes of each individual patient will in general guide selection. When the patient's anginal threshold is relatively fixed, it may be presumed that myocardial ischemia is caused primarily by an increase in myocardial oxygen needs during exercise in the face of a fixed supply, and a beta blocker would be considered the drug of choice. On the other hand, in patients with variable threshold angina in whom reduction of myocardial blood supply caused by coronary vasoconstriction plays a role in the development of ischemia, a calcium antagonist may be a more effective choice.[1]

In the examples chosen, for various reasons one drug may be better than the other. Thus, in patients with significant sinus bradycardia or AV block, nifedipine would be preferable to a beta blocker or the other calcium channel antagonists, which depress specialized cardiac tissue. Conversely, in patients with supraventricular

tachycardia or rapid atrial fibrillation, a beta blocker (or verapamil) would be the drug of choice.

In patients with valvular disease, the choice of antianginal medication is made in part on the basis of left ventricular function, the effects of afterload reduction on disease symptoms, and the hemodynamic importance of heart rate control. Thus in patients with mitral stenosis in whom decreasing the heart rate may improve left ventricular filling, a beta blocker would be indicated. Conversely, patients with either aortic or mitral regurgitation may do better with an agent such as nifedipine, which causes a reduction in afterload.

There are obvious difficulties with beta blockers in the presence of concomitant peripheral vascular disease; thus, nifedipine would be the drug of choice in patients with intermittent claudication, or Raynaud's phenomenon. Nifedipine would also be the drug of choice in patients with bronchial spasm, asthma, and insulin-dependent diabetes mellitus because of potential side effects from beta blockade in these conditions.

REFERENCE

1. Shub, C., Vlietstra, R.E., and McGoon, M.D.: Selection of optimal drug therapy for the patient with angina pectoris. Mayo Clin. Proc. 60:539, 1985.

534-B, 535-A, 536-B, 537-B, 538-D (Braunwald, pp. 918–920; 923–925)

A complete atrioventricular canal defect includes a constellation of findings including an ostium primum atrial septal defect, a ventricular septal defect in the posterior basal portion of the ventricular septum, and a common atrial-ventricular orifice. This latter structure usually has six leaflets. In approximately 35 per cent of cases, accompanying cardiovascular lesions are present, including tetralogy of Fallot, transposition of the great arteries, total anomalous pulmonary venous connection, pulmonic stenosis, double-outlet RV, and persistent left superior vena cava. The malformation is commonly associated with Down syndrome. Patients usually present during the first year of life with a history of poor weight gain and frequent respiratory infections. Heart failure in infancy is extremely common and often requires aggressive medical therapy. Two-dimensional echocardiography is usually diagnostic (see Braunwald, Fig. 30–15, p. 919). However, hemodynamic study is frequently indicated in patients with common AV canal because the level of pulmonary vascular resistance has important prognostic implications. Infants with the complete form of the AV canal defect are at high risk for obstructive pulmonary vascular disease. The diagnosis may also be established during LV angiography, at which time the relationship between the anterior components of the left atrioventricular valve and the aorta leads to a "gooseneck" deformity (see Braunwald, Fig. 30–16, p. 919). In most medical centers, primary repair of the abnormality is the preferred therapeutic approach, especially in patients with growth failure, severe pulmonary hypertension, or intractable heart failure.[1]

In the fetal circulation, most of the output of the RV

bypasses the unexpanded lungs and travels from the pulmonary trunk through the ductus arteriosus to the descending aorta just distal to the left subclavian artery. Patency of the ductus arteriosus after birth occurs most commonly in females, and in the offspring of pregnancies in which the mother had rubella infection in the first trimester. While the lesion may coexist with coarctation of the aorta, ventricular septal defect, pulmonic stenosis, or aortic stenosis, it is most commonly seen in an isolated form. A characteristic continuous "machinery" murmur and thrill are noted on physical examination at the upper left sternal border. However, the presence of a diastolic, high-pitched decrescendo murmur, characteristic of aortic regurgitation, is not heard in either this disorder or in complete atrioventricular canal defect.

The clinical diagnosis of persistent patent ductus arteriosus may be subtle, and full-term infants not uncommonly survive for a number of years, either undiagnosed or with minimal symptoms. The leading causes of death in children with this anomaly as they progress are infective endocarditis and heart failure. The lesion may be visualized directly by two-dimensional echocardiography. If accompanying lesions are suspected, or pulmonary vascular disease needs evaluation, cardiac catheterization may be indicated. Operative ligation of the ductus is a low-risk procedure and may be made safer by aggressive medical therapy of any accompanying heart failure prior to the operation.

REFERENCE

1. Clapp, S.K., Perry, B.L., Farooki, Z.O., Jackson, W.L., Karpawich, P.P., Hakimi, M., Arciniegas, E., and Green, E.W.: Surgical and medical results of complete atrioventricular canal: a ten-year review. Am. J. Cardiol. 59:454, 1987.

539-A, 540-C, 541-B, 542-A, 543-D *(Braunwald, pp. 1471–1477)*

Cardiac myxomas are benign cardiac tumors that comprise the most common type of primary cardiac tumor, accounting for 30 to 50 per cent of the total in most pathological series. The vast majority of myxomas occur sporadically,[1] and three-quarters of myxomas occur in females. Approximately 86 per cent of myxomas occur in the left atrium, and over 90 per cent are solitary.[2] In general, the clinical symptoms and signs produced by myxomas are nonspecific or are related to embolization or mechanical interference with cardiac function (see Braunwald, Table 43–1, p. 1471). Signs and symptoms suggestive of mitral valve disease or embolic phenomena are among the more common clinical presentations of cardiac myxoma. However, a significant number of cases will be appreciated as an incidental finding in the absence of cardiac symptoms. In addition, a number of other conditions may be mimicked by or confused with atrial myxoma; therefore, a heightened degree of suspicion for this lesion is often necessary to make the diagnosis. Pathologically, the vast majority of myxomas are pedunculated with a fibrovascular stalk.

Approximately 7 per cent of all cardiac myxomas occur in an autosomal dominant manner and may be present as part of a syndrome that involves a complex of abnormalities, including lentigines or blue nevi or both and a variety of endocrine tumors.[3] Patients presenting with the familial form of myxoma are in general younger, more likely to have multiple myxomas involving chambers other than the left atrium, and more likely to have recurrence of myxomas postoperatively. It is believed that most sessile myxomas in fact represent the base of a pedicle that remains following embolization of the body of the tumor. The treatment of choice in this disorder is primary excision, which usually is curative.

Approximately 25 per cent of all cardiac tumors are malignant, and the vast majority of these are part of the sarcoma family. While cardiac sarcomas may occur at any age, they are more commonly seen between the third and fifth decades, show no sex preference, and are found most frequently in the right atrium. The prognosis for patients with these tumors is grave, and death usually occurs in less than 2 years following the onset of symptoms. These tumors are in general quite aggressive, and infiltrate the myocardium in a widespread manner, with distant metastases and obstruction of cardiac flow as frequent complications. Approximately 80 per cent of malignant cardiac tumors are pedunculated, with only a minority being sessile or polypoid. Because the right side of the heart is most frequently affected, presentations for cardiac sarcoma may include signs of right heart failure or obstruction of the superior vena cava leading to swelling of the face or upper extremities. In general, surgical removal is not an effective treatment for primary malignant tumors of the heart. Combinations of chemotherapy and radiation therapy along with partial resection have been attempted. These have produced few long-term survivors, although occasionally such combined modality therapy may alleviate symptoms.

REFERENCES

1. McCarthy, P.M., Piehler, J.M., Schaff, H.V., Pluth, J.R., Orszulak, T.A., Vidaillet, H.J., Jr., and Carney, J.A.: The significance of multiple, recurrent, and "complex" cardiac myxomas. Thorac. Cardiovasc. Surg. 91:389, 1986.
2. Carney, J.A.: Differences between nonfamilial and familial cardiac myxoma. Am. J. Surg. Pathol. 9:53, 1985.
3. Rhodes, A.R., Silverman, R.A., Harris, T.J., and Perez-Atayde, A.R.: Mucocutaneous lentigines, cardiomucocutaneous myxomas, and multiple blue nevi: The LAMB syndrome. Am. Acad. Dermatol. 10:72, 1984.

544-B, 545-A, 546-D, 547-D *(Braunwald, p. 1330–1332)*

The beta blockers constitute a cornerstone of therapy for chronic stable angina.[1] Their widespread use is partially explained by the wide variety of agents available and the ability to select for particular characteristics important to individual patient management. The beta blockers can be characterized on the basis of several of their actions. There are two types of beta receptors, designated beta₁ and beta₂, which are present in different proportions in different tissues. Beta₁ receptors predominate in the heart and their stimulation leads to an increase in heart rate and AV conduction and contractility. Beta$_2$ stimulation results in bronchial dilation, vaso-dilation, and glycogenolysis. The beta blockers currently available have been classified according to their relative cardioselectivity: the nonselective beta blocking drugs (propranolol, timolol, pindolol, and nadolol) block both beta$_1$ and beta$_2$ receptors, whereas relatively cardioselective beta blockers (atenolol, metoprolol, and acebutolol) produce selective blockade of beta$_1$ receptors. There are no commercially available beta$_2$ selective blockers.

These drugs can also be characterized by their membrane-stabilizing ability—a quinidine-like effect—measured by the reduction in the rate of rise of the cardiac action potential (of uncertain clinical significance).

The presence of intrinsic sympathomimetic activity may also distinguish types of beta blockers and is characteristic of pindolol and acebutolol, which are partial agonists and produce blockade by shielding beta receptors from more potent beta agonists. Thus, these agents produce low-grade beta stimulation when sympathetic activity is low (for instance, at rest), while during stress and exercise, the agonists behave more like conventional beta blockers.

The major determinant of absorption and metabolism of the beta blockers is their lipid solubility or hydrophobicity. The lipid-soluble beta blockers (propranolol, metoprolol, and pindolol) are readily absorbed from the gastrointestinal tract, are metabolized predominantly by the liver, have a relatively short half-life, and are more likely to cause central nervous system side effects. The water-soluble beta blockers (atenolol, metoprolol, and nadolol) are not as readily absorbed from the gastrointestinal tract, are not as extensively metabolized in the liver, have relatively long plasma half-lives, and therefore accumulate in renal failure. Finally, a beta blocker, labetolol, is now available that also possesses alpha adrenergic receptor blocking activity; this may make it particularly useful as an antihypertensive agent.

REFERENCE

1. Rogers, W.J.: Use of beta blockers in the treatment of ischemic heart disease: A comparison of the available agents. Cardiovasc. Rev. Rep. 5:311, 1984.

PARTS IV AND V: BROADER PERSPECTIVES ON HEART DISEASE AND RELATION BETWEEN HEART DISEASE AND DISEASE OF OTHER ORGAN SYSTEMS

CHAPTERS 49 THROUGH 62

DIRECTIONS: Each question below contains five suggested responses. Select the ONE BEST response to each question.

548. True statements about the blood coagulation system include all of the following EXCEPT:

 A. Hageman factor (factor XII) is a participant in the intrinsic or "contact activation" pathway of coagulation
 B. Tissue factor initiates the extrinsic coagulation pathway by interacting with another protein, factor BII
 C. Prothrombin is converted to thrombin by factor Xa
 D. Thrombin is responsible for cross-linking fibrin polymers
 E. Thrombin activates factors V and VIII

549. True statements about the use of nonimaging modalities in the diagnosis of pulmonary embolism include all of the following EXCEPT:

 A. Arterial blood gases may be misleading in the diagnosis of pulmonary embolism
 B. Thoracentesis may be useful in the diagnosis of pulmonary embolism in patients with pleural effusions
 C. The electrocardiogram often shows characteristic abnormalities in patients with large or massive pulmonary embolism
 D. Pulmonary infarction due to pulmonary embolism may lead to a "Hampton's hump" on the chest x-ray
 E. While fibrin degradation products have been found to be elevated in some patients with pulmonary embolism, there is no rapid, inexpensive, and accurate blood test for the diagnosis of this condition

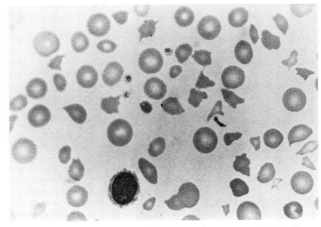

From Jandl, J.H.: Blood Textbook of Hematology. Boston, Little, Brown and Co., 1987.

550. The peripheral blood smear displayed *above* is consistent with each of the following EXCEPT:

 A. mitral valve regurgitation
 B. aortic valve stenosis
 C. coarctation of the aorta
 D. a porcine bioprosthetic valve associated with a perivalvular leak
 E. a Starr-Edwards valve

551. A 15-year-old boy is brought to the office by his grandmother for evaluation of a loud heart murmur. His growth and development have been normal. He has participated in school sports without incident. On examination, he is of normal height and weight. Lungs are clear; carotids have normal volume and upstroke. The cardiac impulse is nondisplaced.

There is a normal S_1, but S_2 is widely split and fixed. A Grade III/VI systolic ejection murmur is loudest over the second left intercostal space. The remainder of the examination is unremarkable except for the presence of "finger-like thumbs." When you tell the grandmother your diagnosis, she tells you that the boy's father was unable to enlist in the Army because of a similar problem. The most likely diagnosis is:

A. Noonan syndrome
B. Holt-Oram syndrome
C. Turner syndrome
D. LEOPARD syndrome
E. Kartagener syndrome

552. A 32-year-old woman has a long history of mitral regurgitation secondary to myxomatous degeneration of the valve. She undergoes uneventful mitral valve replacement with a porcine bioprosthesis. One year later, she returns because of recurrent symptoms of dyspnea. She also complains of polyuria, nocturia, and two episodes of renal colic. On examination, she has a Grade IV/VI murmur of mitral regurgitation and mild hypertension. An echocardiogram demonstrates advanced calcification of the prosthetic valve with a probable tear of one of the leaflets. The most likely associated disease would be:

A. hyperthyroidism
B. hypothyroidism
C. hyperparathyroidism
D. Cushing's syndrome
E. acromegaly

553. Each of the following lesions may be considered amenable to a *reparative* cardiac operation EXCEPT:

A. patent ductus arteriosus
B. ventricular septal defect
C. aortopulmonary window
D. tetralogy of Fallot
E. ventricular aneurysm

554. Treatment of tricyclic antidepressant overdose may include all of the following EXCEPT:

A. sodium bicarbonate therapy to achieve blood alkalinization
B. procainamide or quinidine therapy for atrial arrhythmias
C. lidocaine or phenytoin therapy for ventricular arrhythmias
D. physostigmine to reverse coma and delirium
E. norepinephrine for severe hypotension

555. Preoperative factors associated with a significantly increased risk for development of cardiac complications after major noncardiac surgery in patients over 40 years of age include all of the following EXCEPT:

A. presence of an S_3
B. stable Class II angina
C. myocardial infarction within 3 months
D. severe mitral stenosis
E. more than 5 PVCs/min on the preoperative ECG

556. True statements about the role of platelets in hemostasis include all of the following EXCEPT:

A. Platelet adhesion is the initial event in "primary hemostasis"
B. Platelets initially adhere to collagen fibrils on the endothelial lining of the vessel
C. Activation of platelets leads to release of granular constituents
D. Specific platelet membrane receptors participate in the processes of platelet adhesion and aggregation
E. Arachidonic acid derivatives formed in platelets may recruit additional circulating platelets for the developing platelet aggregate

557. True statements with regard to metastatic disease involving the heart include all of the following EXCEPT:

A. Metastases rarely involve the valves or endocardium
B. The most common primary tumor producing cardiac metastases is bronchogenic carcinoma
C. A chylous pericardial effusion is characteristic of metastatic breast carcinoma
D. More than 50 per cent of patients with malignant melanoma have cardiac metastases that are usually clinically silent
E. A solitary cardiac mass is more likely to be benign than metastatic

DIRECTIONS: Each question below contains five suggested answers. For EACH of the FIVE alternatives listed you are to respond either YES (Y) or NO (N). In a given item ALL, SOME, OR NONE OF THE ALTERNATIVES MAY BE CORRECT.

558. Signs and symptoms of acute rheumatic fever that have been designated "major manifestations" because of their diagnostic utility include which of the following?

    A. heart block
    B. erythema marginatum
    C. chorea
    D. arthritis
    E. fever

559. Which of the following cardiac disorders may be accompanied by hemostatic defects?

    A. chronic right-sided heart failure
    B. mitral stenosis
    C. cyanotic congenital heart disease
    D. peripartum cardiomyopathy
    E. acute infective endocarditis

560. Which of the following cardiovascular drugs is (are) relatively safe to use during pregnancy?

    A. methyldopa
    B. hydralazine
    C. digitalis glycosides
    D. warfarin
    E. procainamide

561. True statements with respect to *heterozygous* familial hypercholesterolemia include which of the following?

    A. It is a relatively common disorder with a gene frequency of 1/500 persons in the population
    B. It is inherited as a recessive trait
    C. Tendon xanthomas and arcus corneae are common but nonspecific findings

    D. Cutaneous planar xanthomas are a specific finding that occur in one-third of patients
    E. The fundamental defect is the presence of only half the normal number of LDL receptors in the individual's cells

562. Which of the following statements pairing anesthetic agents with a side effect is (are) correct?

    A. Halothane–decreased blood pressure
    B. Thiopental–depressed myocardial contractility
    C. Succinylcholine–bradycardia
    D. Ketamine–depressed myocardial contractility
    E. Morphine–venodilation

563. Risk factors for development of doxorubicin cardiotoxicity include:

    A. age greater than 65
    B. preexisting coronary artery disease
    C. administration of more than 250 mg/m^2
    D. prior mediastinal irradiation
    E. hypertension

564. True statements with respect to the cardiovascular effects of tricyclic antidepressants (TCAs) include:

    A. Almost all patients experience increased resting heart rates (10 to 20 beats/min)
    B. Postural changes in blood pressure are common
    C. Desipramine is the most anticholinergic TCA
    D. Patients with atrial tachyarrhythmias may develop a rapid ventricular response
    E. Shortening of the Q-T$_c$ interval is indicative of potential TCA toxicity

DIRECTIONS: Each question below contains four suggested responses of which ONE OR MORE are correct. Select

A if 1, 2, and 3 are correct
B if 1 and 3 are correct
C if 2 and 4 are correct
D if 4 is correct
E if 1, 2, 3, and 4 are correct

565. True statements with regard to cardiac involvement in systemic lupus erythematosus (SLE) include:

1. Pericarditis is the most common cardiac finding
2. Libman-Sacks lesions are caused by active myocarditis
3. Libman-Sacks lesions rarely produce serious valvular regurgitation during the acute phase of the disease
4. In pregnant women with active SLE, fetal tachycardia and atrial fibrillation are caused by transplacental transfer of abnormal antibodies

566. Characteristics of familial hypertriglyceridemia include which of the following?

1. Inheritance as an autosomal dominant trait
2. Development of eruptive xanthomas and pancreatitis following alcohol ingestion
3. Normal cholesterol levels
4. A 5- to 10-fold increased incidence of atherosclerosis

567. Compensatory adaptations to chronic anemia which occur in the cardiovascular system include:

1. increased left ventricular end-diastolic volume
2. decreased left ventricular afterload
3. increased levels of catecholamine and noncatecholamine inotropic factors in plasma
4. increased affinity of red cell hemoglobin for oxygen with a shift in the hemoglobin oxygen dissociation curve to the left

568. True statements with respect to alterations in cardiovascular function with aging include:

1. There is a steady 1 to 2 per cent increase in the number of myocardial cells each year
2. There is moderate hypertrophy of left ventricular myocardium

3. In healthy elderly individuals there is a significant fall in stroke volume and ejection fraction due to a decrease in peak contractile force
4. During exercise, heart rate increases less in older individuals, probably because of decreased catecholamine responsiveness

569. The effects of amiodarone on thyroid function include:

1. inhibition of peripheral conversion of T_4 to T_3
2. decrease in thyroid-stimulating hormone levels
3. inhibition of thyroid organification with a decrease in thyroid clearance of iodide
4. development of hyperthyroidism in 25 per cent of patients on therapy for longer than 12 weeks

570. True statements with regard to the auscultatory examination of acute rheumatic carditis include:

1. Pericardial friction rubs are audible in at least 50 per cent of patients
2. The Carey-Coombs murmur is an apical mid-diastolic murmur heard with mitral valve involvement
3. A loud S_3 is more likely to occur with the first attack of carditis than with a rheumatic recurrence
4. The systolic murmur of mitral regurgitation is commonly heard

571. Development of rheumatic fever following streptococcal infection requires which of the following?

1. A streptococcal antibody response indicative of actual recent infection
2. Persistence of the organism in the pharynx for several days
3. Localization of the infection to the oropharynx
4. Presence of group D streptococci

DIRECTIONS: The group of questions below consists of lettered headings followed by a set of numbered items. For each numbered item select the ONE lettered heading with which it is MOST closely associated. Each lettered heading may be used ONCE, MORE THAN ONCE, OR NOT AT ALL.

A. Kartagener syndrome
B. Holt-Oram syndrome
C. LEOPARD syndrome
D. Noonan syndrome

572. Webbed neck, pulmonic stenosis, left anterior hemiblock

573. Deafness, pulmonic stenosis, complete heart block

574. Lentigines, pulmonic stenosis, P-R prolongation

575. Sinusitis, dextrocardia, bronchiectasis

576. Abnormal scaphoid bone, ventricular septal defect, right bundle branch block

A. Duchenne muscular dystrophy
B. Kearns-Sayre syndrome
C. Facioscapulohumeral dystrophy
D. Myotonic muscular dystrophy

577. Tall, R waves in the right precordium with deep, narrow, Q waves in the lateral precordium are characteristic of the 12 lead ECG in this disorder

578. Pseudohypertrophy of the calves is common

579. Paralysis of the atria is characteristic

580. ECG commonly shows P-R prolongation, left anterior fascicular block, and prolonged QRS duration

581. External ophthalmoplegia is usually present

See illustrations below for Questions 582–585

A. Familial hypercholesterolemia
B. Type III hyperlipoproteinemia (familial dysbetaliproteinemia)
C. Both
D. Neither

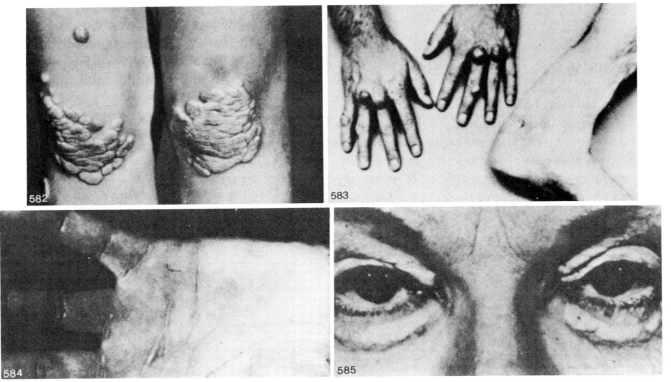

582–585, From Stanbury, J.B., et al. (eds.): The Metabolic Basis of Inherited Disease. 5th ed. New York, McGraw-Hill, 1983, pp. 659, 676–677.

For each inherited disease, match the mode of transmission.

    A. Autosomal dominant with variable penetrance
    B. X-chromosome linked
    C. Autosomal recessive
    D. Y-chromosome linked
    E. Unknown mode of inheritance

586. Familial hypertrophic obstructive cardiomyopathy

587. Duchenne muscular dystrophy

588. Marfan syndrome

589. Homocystinuria

Match the photograph *below* with the condition it represents

590. Fabry's disease

591. Subacute infective endocarditis

592. Amyloidosis

593. Scleroderma

For each disease state, match the appropriate associated cardiac finding or anomaly.

    A. Hypothyroidism
    B. Pheochromocytoma
    C. Hyperthyroidism
    D. Hyporeninemic hypoaldosteronism
    E. Acromegaly

594. Administration of beta blockers leading to hyperkalemia

595. Failure to respond to conventional doses of cardiac glycosides

596. Myocarditis and contraction band necrosis

597. Cardiomegaly and readily treatable hypertension

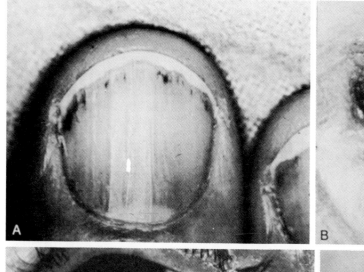
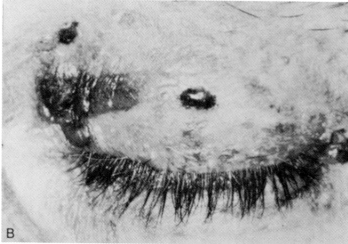
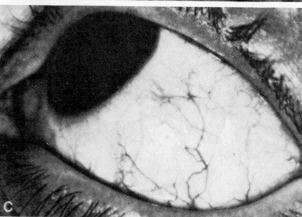
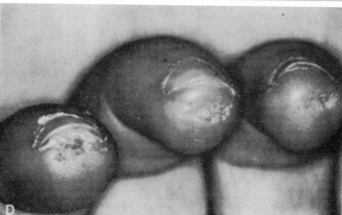

A, From Swartz, M.N., and Weinberg, A.N.: *In* Fitzpatrick, T.B., et al. (eds.): Dermatology in General Medicine. New York, McGraw-Hill, 1979, p. 436.

B, From Calkins, E.: *In* Fitzpatrick, T.B., et al. (eds.): Dermatology in General Medicine. New York, McGraw-Hill, 1979, p. 1065.

C, From Frost, P., and Spaeth, G.L.: *In* Fitzpatrick, T.B., et al. (eds.): Dermatology in General Medicine. New York, McGraw-Hill, 1979, p. 1129.

D, Eisen, A.Z., Uitto, J.J., and Bauer, E.A.: *In* Fitzpatrick, T.B., et al.: Dermatology in General Medicine. New York, McGraw-Hill, 1979, p. 1307.

DIRECTIONS: The group of questions below consists of four lettered headings followed by a set of numbered items. For each numbered item select

A if the item is associated with (A) *only*
B if the item is associated with (B) *only*
C if the item is associated with *both* (A) and (B)
D if the item is associated with *neither* (A) nor (B)

Each lettered heading may be used ONCE, MORE THAN ONCE, OR NOT AT ALL.

A. The Marfan syndrome
B. Pseudoxanthoma elasticum
C. Both
D. Neither

598. A specific abnormality in elastin has been documented

599. Subendocardial fibrosis may be present

600. A predilection for involvement of the aorta is noted

601. Cardiovascular complications lead to death in one-half of affected patients by the fourth decade

602. Angina is one part of the clinical spectrum of the illness

A. Turner syndrome
B. Noonan syndrome
C. Both
D. Neither

603. Coarctation of the aorta

604. Normal karyotype

605. Pulmonic stenosis

606. Short stature, webbing of the neck, skeletal anomalies, and renal anomalies

See illustrations below
A. *See below*
B. *See below*
C. Both
D. Neither

607. A ventricular septal defect may accompany this anomaly

608. D-transposition of the great arteries may accompany this anomaly

609. The coronary arteries in this condition may have surgically important variations

610. Cyanosis and an ECG finding of left ventricular hypertrophy may be found in this condition

611. The Fontan procedure may be useful in this condition

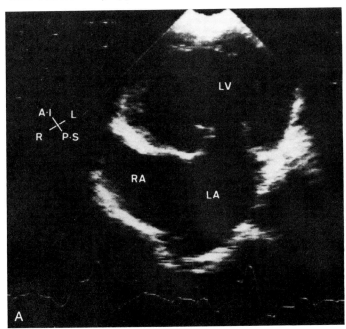

From Fulton, D.R., Geggel, R.L., and Pandian, N.G.: Two dimensional and Doppler echocardiographic evaluation. *In* Miller, D.D., et al. (eds.): Clinical Cardiac Imaging. New York, McGraw-Hill, 1988, p. 562.

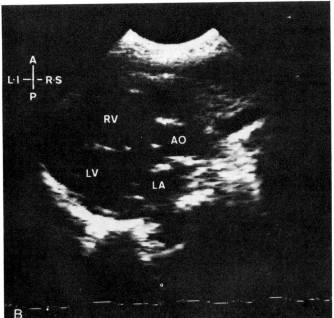

From Fulton, D.R., Geggel, R.L., and Pandian, N.G.: Two dimensional and Doppler echocardiographic evaluation. *In* Miller, D.D., et al. (eds.): Clinical Cardiac Imaging. New York, McGraw-Hill, 1988, p. 561.

A. Sickle cell anemia
B. Thalassemia
C. Both
D. Neither

612. Pericarditis

613. Pulmonary infarction

614. Second-degree heart block

615. Transfusional hemosiderosis

616. Chordae tendineae calcification

A. Ankylosing spondylitis
B. Rheumatoid arthritis
C. Both
D. Neither

617. Associated with histocompatibility antigen B27

618. Classic presentation is progressive mitral regurgitation with varying degrees of AV block

619. Most common finding on echocardiography is a pericardial effusion

---

A. Tissue plasminogen activator (tPA)
B. Alpha$_2$-plasmin inhibitor
C. Both
D. Neither

620. Structurally homologous to other serine proteases

621. Synthesized in renal tubular epithelial cells as well as endothelial cells

622. Activity for plasmin bound to fibrin is inhibited

623. Both single- and double-chain forms demonstrate proteolytic activity

---

PARTS IV AND V: BROADER PERSPECTIVES ON HEART DISEASE AND RELATION BETWEEN HEART DISEASE AND DISEASE OF OTHER ORGAN SYSTEMS

CHAPTERS 49 THROUGH 62

ANSWERS

548-D *(Braunwald, pp. 1761–1763)*

Several steps in blood coagulation occur on vascular subendothelium or on phospholipid-rich surfaces such as the plasma membrane of platelets or endothelial cells. Surface-bound enzyme-cofactor complexes, which are precursor proteins or zymogens, are converted to active enzymes by limited proteolysis. The rate of these activation reactions is controlled by certain higher molecular weight protein cofactors, such as factors V and VIII. The intrinsic, or contact-activation, pathway of coagulation is initiated by the formation of such a complex, which involves three plasma proteins: Hageman factor (factor XII), high molecular weight kininogen (HMWK), and prekallikrein (PK). The resulting complex is capable of activating factor XII, which in turn leads to the active form of factor XI. It is factor XI that subsequently activates factor IX to factor IXa. This factor then participates with factor VIII, calcium, and phospholipids to create a complex that leads to the activation of factor X. It is at this point that the common coagulation pathway has been entered.

A second route that leads to the activation of factor X involves a ubiquitous cellular lipoprotein called tissue factor. This pathway is known as the extrinsic coagulation pathway. In this pathway, tissue factor, which is found in endothelial cells and circulating leukocytes, forms a calcium-dependent complex with factor VII in the presence of phospholipid. This complex subsequently activates factor IX, which, as already discussed, leads to activation of factor X and again initiates the sequence of events in the common coagulation pathway.

Activated factor X converts prothrombin to thrombin in conjunction with factor Va, calcium, and phospholipid. This process occurs on activated platelets or endothelial surfaces and releases an extremely potent protease that participates in hemostasis at a variety of points. Thus thrombin activates factors V, VIII, and XIII, as well as performing the important role of cleaving peptides from the A and B chains of fibrinogen to form fibrin monomers that may then polymerize into larger fibrillar polymers. While these polymers are initially held together by weak chemical bonds, they are cross-linked by factor XIIIa (not

by thrombin), which leads to the mature fibrin complex (see also Braunwald, Fig. 56–8, p. 1763).

549-B *(Braunwald, pp. 1581–1582)*

In general, nonimaging modalities are not of great value in the diagnosis of pulmonary embolism. While arterial blood gas studies may be useful in managing a patient's respiratory status, they do not tend to be of great value in the diagnosis of pulmonary embolism. For example, patients with proven pulmonary embolism may have a normal or high arterial PO_2, and conversely, those suspected of having pulmonary embolism with hypoxemia may prove to have normal lung scans and pulmonary angiograms.[1] The finding of a pleural effusion is a nonspecific sign, and analysis of the pleural fluid is variable to the point of being useless in the diagnosis of suspected pulmonary embolism. (It should also be emphasized that a prior thoracentesis is a contraindication to the administration of thrombolytic agents in the 10 to 14 days after the procedure.)

The classic manifestations of acute cor pulmonale secondary to pulmonary embolism seen on the ECG, such as $S_1Q_3T_3$, right bundle branch block, P pulmonale, or right-axis deviation, occur in only about one-fourth of pulmonary embolism patients.[2] In general, these findings are present in patients who have had large or massive embolism, in whom the diagnosis has been apparent for other reasons. At the present time, no rapid, accurate, inexpensive blood test to screen for pulmonary embolism is available. Recently, measurement of fibrin split products or fibrin degradation products has shown some correlation with the presence of pulmonary embolism, but their utility in diagnosis has not been proven. The chest x-ray may provide some clues to the diagnosis but more often than not is normal. Markedly diminished vascular markings, an engorged major hilar artery, the sudden appearance of a "plump" vessel, and the presence of a homogeneous wedge-shaped density in the peripheral region of the lung with the rounded, convex apex pointing toward the hilum ("Hampton's hump") (see Braunwald, Fig. 47–6, p. 1582) all may indicate the presence of underlying pulmonary embolism and/or pulmonary infarction. The major value of the chest x-ray is its utility in bringing to mind diagnoses other than pulmonary embolism.

REFERENCES

1. Branch, W.T., Jr., and McNeil, B.J.: Analysis of the differential diagnosis and assessment of pleuritic chest pain in young adults. Am. J. Med. 75:671, 1983.
2. Stein, P.D., Dalen, J.E., McIntyre, K.M., Sasahara, A.A., Wenger, N.K., and Willis, P.W., III: The electrocardiogram in acute pulmonary embolism. Prog. Cardiovasc. Dis. 17:247, 1975.

550-A   *(Braunwald, p. 1739)*

The peripheral blood smear shown demonstrates the classic findings of microangiopathic hemolytic anemia (HA) with many fragmented blood forms and schistocytes. This condition has been reported in association with many cardiac defects, including intracardiac and intravascular prostheses, following unsuccessful mitral valvuloplasty, following patch repairs of ostium primum defects, following repair of tetralogy of Fallot, in association with severe aortic valve disease (particularly aortic stenosis), following rupture of an aneurysm of the sinus of Valsalva, and in association with coarctation of the aorta and hypertrophic obstructive cardiomyopathy.

Microangiopathic HA is thought to be due to turbulence. For example, following insertion of a prosthetic valve, if perivalvular regurgitation develops, the increase in stroke volume may lead to turbulent flow with shear stresses in excess of 3000 dynes per cm^2. Findings of microangiopathic HA may also occur in situations in which the lumen of an aortic valve prosthesis is small in relationship to stroke volume or when the ball of a ball-in-cage prosthesis is large in relationship to the diameter of the aorta. Both abnormalities may occur with a Starr-Edwards prosthetic valve, especially in the aortic position. Microangiopathic HA is much less common in association with prosthetic mitral valves because the valve area is usually much larger. In uncomplicated mitral regurgitation, microangiopathic HA would be unlikely to occur because velocity and shear stress abnormalities in this circumstance are not substantial. The only definitive treatment of the hemolytic syndrome secondary to turbulence consists of surgical repair (either replacement or correction) of the cardiac abnormality.

551-B   *(Braunwald, pp. 1626–1628)*

This 15-year-old boy presents with a cardiac murmur consistent with an atrial septal defect. The fact that his father had a similar cardiac anomaly suggests the presence of a hereditary syndrome. The most common cause of familial atrial septal defect is the *Holt-Oram syndrome.* This diagnosis is further supported by the boy's skeletal abnormality (deformed thumbs). The classic clinical presentation of the Holt-Oram syndrome is an upper limb deformity in a patient with congenital heart disease. Atrial septal defect of the secundum type is the most frequently encountered cardiac abnormality, usually accompanied by electrocardiographic abnormalities, including first-degree AV block, right bundle branch block, and bradycardia. Ventricular septal defect is the second most commonly encountered congenital heart lesion. Many different upper limb deformities have been observed, which are typically bilateral and most characteristically involve the thumbs. The thumbs may be absent, hypoplastic, triphalangeal, or finger-like. The radius and the wrist are also frequently involved; diagnosis may be made on x-ray, which shows an abnormal scaphoid bone and/or accessory carpal bones. There frequently are also deformities of the humerus and rotation of the scapula. The gene is transmitted as an autosomal dominant; therefore, 50 per cent of first-degree relatives will be affected, making recognition and diagnosis of this syndrome important.

The *Noonan syndrome* is another autosomal dominant syndrome characterized by an abnormal short stature, mild mental retardation, unique facial appearance with webbing of the neck, cryptorchidism, renal anomalies, and congenital heart disease (most commonly pulmonary stenosis).

The *Turner syndrome* superficially resembles Noonan syndrome but most commonly involves a 45,X karyotype, and occurs only in females. These females have short stature, amenorrhea due to gonadal dysgenesis, shield-shaped chest, pigmented nevi, webbing of the neck, abnormal metacarpals, renal abnormalities, and cardiovascular abnormalities (most typically coarctation of the aorta and hypertension).

The *LEOPARD syndrome* is a rare condition, inherited as an autosomal dominant trait. The cardinal features are embodied in the mnemonic device LEOPARD: *L*, lentigines; *E*, electrocardiographic conduction defects; *O*, ocular hypertelorism; *P*, pulmonic valve stenosis; *A*, abnormality of the genitals; *R*, retardation of growth; and *D*, deafness of the sensorineural type. The most striking feature of this syndrome and one that is diagnostic is the occurrence of numerous lentigines.

The *Kartagener syndrome* consists of a triad of sinusitis, bronchiectasis, and situs inversus with dextrocardia. The disease is inherited as an autosomal recessive with equal distribution among males and females. In most individuals dextrocardia is the only cardiovascular anomaly.

552-C   *(Braunwald, pp. 1814–1815)*

This patient presents with unusually rapid calcification of the prosthetic valve in the setting of mild hypertension and signs of renal disease. The most likely diagnosis encompassing these findings is hyperparathyroidism. In the most common form of this disease, primary hyperparathyroidism, excess production of parathyroid hormone (PTH) is caused by a solitary parathyroid adenoma. Signs and symptoms are related to the direct effects of PTH on kidney and bone, including signs and symptoms of renal dysfunction, such as polyuria, nocturia, renal stones, and in severe cases nephrocalcinosis and renal failure. This woman has probably had an elevated serum calcium level in association with elevated levels of PTH, and this has led to accelerated calcification and dysfunction of her prosthetic valve.

PTH may also have other primary effects on the cardiac

system, including hypertension. A common presentation of hyperparathyroidism may be a rise in serum calcium following initiation of thiazide therapy.

553-E (Braunwald, pp. 1663–1664)

In current cardiac surgery, most procedures have a low hospital mortality. Reparative operations in general are ones that are most likely to yield excellent or prolonged palliation or cure and are least likely to require repeat operation. Included among these are closure of patent ductus arteriosus, closure of aortopulmonary windows, closure of atrial septal and ventricular septal defects, simple repair (opening) of mitral stenosis, and simple repair of tetralogy of Fallot. (A more complicated reconstruction of tetralogy of Fallot, such as use of a transannular patch, is not considered a simple repair.)

Excisional procedures are less common in cardiac surgery than in most other fields of surgery; they include removal of atrial myxomas as well as excision of left ventricular aneurysms. In many cases, such excisional procedures are accompanied by a reconstructive process. However, surgical treatment of ventricular aneurysm cannot be considered a simple reparative operation.

In some institutions simple cardiac repairs, including pulmonary, aortic, and mitral valvotomy, as well as closure of patent ductus arteriosus, are now successfully carried out via percutaneous approaches in the cardiac catheterization laboratory.

554-B (Braunwald, pp. 1894–1896)

Overdosage with tricyclic antidepressants can result in severe cardiovascular complications. Toxic effects of these drugs, which include amitriptyline, imipramine, desipramine, nortriptyline, doxepin, and protriptyline, are due to three mechanisms: inhibition of acetylcholine (anticholinergic effect); blockade of norepinepherine reuptake by adrenergic nerve terminals (sympathomimetic effect); and a direct, quinidine-like myocardial effect. Major overdosage is associated with acute prolongation of the QRS interval to ≥ 0.10 second, the QTC_c to greater than 0.48 sec, and plasma levels greater than 1000 nanograms/ml.

Treatment includes supportive care and cardiac monitoring as well as specific treatments as follows: Sodium bicarbonate, given intravenously, is the drug of choice for reversing the cardiovascular complications, since alkalinization of the blood to a pH of 7.5 has been shown to be effective in correcting hypotension, dysarrhythmias, and conduction disturbances.[1] For hypotension unresponsive to alkalinization and fluid challenge, norepinephrine is considered the vasopressor of choice. Physostigmine may reverse the central nervous system effects such as coma. Propranolol is the drug of choice to treat supraventricular tachyarrhythmias, but in general it should be avoided because of the coexisting presence of conduction disturbances and hypotension. Lidocaine or phenytoin may be used to manage ventricular arrhythmias. Procainamide and quinidine, however, are contraindicated because they have anticholinergic and antiarrhythmic effects similar to those of the tricyclics. Temporary cardiac pacing may be required to manage bradycardia and high-degree

heart block in particularly severe overdoses. Finally, because the tricyclics are highly protein-bound and tissue-bound, their volume of distribution is very large and dialysis or hemoperfusion is generally not useful. Efforts should be made using activated charcoal to eliminate any residue of tricyclics that is still present in the gastrointestinal tract.

REFERENCE

1. Marshall, J.B., and Forker, A.D.: Cardiovascular effects of tricyclic antidepressant drugs. Therapeutic usage, overdose, and management of complications. Am. Heart J. 103:401, 1982.

555-B (Braunwald, p. 1702)

Because many patients over the age of 40 who are scheduled for elective surgery are likely to have coronary artery disease and other cardiac illnesses, it is useful to estimate their preoperative risk for a cardiac event. Certain cardiovascular problems, such as recent myocardial infarction (less than 3 months), inadequately treated congestive heart failure, and severe mitral or aortic stenosis, are absolute contraindications to *elective* surgery. Relative contraindications to surgery include a history of MI (within 3 to 6 months of the surgery), angina pectoris, mild heart failure, cyanotic congenital heart disease, and coagulation abnormalities. Several criteria have been suggested for estimation of cardiac risk.[1, 2] Included are age greater than 70 years, recent myocardial infarction, signs of congestive heart failure, S_3 gallop, jugular venous distention, abnormal ECG (including rhythm other than sinus or more than 5 PVCs/min), and abnormal arterial blood gases with PCO_2 greater than 50 mm Hg, BUN greater than 50 mg/dl, and creatine greater than 3 mg/dl. Notably, statistically nonsignificant factors include smoking, glucose intolerance, hyperlipidemia, hypertension, peripheral atherosclerotic vascular disease, stable class I or II angina, and a remote MI.[1]

It should be noted that these criteria are useful only for risk stratification. The history and examination of the patient, including prior responses to surgery, development of unstable angina, and abnormalities on chest x-ray consistent with heart failure, should initially alert the clinician to cardiac risk. Furthermore, it is clear that any correctable abnormality, including anemia, hypovolemia, polycythemia, hypoxemia, electrolyte abnormalities, hypertension, and arrhythmias, should be treated preoperatively when identified.

REFERENCES

1. Goldman, L., Caldera, D.L., Nussbaum, S.R., Southwick, F.S., Krogstad, D., Murray, B., Burke, D.S., O'Malley, T.A., Gorroll, A.H., Caplan, C.H., Nolan, J., Carabello, B., and Slater, E.E.: Multifactorial index of cardiac risk in noncardiac surgical procedures. N. Engl. J. Med. 297:845, 1977.
2. Zeldin, R.A.: Assessing cardiac risk in patients who undergo noncardiac surgical procedures. Can. J. Surg. 27:402, 1984.

556-B (Braunwald, pp. 1758–1761)

In their unactivated state, platelets circulate as smooth-surfaced discs that do not interact with the endothelial cells lining blood vessels. The events of primary hemostasis may be initiated by exposure of *subendothelium* by vascular injury. Platelet adhesion is the initial event in primary hemostasis and is a complex process that involves the interaction of specific platelet membrane receptors, subendothelial collagen, and adhesive glycoproteins (including von Willebrand's factor), and fibronectin. The process of platelet activation and secretion is complex and culminates in both phosphorylation of intraplatelet regulatory proteins and the formation of specific eicosanoids derived from arachidonic acid. These eicosanoids are capable of extending the processes of platelet activation and vasoconstriction during hemostasis. Degranulation of platelets occurs following activation. It leads to the release of further constituents and mediators such as ADP, which are capable of recruiting circulating platelets to the developing platelet aggregate.

These events, known as "primary hemostasis," serve as an initial defense against hemorrhage following vascular injury. They are especially important in capillaries and arterioles, in which shear forces are higher and the formation of a platelet plug is therefore critical for effective hemostasis. The "secondary hemostatic" system includes the plasma coagulation system, which leads to the generation of fibrin strands capable of interdigitating with the platelet plug and further strengthening the local hemostatic response.

557-C *(Braunwald, pp. 1744–1746)*

Metastatic tumors to the pericardium or heart are much more common than are primary tumors of the heart. Cardiac metastases are present at autopsy in approximately 6 per cent of patients with malignant disease, while primary cardiac tumors occur in less than 0.1 per cent of autopsies. Usually the metastases involve the pericardium and the myocardium, with the valves and endocardium rarely affected. Solitary metastases to the heart are rare, and a solitary cardiac tumor is usually a benign tumor. Many cardiac metastases are clinically silent. For instance, in malignant melanoma, approximately 60 per cent of patients have cardiac metastases, yet cardiac symptoms are rare. The most common clinical manifestations of metastatic disease are secondary to the effects of pericardial effusion, such as tamponade, tachyarrhythmias, AV block, and congestive heart failure. The most common primary tumor producing cardiac metastases is carcinoma of the bronchus, with carcinoma of the breast, malignant melanoma, lymphoma, and leukemias following in order of frequency.[1]

Signs and symptoms of pericarditis, pericardial effusion, and tamponade are typical in patients with carcinoma of the lung and breast as well as in Hodgkin's disease, non-Hodgkin's lymphoma, and leukemia involving the heart. The finding of a chylous pericardial effusion is usually characteristic of lymphomatous involvement.

Pericardial symptoms are best treated by effective therapy of the primary tumor with chemotherapy or radiation therapy. When ineffective, recurrent pericardiocentesis or surgical construction of a pericardial window may provide symptomatic relief. In rare cases, analysis of pericardial fluid may help produce the diagnosis in otherwise unexpected situations. Pericardial fibrosis secondary to radiation therapy may mimic chronic constrictive pericarditis or chronic effusive pericardial disease, especially in patients with carcinoma of the lung, Hodgkin's disease, or non-Hodgkin's lymphoma, who commonly undergo radiation to the thorax. It has become clear that radiation-induced pericarditis may occur eight years or more following therapy. Therefore, in patients with recurrent symptoms of pericardial disease who have also received radiation, differentiation from recurrent disease is sometimes difficult.

REFERENCE

1. Schoen, F.J., Berger, B.M., and Guerina, N.G.: Cardiac effects of noncardiac neoplasms. Cardiol. Clin. 2:657, 1984.

558   A-N, B-Y, C-Y, D-Y, E-N   *(Braunwald, pp. 1711–1712)*

The five *major* manifestations of acute rheumatic fever are carditis, arthritis, chorea, subcutaneous nodules, and erythema marginatum. *Minor* manifestations which are frequently present but which are too nonspecific to be critical in the diagnosis include fever, arthralgia, acute phase reactants in the blood, heart block, and a history of previous acute rheumatic fever or rheumatic heart disease.

Arthritis occurs in about 75 per cent of patients during the acute stage of the disease, and usually involves the large joints—particularly the knees, ankles, elbows and wrists. Each joint remains active less than a week before the inflammation begins to subside. Acute polyarthritis rarely occurs more than 35 days *after* the onset of the streptococcal infection and therefore is almost always associated with a rising or peak titer of streptococcal antibodies.

Carditis is the most important manifestation of acute rheumatic fever and causes the vast majority of deaths, usually due to acute cardiac failure. Cardiac manifestations are multiple. The four major criteria for the clinical diagnosis of rheumatic carditis are (1) an organic heart murmur or murmurs not previously present, (2) enlargement of the heart, (3) congestive heart failure, and (4) pericardial friction rub or signs of effusion. Among the murmurs, the mitral valve is the most common site of rheumatic inflammation; it is involved about three times as frequently as the aortic valve. Congestive heart failure is the least common and most serious manifestation of rheumatic carditis, occurring in 5 to 10 per cent of first attacks. Clinically evident pericarditis occurs in approximately 5 to 10 per cent of patients. Among the arrhythmias, delayed AV conduction is the most common manifestation.

Subcutaneous nodules similar to those in acute rheumatic fever may also occur in rheumatoid arthritis and systemic lupus erythematosus. The nodules are round, firm, painless subcutaneous lesions varying in size from 0.5 to 2.0 cm. They occur in crops of up to 3 or 4 dozen, are evanescent, and tend to be much smaller and less persistent than rheumatoid nodules.

Erythema marginatum is uncommon but is nearly pathognomonic of acute rheumatic fever. Erythema marginatum appears as a bright pink "smoke ring," spreading in a serpentine fashion through pale skin. It is nonpruritic, nonpainful, and neither indurated nor raised. Sydenham's chorea, also called St. Vitus' dance, is a neurological disorder characterized by involuntary, purposeless, choreiform movements, with muscular weakness and emotional lability. The chorea lasts for about 8 to 15 weeks and is not seen in association with arthritis but often coexists with carditis.

These manifestations have been formulated as the Jones criteria. Diagnostically, documentation of a preceding streptococcal infection is cardinal, including a history of recent scarlet fever, positive throat culture for group A streptococcus, and increased ASO titer or other streptococcal antibodies. If supported by such evidence, the presence of two major (carditis, polyarthritis, chorea, erythema marginatum, and subcutaneous nodules), or one major and two minor (fever, arthralgia, previous rheumatic fever or heart disease, elevated ESR or C-reactive protein, prolonged P-R interval) criteria indicates a high probability of acute rheumatic fever.

559   A-Y, B-N, C-Y, D-N, E-Y   (Braunwald, p. 1679)

Impaired hemostasis may be seen in certain cardiovascular disorders. Patients with chronic right-sided heart failure may develop liver dysfunction and cardiac cirrhosis. This may lead to an impaired absorption of vitamin K, a decreased or impaired production of prothrombin complex proteins, thrombocytopenia, splenomegaly, and platelet sequestration, and an overall increase in the tendency to bleed. In patients who have a markedly expanded red cell volume and increased whole blood viscosity such as those with severe cyanotic congenital heart disease, a syndrome may develop resembling disseminated intravascular coagulation (DIC) characterized by thrombocytopenia, shortened platelet survival, and increased consumption of fibrinogen and other coagulation proteins. While the precise etiology of the DIC syndrome in this setting is unknown, reduced blood flow and increased viscosity due to the marked increase in red cell mass are implicated. Such coagulation abnormalities may be corrected by decreasing the red cell mass directly and by replacing removed plasma.[1] In addition, patients who have acute infective endocarditis may develop a subclinical form of DIC. This process may be exacerbated by the insertion of a prosthetic valve in select instances. Neither mitral stenosis nor peripartum cardiomyopathy has been associated with specific hemostatic defects.

REFERENCE

1. Milan, J.D., Austin, S.F., Nihill, M.R., Keats, A.S., and Cooley, D.A.: Use of sufficient hemodilution to prevent coagulopathies following surgical correction of cyanotic heart disease. J. Thorac. Cardiovasc. Surg. 89:623, 1985.

560   A-Y, B-Y, C-Y, D-N, E-Y   (Braunwald, pp. 1864–1865)

A number of antihypertensive agents have proven useful and relatively safe in pregnant patients. *Methyldopa* crosses the placenta, achieving concentrations in fetal serum similar to those in the mother. The drug is excreted into breast milk in small amounts, but a large experience has not revealed any adverse effects when it is used during pregnancy, and it is considered to be a safe agent for the treatment of hypertension in pregnancy.[1] *Hydralazine* has also been used safely during pregnancy, and there are no reports of this agent being excreted directly into breast milk. In addition, *beta-adrenoreceptor blocking agents* can be used during pregnancy not only for hypertension but also for management of arrhythmias and hypertrophic cardiomyopathy. While these drugs readily cross the placenta, they are not considered teratogens, although there has been some evidence of fetal growth retardation in the children of mothers using propranolol. In addition, neonatal bradycardia, respiratory depression, and hypoglycemia have all been reported.[2] In patients receiving propranolol, it may be desirable to discontinue the drug toward the end of term in order to restore the fetus' cardiovascular response to prepare it for stress of labor and delivery that may be attenuated by fetal beta blockade.

A large experience using *digitalis glycosides* in pregnant patients has demonstrated that this class of agents is safe to use during pregnancy. While these drugs rapidly cross the placenta and enter the fetal circulation, they are well tolerated. On occasion they may be used to treat fetal tachycardia and congestive heart failure via maternal administration.[3] While digitalis may exert an inotropic effect on the myometrium, there is no evidence that this effect leads to a shortening of labor. *Quinidine* also crosses the placenta, achieves concentrations in fetal serum similar to those in the mother, and has been used extensively without problems during pregnancy.[4] *Procainamide*, too, appears to be relatively safe during pregnancy, although it is often regarded as a second-line agent in view of the incidence of antinuclear antibodies and the lupus-like syndrome that may occur during chronic procainamide therapy.

Phenytoin is a known teratogen, which may lead to abnormalities in fetal growth and development (the "hydantoin syndrome") and which must therefore be avoided in the therapy of arrhythmias during pregnancy. Similarly, the use of *warfarin* anticoagulants such as coumadin during pregnancy is associated with a variety of complications, including a fetal mortality rate of approximately 30 per cent. A constellation of findings make up warfarin embryopathy, including saddlenose and hypoplastic development of the nares, hypoplasia of the air passages causing upper airway obstruction, hypertelorism, shortened stature, and stippled epiphyses.[5] This abnormality occurs when the drug is given during the time of conception or the first trimester. The risks of warfarin extend into the second trimester, at which time they include optic atrophy, deafness, mental retardation, microcephaly, and even cerebral agenesis.[6] It is because of these grave effects that heparin is usually employed during pregnancy—especially during the first and second trimesters—in patients who have an absolute indication for anticoagulation.

REFERENCES

1. Tamari, I., Eldar, M., Rabinowitz, B., and Neufeld, H.N: Medical treatment of cardiovascular disorders during pregnancy. Am. Heart J. 104:1357, 1979.

2. Pruyn, S.C., Phelan, J.P., and Buchanan, G.C.: Long-term propranolol therapy in pregnancy: Maternal and fetal outcome. Am. J. Obstet. Gynecol. 135:485, 1979.

3. Rotmensch, H.H., Elkayam, U., and Frishman, W.: Antiarrhythmic drug therapy during pregnancy. Ann. Intern. Med. 98:487, 1983.

4. Briggs, G.G., Bodendorfer, T.W., Freeman, R.K., and Yaffe, J. (eds.): Drugs in Pregnancy and Lactation. Baltimore, Williams and Wilkins, 1983.

5. Hall, J.G., Pauli, R.M., and Wilson, K.M.: Maternal and fetal sequelae of anticoagulation during pregnancy. Am. J. Med. 68:122, 1980.

6. Pettifor, J.M., and Benson, R.: Congenital malformations associated with the administration of oral anticoagulants during pregnancy. J. Pediatr. 86:459, 1975.

561   A-Y, B-N, C-Y, D-N, E-Y   (Braunwald, pp. 1638–1640)

Familial hypercholesterolemia is one of the few examples of an autosomal dominant disorder in which homozygotes survive infancy. Heterozygotes number about 1/500 persons in the population, making this disease one of the most common caused by a single mutant gene. The inherited defect in familial hypercholesterolemia involves the gene coding for the cell surface low-density lipoprotein (LDL) receptor. Heterozygotes inherit one mutant gene and one normal gene and therefore produce only half the normal number of receptors. Homozygotes inherit two copies of the mutant gene and so have virtually no LDL receptors. Physicians rarely see homozygotes, who occur at a frequency of 1/1,000,000.[1]

Familial hypercholesterolemia heterozygotes commonly present with tendon xanthomas, which are nodules that may involve the Achilles tendon and various extensor tendons of the forearm and leg. They consist of deposits of cholesterol derived from deposition of LDL particles. Cutaneous planar xanthomas occur only in homozygotes and usually present within the first 6 years of life. These particular xanthomas are yellow to bright orange and occur over areas of trauma. Both the heterozygous and homozygous forms of familial hypercholesterolemia are associated with an increased incidence of a coronary artery disease due to the elevated levels of LDL, the latter far more severe than the former.

REFERENCE

1. Goldstein, J.L., and Brown, M.S.: Familial hypercholesterolemia. In Stanbury, J.B., Wyngaarden, J.B., Fredrickson, D.S., Goldstein, J.L., and Brown, M.S. (eds.): The Metabolic Basis of Inherited Disease. 5th ed. New York, McGraw-Hill Book Co., 1983, p. 672.

562   A-Y, B-Y, C-Y, D-N, E-Y   (Braunwald, p. 1694)

Changes in cardiovascular function during general anesthesia are due to many factors, including direct effects of the anesthetic agents on the heart and indirect effects mediated primarily by the nervous system. In addition, depending on the anesthetic's effects on respiration, there may be resulting changes in oxygen and CO_2 content, which exert indirect effects on myocardial contractility and cardiac irritability. In general, the dominant effects of all the anesthetic agents are to decrease cardiac contractility and lower blood pressure. Specifically, inhalation agents, which enter the bloodstream by way of the alveoli, are known to cause moderate decreases in cardiac function. Nitrous oxide causes about a 15 per cent decrease in cardiac output but does not cause significant hypotension because there is reflex vasoconstriction. Halothane also causes a reduction in myocardial contractility but is not associated with substantial reflex vasoconstriction so that it is commonly associated with falls in arterial pressure.

Of the narcotic analgesics, morphine is well tolerated, although it can cause venodilatation, thus decreasing preload and cardiac output. It does not have major effects on myocardial contractility per se. The short-acting barbiturates, including thiopental, cause a fall in blood pressure because of the combination of depressive actions on myocardial contractility and sympathetic tone. Ketamine, another intravenous anesthetic, is useful because it does *not* cause cardiovascular depression.

Frequently, in addition to inhalation and intravenous anesthetics, a muscle relaxant is added. Succinylcholine can cause bradycardia, while tubocurarine and metocurine result in falls of mean arterial pressure, mild elevations in heart rate, and little if any change in cardiac output.

By skillful adjustment of the relative proportions of inhalation anesthetics, narcotic analgesics, and muscle relaxants, the anesthesiologist can modify the effects of anesthesia on the cardiovascular system. It should be noted that the level of anesthesia determines the sympathetic responses that are possible. In patients with cardiovascular disease, the depth of anesthesia is very important to the long-term outcome of surgery. Thus, increases in blood pressure during lightening of anesthesia can lead to dangerous effects on cardiac function, and it is important to monitor the potential interplay between anesthetic drugs.

563   A-Y, B-Y, C-N, D-Y, E-Y   (Braunwald, pp. 1749–1751)

The advent of the anthracyclines for treatment of many tumors has resulted in an increased incidence of cardiac toxicity. Doxorubicin is a glycoside antibiotic with potent antitumor effects, particularly for patients with solid tumors and hematological malignancies. However, it is associated with dose-related cardiotoxicity. Early or acute manifestations include arrhythmias, ECG changes, LV dysfunction, pericarditis, myocardial infarction, and sudden death. Late complications, which are more common, include cardiomyopathy, pericardial effusions, and development of low-output heart failure. Several risk factors have been established for development of doxorubicin cardiotoxicity, including the four listed in the question. In addition, cumulative doses of *more than* 550 mg/m^2 in healthy individuals have been associated with cardiotoxicity. Other risk factors include the presence of metastatic pericardial or myocardial disease, and coexisting chemotherapy with alkylating agents.

It has been suggested that in high-risk patients careful monitoring be performed with serial exercise radionuclide ventriculograms. If these show an abnormality, cardiac catheterization and endomyocardial biopsy should be performed. These should be repeated for each 100 mg/m² increase in dose. Altering the mode of delivery to a slow continuous intravenous effusion may decrease cardiac toxicity. However, once toxicity has developed, there is no effective therapy other than ceasing drug administration.[1]

REFERENCE

1. Young, R.C., Oxols, R.F., and Myers, C.E.: The anthracycline antineoplastic drugs. N. Engl. J. Med. 305:139, 1981.

564 A-Y, B-Y, C-N, D-Y, E-N (*Braunwald, pp. 1894–1895*)

The tricyclic antidepressants (TCAs) provide a significant benefit in 60 to 80 per cent of severe depressions but have several cardiac side effects. The most prominent side effect, an increase in heart rate, is due to their anticholinergic activity. These increases are usually small (10 to 20 beats/min) and clinically unimportant, except in patients with moderate to severe congestive heart failure or coronary artery disease. Among the TCAs, amitriptyline is the most anticholinergic, followed in order by doxepin, imipramine, nortriptyline, and desipramine.

TCAs resemble type 1 antiarrhythmic drugs such as quinidine and procainamide in their ability to delay cardiac conduction. This most commonly is manifested as an increase in the QT_c interval. In patients with preexisting second- or third-degree heart block, TCAs may exacerbate the AV conduction disturbance. Furthermore, because of quinidine-like effects, patients on TCAs with atrial arrhythmias have the potential to develop rapid ventricular responses. Therefore, digitalization should be carried out in patients with atrial tachyarrhythmias prior to beginning TCA therapy.

Postural hypotension is a common complication of TCA treatment. Although up to 25 per cent of patients experience postural hypotension, this is markedly increased in those with left ventricular impairment or those receiving other cardiac medications.[1] The symptoms of orthostatic hypotension usually lessen with chronic therapy and can also be reduced by maintaining lower dosages.

Finally, it has been suggested that these drugs exert a direct depressant effect on the myocardium, but recent studies have shown that a negative inotropic response may occur only after toxic doses. Therefore, with appropriate preselection of patients and monitoring of those patients at increased risk for side effects, TCAs can be used in patients with coexistent cardiac disease.

REFERENCE

1. Glassman, A.H.: Cardiovascular effects of tricyclic antidepressants. Annu. Rev. Med. 35:503, 1984.

565-B (1 and 3 are correct) (*Braunwald, p. 1721*)

Systemic lupus erythematosus (SLE) is an autoimmune disease causing a diffuse microvasculitis, so that the heart is almost always involved at autopsy. Cardiac manifestations are frequently overshadowed by associated renal and dermatological findings. Pericarditis is found in ap-

proximately 70 per cent of cases at autopsy and is the most common cardiac lesion of SLE. During acute disease flares, pericardial inflammation may extend into the sinoatrial and AV nodes, causing acute heart block, while massive inflammation may lead to large effusions and tamponade.

Myocarditis is proportional to the severity of the systemic disease process but is usually subclinical. The myocarditic lesions consist of fibrinoid necrosis of interstitial tissues and blood vessels. There is rarely gross myocardial dysfunction except in the setting of hypertension and edema secondary to renal disease.

Endocarditis is a common cardiac manifestation of SLE. The most characteristic finding is the Libman-Sacks lesion, which is a wart-like collection of degenerating valve tissue which extrudes beyond the endothelium. These lesions are found most commonly in the angles of the AV valves and on the underside of the base of the mitral valve. They may lead to marked scarring or deformity, and can be distinguished from the fibrinoid necrosis that is common in myocarditis. Clinically important valvular disease in SLE is not uncommon, however, especially in a subset of patients with valvular thickening and deformity of a nonspecific nature.[2]

Infants born to women with active SLE may demonstrate congenital complete heart block. Several observations indicate that transplacental transfer of abnormal antibodies may be of pathogenic importance in these cases.[3] Thus, during examination of pregnant women with SLE, fetal bradycardia should be recognized as a possible complication of maternal SLE rather than fetal distress from other causes. Arrhythmias such as atrial flutter and fibrillation are rare, both in mothers with SLE and in their fetuses.

REFERENCES

1. Doherty, N.E., and Siegal, R.J.: Cardiovascular manifestations of systematic lupus erythematosus. Am. Heart J. 110:1257, 1985.
2. Galve, E., et al.: Prevalence, morphologic types, and evolution of cardiac valvular disease in systemic lupus erythematosus. N. Engl. J. Med. 319:817, 1988.
3. Litsey, S.E., Noonan, J.A., Connor, W.N., Cottrell, C.M., and Mitchell, B.: Maternal connective tissue disease and congenital heart block. N. Engl. J. Med. 309:209, 1983.

566-A (1, 2, and 3 are correct) (*Braunwald, pp. 1642–1643*)

Familial hypertriglyceridemia is a relatively common autosomal dominant disorder, in which the concentration of very low density lipoprotein (VLDL) is elevated in the plasma. These patients do not usually exhibit hypertriglyceridemia until puberty or early adulthood, at which time plasma triglyceride levels are moderately elevated in the range of 200 to 500 mg/dl. Associated conditions include obesity, hyperglycemia, hyperinsulinemia, hypertension, and hyperuricemia. Xanthomas are not a characteristic feature of this disorder. These individuals exhibit only a slightly increased incidence of atherosclerosis, and it is unclear whether or not this is caused by the hypertriglyceridemia, by associated decreases in HDL cholesterol, or by the associated illnesses. Patients with hypertriglyceridemia can develop severe exacerbations, with increases in plasma triglyceride levels as high as 1000 mg/dl, when they are exposed to a variety of precipitating factors. These include excessive alcohol ingestion, poorly controlled diabetes, ingestion of birth control pills containing estrogen, and development of hypothyroidism.[1] These high levels of triglycerides may lead to pancreatitis and eruptive xanthomas.

The disorder appears to be genetically heterogeneous in that patients from different families may have different mutations. No consistent abnormalities of lipoprotein structure or receptor function have been described at this time. The cardinal diagnostic feature is the presence of a moderate elevation in plasma triglyceride levels, with a normal cholesterol level. Lipoprotein electrophoresis shows an increase in the pre-beta fraction (Type IV lipoprotein pattern). These individuals can be treated by controlling the exacerbating conditions, such as obesity, and restricting intake of fats and alcohol.

REFERENCES

1. Chart, A., and Brunzell, J.D.: Severe hypertriglyceridemia: Role of familial and acquired disorders. Metabolism 32:209, 1983.
2. Schonfeld, G., and Kudzma, D.J.: Type IV hyperlipoproteinemia. Arch. Intern. Med. 132:55, 1973.

567-A   (1, 2, and 3 are correct)   *(Braunwald, pp. 1734–1735)*

Anemia is one of the most common causes of increased cardiac output and sometimes results in heart failure due to a high-output state. Several compensatory adaptations occur which result in maintenance of normal cardiac function in association with cardiac anemia. These include an increase in left ventricular end-diastolic volume due to an increase in preload, a reduction in systemic vascular resistence due to the decrease in blood viscosity resulting in a lowered afterload, and an increase in the levels of catecholamine and noncatecholamine inotropic factors in the plasma.[1–3]

There are also changes in the affinity of red blood cells for oxygen with a shift in the hemoglobin oxygen dissociation curve *to the right*, so that more oxygen is released from hemoglobin as the PO_2 declines. This is thought to be due to an increase in the production of 2,3-diphosphoglycerate (2,3-DPG). At normal arterial PO_2, arterial oxygen saturation remains high, despite the reduction in oxygen affinity. However, at lower PO_2 in the venous system, the elevated 2,3-DPG displaces the hemoglobin dissociation curve to the right, causing greater release of oxygen from the cells at any level of PO_2. In terms of actual numbers, the position of the hemoglobin oxygen dissociation curve can be expressed by the value of P_{50}; i.e., the partial pressure of oxygen at which hemoglobin is 50 per cent saturated. A shift of the dissociation curve to the right as occurs with anemia increases the P_{50} value. As a consequence, an anemic individual with a 50 per cent reduction in red cell mass may suffer only a 27 per cent reduction in oxygen delivery.[4]

REFERENCES

1. Quinones, M.A., Gaasch, W.H., and Alexander, J.K.: Influence of acute changes in preload, afterload, contractile state and heart

rate on ejection and isovolumic indices of myocardial contractility in man. Circulation 53:293, 1976.
2. Rossi, M.A., Carello, S.V., and Oliveria, J.S.M.: The effect of iron deficiency anemia in the rat on catecholamine levels and heart morphology. Cardiovas. Res. 15:313, 1981.
3. Duke, M., and Abelmann, W.H.: The hemodynamic response to chronic anemia. Circulation 39:503, 1969.
4. Oski, FA., Marshall, B.D., Cohen, P.J., Sugerman, H.J., and Miller, L.D.: Exercise with anemia. The role of the left or right shifted oxygen-hemoglobin equilibrium curve. Ann. Intern. Med. 74:44, 1971.

568-C   (2 and 4 are correct)   *(Braunwald, pp. 1650–1656)*

Aging involves all organs of the body, including the heart. However, study of the normal aging process is difficult because of the high prevalence of cardiovascular disease in the American population. Recent studies in which coronary artery disease and other common cardiovascular diseases have been carefully screened out have revealed several interesting findings. First, there is moderate hypertrophy of left ventricular myocardium, probably in response to increased arterial stiffness and loss of cardiac myocytes with age. Although myocardial cells are unable to proliferate or increase in number, they can increase in size; this appears to be an adaptive response. Careful studies have shown that despite alterations in the contractile proteins leading to reductions in the velocity of contraction and lengthening of contraction and relaxation times, peak contractile force production is maintained at normal levels.

However, there are changes in beta adrenoceptor–mediated inotropic and chronotropic cardiovascular responses with aging due to a generalized desensitization. Thus, maximal heart rate during exercise and other cardiovascular responses to exercise are blunted. Maximal heart rate at peak exercise can be determined by the formula: 200 minus patient age in years. In summary, there appears to be no change in cardiac output, stroke volume, or ejection fraction at rest with aging.[1] Preservation of these functions is due to adaptive responses in contraction time and calcium transients. These adaptations compensate for the increased LV stiffness secondary to hypertrophy and loss of elasticity of pericardium and other supporting structures.

REFERENCE

1. Gerstenblith, G., et al.: Echocardiographic assessment of a normal adult aging population. Circulation 56:273, 1977.

569-B   (1 and 3 are correct)   *(Braunwald, pp. 1807–1808)*

Amiodarone, a potent antiarrhythmic agent, has two primary effects on thyroid function. First, it inhibits the peripheral conversion of T_4 to T_3, causing reduction in serum T_3 levels and a transient rise in TSH. Within a few days to weeks, however, a compensatory increase in serum T_4 levels occurs and TSH returns to normal. Clinically, these patients are euthyroid, even when the T_4 levels are elevated.[1] Amiodarone's second effect occurs because it contains a large amount of iodine (35 per cent by weight) so that when it is metabolized, there is a significant increase in the available inorganic iodide. This results in acute inhibition of thyroid organification and a decrease in clearance of iodide. In the United States, where there is a high level of iodide uptake, patients may develop hypothyroidism. In one study of 45 patients,[1] nearly 50 per cent of the patients had an increase in T_4, with 25 per cent having an elevated TSH level. Of these, 7 per cent also had a low level of T_4. In this series no subject developed hyperthyroidism, but 9 per cent developed clinical hypothyroidism.

REFERENCE

1. Borowski, G.D., Garofano, C.D., Rose, L.L., Spielman, S.R., Rotmensch, H.R., Greenspan, A.M., and Horowitz, L.N.: Effect of long-term amiodarone therapy on thyroid hormone levels and thyroid function. Am. J. Med. 78:443, 1985.

570-C (2 and 4 are correct) *(Braunwald, p. 1712)*

The presence of cardiac murmurs in association with acute rheumatic carditis is almost universal. However, the murmur may be difficult to hear when the heart rate is too rapid, when cardiac output is extremely low, or in the presence of a loud pericardial rub. The mitral valve is the most common site of rheumatic inflammation, about three times more frequently involved than the aortic valve, so that the murmur of mitral regurgitation is quite commonly heard. This systolic murmur, which is heard best at the apex, frequently has a high-pitched blowing quality. The Carey-Coombs murmur is the name given to an apical mid-diastolic murmur, which characteristically begins directly after the onset of a third heart sound and ends before the first heart sound. The presence of this murmur makes the diagnosis of mitral valve involvement more definite. This condition usually occurs in patients with significant congestive heart failure, indicating a more serious illness. Aortic diastolic murmurs may also occur early in the course of disease as a consequence of aortic valve inflammation, usually audible as a soft, high-pitched decrescendo blow immediately after the second heart sound.

Congestive heart failure is the least common presentation of rheumatic carditis, occurring in 5 to 10 per cent of first attacks of rheumatic fever. Severe heart failure and findings such as a loud S_3 are more common manifestations of rheumatic recurrence than of a primary attack.

Pericarditis occurs in approximately 5 to 10 per cent of patients in most large series of acute rheumatic fever. In these studies, diagnosis was made on the basis of clinical examination. With modern echocardiographic techniques it is likely in the future that small pericardial effusions will be found at a much higher frequency. Nonetheless, pericardial friction rubs are a relatively uncommon cardiac finding.

571-A (1, 2, and 3 are correct) *(Braunwald, pp. 1707–1710)*

Although the incidence of acute rheumatic fever in the United States has decreased dramatically during the last 20 years, it still remains an important problem in many developing nations. In recent immigrants to the United States the sequelae of rheumatic fever are not uncommon. The pathogenesis of rheumatic fever has remained elusive. However, there are a few well-established requirements for development of the disease, including the presence of a group A streptococcus, its persistence in the organism in the pharynx for a sufficient period of time, and development of an antibody response.

The most widely accepted pathogenic theory for rheumatic fever is that it results from some type of hyperimmune or autoimmune reaction to a streptococcal antigen. There is a good correlation between development of an immune response and appearance of the disease. Group A streptococci contain a number of components such as hyaluronidase, certain cell wall polysaccharides, and membrane antigens which are related to components of mammalian tissues. The molecular structure of several streptococcal M proteins has revealed shared epitopes with myosin.[1]

Regardless of the pathogenesis, the most convincing evidence for the role of pharyngeal streptococcal infection is that both the initial and recurrent attacks of rheumatic fever can be prevented by the use of penicillin therapy and continuous prophylaxis with penicillin.

REFERENCE

1. Dale, J.B., and Beachey, E.H.: Epitopes of streptococcal M proteins shared with cardiac myosin. J. Exp. Med. 162:583, 1985.

572-D, 573-C, 574-C, 575-A, 576-B *(Braunwald, pp. 1625–1629)*

Noonan syndrome is a genetic disorder with an inheritance that is consistent with autosomal dominant pattern.[1] The entity is relatively common, and is characterized phenotypically by short stature, a unique facial appearance (see Braunwald, Fig. 49–1, p. 1625), mild mental retardation, webbing of the neck, cryptorchidism, and renal anomalies. Approximately half of all patients with Noonan syndrome have congenital heart disease, the most common lesion of which is valvular pulmonic stenosis, present in about 60 per cent of patients with cardiac involvement. Because of the relatively high frequency of Noonan syndrome, cardiologists encountering patients with congenital pulmonic stenosis should have a high index of suspicion regarding the possibility of underlying Noonan syndrome. The ECG in pulmonic stenosis associated with Noonan syndrome is often different from the pattern seen in usual pulmonary valve stenosis, and commonly displays left anterior hemiblock with a deep S wave in precordial leads. Approximately 20 per cent of patients with Noonan syndrome have an atrial septal defect or hypertrophic cardiomyopathy, primarily involving the LV.

The *LEOPARD syndrome*[2] is a rare, single-gene complex of congenital malformations for which the acronym LEOPARD was formed. The mnemonic includes *L*, lentigines; *E*, electrocardiographic conduction defects; *O*, ocular hypertelorism; *P*, pulmonic valve stenosis; *A*, abnormalities of the genitals; *R*, retardation of growth; and *D*, deafness. The most common structural cardiac feature in this disorder is pulmonic stenosis, which may exist as an isolated anomaly, or in combination with aortic stenosis. In addition, endocardial fibroelastosis and hypertrophic cardiomyopathy have been reported in the syndrome. The electrocardiographic conduction defects which are most commonly noted in the LEOPARD syndrome include P-R interval prolongation, QRS widening, left anterior hemiblock, and complete heart block. The most striking feature of the syndrome is the presence of diagnostic small, dark-brown spots, known as lentigines, which are concentrated over the neck and upper extremities (see Braunwald, Fig. 49–3, p. 1627). LEOPARD syndrome is transmitted in an autosomal dominant fashion, with cardiovascular abnormalities in at least 95 per cent of affected subjects. Approximately 80 per cent of patients have lentigines, while deafness and abnormalities of the genitals occur in about 20 per cent of patients.

Kartagener syndrome is an autosomal recessive disorder with a primary genetic defect that has been elucidated by electron microscopic investigation of cilia from affected individuals' bronchial mucosa or sperm. Dynein arms, which are protein structures that normally form cross bridges between adjacent microtubules in cilia and sperm tails, are abnormal in this disorder.[3] Several different mutations capable of producing the syndrome are recognized, and in each case, the mutant gene disrupts the synthesis either of the dynein protein itself or of a protein that binds dynein to the microtubules. Clinically, the syndrome consists of the triad of sinusitis, bronchiectasis, and situs inversus with dextrocardia. Cases of Kartagener syndrome usually come to attention in infancy due to recurrent upper respiratory infections or pneumonia, and development of classic sinusitis and chronic bronchiectasis occurs as childhood progresses. The majority of individuals with Kartagener syndrome have dextrocardia as the only cardiac manifestation, which leads to an abnormal 12-lead ECG when the leads are routinely placed, but has no other clinical consequences. On rare occasions associated cardiac anomalies may be present, including transposition of the great vessels or trilocular or bilocular heart.

Holt-Oram syndrome is a rare autosomal dominant disorder with varying degrees of clinical involvement and some constellation of clinical abnormalities in all affected individuals. The classic clinical manifestation of the syndrome is the simultaneous occurrence of congenital heart disease and an upper limb deformity. The most common cardiovascular abnormality is an atrial septal defect of the secundum type, with ventricular septal defect being next most common. While other types of congenital heart disease have been noted in this disorder, 70 per cent of affected individuals have either an atrial septal defect or a ventricular septal defect. Electrocardiographic abnormalities are frequently present as well and may include first-degree AV block, right bundle branch block, or bradycardia. Deformities of the thumb are the best-known features of the Holt-Oram syndrome with "digitalization of the thumbs," hypoplasia, or triphalangeal changes in the thumbs. However, these deformities are not pathognomonic for Holt-Oram syndrome.[4] The most specific upper extremity abnormalities in this disorder, an abnormal scaphoid bone and/or accessory carpal bones, may be detected on wrist radiography.

REFERENCES

1. Mendez, H.M.M., and Opitz, J.M.: Noonan syndrome: A review. Am. J. Med. Genet. 21:493, 1985.
2. Seuanez, H., Mane-Garzon, F., and Kolski, R.: Cardiocutaneous syndrome (the "LEOPARD" syndrome). Review of the literature and a new family. Clin. Genet. 9:266, 1976.
3. Afzelius, B.A.: A human syndrome caused by immotile cilia. Science 193:317, 1976.
4. Lin, A.E., and Perloff, J.K.: Upper limb malformations associated with congenital heart disease. Am. J. Cardiol. 55:1576, 1985.

577-A, 578-A, 579-C, 580-D, 581-B *(Braunwald, pp. 1782–1793)*

Cardiac involvement is noted in a variety of neuromyopathic disorders. Classic *Duchenne muscular dystrophy* is a sex-linked recessive disorder which is transmitted by the mother to half her sons as overt disease and to half her daughters as a carrier state. The overt manifestations of this illness occur early in life and begin with a clumsy waddling gait, with more frequent falls when the child learns to walk. Characteristic early pseudohypertrophy of the calves may be seen (see Braunwald, Fig. 57–1, p. 1782) and may mislead parents and physicians into thinking that good muscle development is present.

Cardiac involvement in Duchenne muscular dystrophy is characterized by a genetically predetermined involvement of the posterobasal and left lateral ventricular walls.[1] This anatomical involvement may lead to posterior papillary muscle dysfunction and a murmur of mitral regurgitation. Characteristically, the ECG is abnormal even in early childhood in patients with Duchenne muscular dystrophy.[2] The specific anatomical involvement mentioned is reflected in tall right precordial R waves, with an increase in the R-S amplitude ratio along with deep, narrow Q waves in leads I, aVL, and V_4–V_6 (see Braunwald, Fig. 57–2, p. 1783). The myocardial dystrophy present in the posterobasal left ventricular wall is thought to lead to anterior shift of the QRS, and the contiguous involvement of the lateral wall creates the deep Q waves noted in lateral leads. Other common findings include inappropriate sinus tachycardia, acceleration of atrioventricular conduction (with a shortened P-R interval, without obvious delta waves), and disorders of atrial rhythm attributed to "dystrophic" sinoatrial node infiltration or fibrosis. While patients with Duchenne muscular dystrophy usually succumb to pulmonary infection during the second decade of life, cardiac disease may be an important and dramatic cause of death.

Kearns-Sayre syndrome is characterized by a triad of progressive, external ophthalmoplegia, pigmentary retinopathy, and heart block[3] (see Braunwald, Fig. 57–19, p. 1792). Cardiac involvement in this disorder occurs due to specific pathological involvement of the specialized conduction pathways, while the myocardium itself is relatively spared. A gradual and progressive impairment of infranodal conduction may be noted, with left anterior hemiblock, right bundle branch block, and eventually, complete heart block. Interestingly, patients may have simultaneous enhancement of AV nodal conduction[4]; therefore, a shortened P-R interval does not discount risk of trifascicular disease in patients with this syndrome.

Facioscapulohumeral dystrophy (*Landouzy-Dejerine*

dystrophy) is a rare autosomal dominant disorder with a variable clinical expression, which typically appears at the end of the first decade of life. The clinical symptomatology is characterized by facial weakness, which may begin with an inability to purse the lips and which progresses to an inability to close the eyes. Scapulohumeral involvement includes loss of muscular function in the arms and shoulders; this may lead to winging of the scapula accompanying the expressionless facies (see Braunwald, Fig. 57–8, p. 1787). The characteristic cardiac involvement in this disorder is permanent paralysis of the atria (atrial standstill).[5] The diagnosis of atrial paralysis is marked by an absence of P waves on the electrocardiogram, a lack of response to direct electrical or mechanical stimulation of the atria, an absence of *a* waves in the jugular venous and right atrial pressure pulses, a supraventricular QRS, and total immobility of the atria on either echocardiography or fluoroscopy.

Myotonic muscular dystrophy *(Steinert disease)* is also an autosomally dominant neuromuscular disorder, the symptoms of which go unnoticed typically until adolescence or early adulthood. The adult phenotype of this disease is characterized by atrophy of the sternocleidomastoid muscles, weakness of the flexor muscles of the neck, and the presence of myotonia, which is easily provoked. The disease has a variety of systemic features, including the presence of cataracts, gonadal atrophy, frontal baldness, and involvement of the upper gastrointestinal tract.[6]

Cardiac involvement in myotonic muscular dystrophy is primarily confined to the His-Purkinje system. This involvement includes atrioventricular and intraventricular conduction defects, most commonly prolongation of the P-R interval, left anterior fascicular block, and increased QRS duration. In addition, prolongation of the H-V interval and the effective refractory period of the right bundle branch may be noted, with the development of right bundle branch block. His-Purkinje disease may progress to fatal Stokes-Adams episodes unless sought and treated. While sudden death from complete or high grade AV block is relatively rare, it is the most serious cardiac threat in this myotonic disorder.[7]

REFERENCES

1. Sanyal, S.K., Johnson, W.W., Thapar, M.K., and Pitner, S.E.: An ultrastructural basis for the electrocardiographic alterations associated with Duchenne's progressive muscular dystrophy. Circulation 57:1122, 1978.
2. Perloff, J.K., Roberts, W.C., deLeon, A.C., and O'Doherty, D.: The distinctive electrocardiogram of Duchenne's progressive muscular dystrophy. Am. J. Med. 42:179, 1967.
3. Lowes, M.: Chronic progressive external ophthalmoplegia, pigmentary retinopathy and heart block (Kearns-Sayre syndrome). Acta Ophthalmol. 53:610, 1975.
4. Roberts, N.K., Perloff, J.K., and Kark, P.: Cardiac conduction in Kearns-Sayre syndrome. Am. J. Cardiol. 44:1396, 1979.
5. Woollescroft, J., and Tuna, N.: Permanent atrial standstill: The clinical spectrum. Am. J. Med. 49:2037, 1982.
6. Kohn, N.N., Faires, J.S., and Rodman, T.: Unusual manifestations due to involvement of involuntary muscle in dystrophia myotonica. N. Engl. J. Med. 271:1179, 1964.
7. Kennel, A.J., Titis, J.L., and Merideth, J.: Pathologic findings in the atrioventricular conduction system in myotonic dystrophy. Mayo Clin. Proc. 49:838, 1974.

582-A, 583-A, 584-B, 585-C *(Braunwald, pp. 1638–1644; 1160–1167)*

Familial hypercholesterolemia is an autosomal dominant trait caused by a single-gene mutation that leads to hypercholesterolemia and atherosclerosis and its complications. Heterozygotes for the condition number about 1 in 500 persons, while the homozygote form of the disease is rare, occurring in approximately 1 in 1 million subjects.[1] The single-gene mutation in this disorder leads to a defect in the production of the cell-surface LDL receptor. Heterozygotes thus produce approximately one-half the normal number of receptors for this lipoprotein particle, while homozygotes with familial hypercholesterolemia produce few if any LDL receptors. These biochemical defects lead to dramatic clinical presentations; heterozygotes with this condition develop MI, typically in their fourth or fifth decades, while homozygotes usually develop MI before the age of 20. Characteristic dermatological lesions are noted in this disorder. Heterozygotes may develop nodular swellings involving the various tendons around the knee, elbow, dorsum of the hand, and ankle, which are known as *tendon xanthomas*, as shown in the figure for Question 583. Microscopically, these consist of large deposits of cholesterol, which apparently is derived from the deposition of LDL particles, both extracellularly and within scavenger macrophage cells. Tendon xanthomas are diagnostic, while deposition of cholesterol in the tissues of the eyelid or within the cornea, known respectively as *xanthelasma* (see figure for Question 585) and *arcus corneae*, may occur in adults with normal plasma lipid levels, as well as in other lipid disorders.

Patients with homozygous familial hypercholesterolemia disease have dramatic elevations in the plasma LDL level from birth, with levels typically in the 6- to 8-fold higher than normal range. In addition, they demonstrate a specific and unique cutaneous xanthoma known as a *planar xanthoma*, which is often present at birth, and always develops within the first 6 years of life (see figure for Question 582).[2] Planar xanthomas are yellow and occur at points of trauma over the knees, elbows, and buttocks. In addition, they may be found in the interdigital webs of the hands, especially between the thumb and index finger. Tendon xanthomas, xanthelasma, and arcus corneae also occur in homozygotes. As already noted, coronary artery atherosclerosis in homozygote familial hypercholesterolemia is rapidly progressive and frequently fatal. Most homozygotes die before the age of 30.[3] The severe atherosclerosis that develops in this disorder occurs throughout the thoracic and abdominal aorta, and in the major pulmonary arteries in addition to the coronary arteries. Deposition of atheromatous material characteristically also involves the aortic valve and may lead to significant aortic stenosis, with subsequent congestive heart failure. It should therefore be noted that subjects with the homozygous form may present in a manner analogous to rheumatic fever or connective tissue disease, with painful joints, a persistently elevated sedimentation rate, and cardiac murmurs.[4]

Diagnosis of the heterozygote form of familial hypercholesterolemia is suggested by the finding of an isolated elevation of plasma cholesterol with a normal fasting concentration of plasma triglycerides. While this pattern is the phenotypical type IIA hyperlipoproteinemia, several features distinguish the heterozygous form of familial hypercholesterolemia from other hyperlipidemias that create a similar plasma lipid pattern (such as polygenic hypercholesterolemia and multiple lipoprotein-type hyperlipidemia). These characteristics include a higher average level of plasma cholesterol (in the 350 to 400 mg/dl range), tendon xanthomas, and a characteristic family history. Diagnosis of the homozygote form is more easily established. The early appearance of cutaneous xanthomas, massive elevations of cholesterol (greater than 600 mg/dl) with a normal triglyceride level, and early symptomatology referable to atherosclerosis all make the diagnosis readily apparent.

The approach to treatment of familial hypercholesterolemia includes specific dietary therapy, bile acid–binding resins, and the use of HMG CoA reductase inhibitors such as lovastatin. Treatment of homozygotes is much more difficult and may require dramatic measures, including plasma exchanges at monthly intervals in addition to the specific drug therapy just mentioned. In selected instances, portacaval anastamosis has been effective. Liver transplantation, which provides the recipient with a normal hepatic complement of LDL receptor, has also been successfully employed.[5]

Type III hyperlipoproteinemia, or familial dysbetalipoproteinemia, is a single-gene disorder that requires both the presence of a mutation in the gene for apolipoprotein E and contributory environmental or genetic factors.[6] In this disorder, the plasma concentrations of both cholesterol and triglycerides are elevated due to the accumulation of remnant-like particles that come from the partial metabolism of both VLDL and chylomicrons. This condition is characterized clinically by severe atherosclerosis involving the coronary arteries, the internal carotids, and the abdominal aorta and its branches. Interestingly, hyperlipidemia or the other clinical features of the disease are usually not seen until after the age of 20 years. Two specific dermatological lesions are characteristic of type III hyperlipoproteinemia. *Xanthoma striata palmaris* appears as orange or yellow discolorations of the palmar and digital creases, as illustrated in Question 584. In addition, bulbous cutaneous xanthomas in a variety of sizes known as tuberous or tuberoeruptive xanthomas are characteristically located over the elbows and knees in this disorder (not shown). Xanthelasmas of the eyelids may also occur in this disease but, as noted, are not unique to familial dysbetalipoproteinemia. While about 1 per cent of Caucasian individuals are homozygotes for the allele of apoprotein E, which confers the biochemical abnormality of this disorder, only 1 in 100 of these homozygous individuals (1/10,000 of the general population) has clear-cut familial dysbetalipoproteinemia. The mechanism by which the remaining homozygotes for this disorder are able to compensate for the defective protein and thus avoid the clinical sequelae mentioned remains obscure. Diagnosis of this disorder is suggested by moderate elevations in both cholesterol and triglyceride levels to approximately 300 to 350 mg/dl. In addition, 80 per cent of patients exhibit palmar or tuberous xanthomas. The diagnosis is strongly supported by a "broad beta"

band on lipoprotein electrophoresis, which results from the presence of the unique remnant particles just described. Definitive confirmation of the diagnosis rests upon specific analysis of the patient's VLDL fraction, which contains an abnormal remnant particle with a relatively high ratio of cholesterol to triglyceride, and specific extraction and analysis of the proteins present in this VLDL particle to confirm that apoprotein E-II is present.

REFERENCES

1. Brown, M.S., and Goldstein, J.L.: A receptor-mediated pathway for cholesterol homeostasis. Science 232:34, 1986.
2. Goldstein, J.L., and Brown, M.S.: Familial hypercholesterolemia. *In* Stanbury, J.B., Wyngaarden, J.B., Fredrickson, D.S., Goldstein, J.L., and Brown, M.S. (eds.): The Metabolic Basis of Inherited Disease. 5th ed. New York, McGraw-Hill, 1983, p. 672.
3. Sprecher, D.L., Schaefer, E.J., and Kent, K.M., Gregg, R.E., Zech, L.A., Hoeg, J.M., Manus, B., Roberts, W.C., and Brewer, H.B., Jr.: Cardiovascular features of homozygous familial hypercholesterolemia: Analysis of 16 patients. Am. J. Cardiol. 54:20, 1984.
4. Glueck, C.J., Levy, R.I., and Fredrickson, D.S.: Acute tendonitis and arthritis: A presenting symptom of familial type II hyperlipoproteinemia. JAMA 206:2895, 1969.
5. Bilheimer, D.W., Goldstein, J.L., Grundy, S.C., Starzl, T.E., and Brown, M.S.: Liver transplantation provides low density lipoprotein receptors and lowers plasma cholesterol in a child with homozygous familial hypercholesterolemia. N. Engl. J. Med. 29:385, 1984.
6. Mahley, R.W., and Angelin, B.: Type III hyperlipoproteinemia: Recent insights into the genetic defect of familial dysbetalipoproteinemia. Adv. Intern. Med. 29:385, 1984.

586-A, 587-B, 588-A, 589-C (*Braunwald, pp. 1630–1635; see also Answers 577–581 above*)

There are many inherited diseases that affect the cardiovascular system. *Marfan syndrome* is a generalized disorder of the connective tissue inherited as an autosomal dominant trait with variable penetrance. Cardiac abnormalities occur in 60 per cent of affected adults. The major cardiac lesion is dilatation of the aortic ring, the sinuses of Valsalva, and the ascending thoracic aorta. Stretching of the aortic valve eventually leads to aortic regurgitation, aortic dissection, or both. In 85 per cent of cases, one of the parents is affected. The other 15 per cent of cases occur sporadically and are likely to represent new mutations. First-degree relatives of affected individuals have a 50 per cent risk for having Marfan syndrome and should be screened, although this is relatively nonspecific because of the incomplete clinical expression of the disease. However, by use of echocardiography (prolapse of the mitral valve and dilatation of the aortic root), anthropometrical evaluation (measurement of upper-to lower-body segment ratio), and ophthalmological examination (presence of ectopia lentis) the diagnosis can be established.

Familial hypertrophic obstructive cardiomyopathy is inherited in an autosomal dominant mode but has more complete clinical expression than that seen with Marfan syndrome. In families with dominantly inherited disease, the mutant gene appears to be fully penetrant; i.e., virtually all individuals who inherit the gene show asymmetric septal hypertrophy. Because of the high level of penetrance, first-degree relatives should be studied by echocardiography, searching for signs of asymmetric septal hypertrophy. Although the underlying biochemial defect is still unknown, this particular disease offers an opportunity to gain insights into the cellular basis of cardiac hypertrophy.

Duchenne muscular dystrophy (DMD) is inherited as an X-linked recessive trait, so that it occurs almost exclusively in males. Characteristically, it manifests during the first 5 years of life, with initial involvement of the pelvic girdle muscles causing lumbar lordosis and a clumsy waddling gait, as well as pseudohypertrophy of the calves. It is a rapidly progressive disease, and most boys are confined to a wheelchair or bed by age 10. There is a characteristic ECG with a tall R wave in lead V1 and deep Q waves in leads I, aVL, V_5, and V_6. Skeletal muscle damage can be detected by release of the muscle enzyme creatine phosphokinase into the serum providing a useful diagnostic test. Recent work has yielded restriction fragment length polymorphisms specific for the DMD gene, which will soon allow prenatal diagnosis. Furthermore, it has been suggested, based on mouse models, that the protein product of the affected gene localizes to the skeletal muscle triad, and this protein has recently been isolated and termed "dystrophin."

Homocystinuria is an autosomal recessive disease characterized by arterial and venous thrombosis, increased incidence of atherosclerosis, myocardial infarction, and pulmonary embolism. It usually occurs in young adults and may also include ectopia lentis, osteoporosis, and mental retardation. Although the biochemical defect is known to be a deficiency of cystathionine synthase, the mechanism for accelerated atherosclerosis is not known. This illness, inherited in an autosomal recessive fashion, is quite rare.

590-C, 591-A, 592-B, 593-D *(Braunwald, pp. 13–15; 1104–1105; 1431–1434; 1723–1724)*

Dermatological manifestations of systemic disorders that have major cardiac involvement are relatively common and may provide specific clues to the underlying diagnosis. A classic example of such a disorder is *subacute infective endocarditis*, which has several lesions involving the skin and its appendages and the eye that have for many years been considered classic peripheral stigmata of the disorder. These include petechiae, Osler nodes, Janeway lesions, Roth spots, and subungual or "splinter hemorrhages"; the last are illustrated in Figure A. Subungual hemorrhages are uncommon but helpful in the diagnosis of infective endocarditis at the bedside. The differential diagnosis of this dermatological finding includes advanced age, trauma, and trichinosis. Osler nodes are small, raised, nodular, and painful red to purple lesions that are present in the pulp spaces of the terminal phalanges of the fingers. They, along with all of the peripheral stigmata of infective endocarditis, are seen much less commonly since the advent of antibiotic ther-

apy for this disorder. Janeway lesions are small, irregular, flat, and nontender macules occurring most often on the thenar and hypothenar eminences of the hands and soles of patients with subacute infective endocarditis. Roth spots, located in the retina, have the appearance of a "cotton wool" exudate and consist of aggregations of cytoid bodies.

Amyloidosis is a systemic illness that is due to deposition of unique fibrils of amyloid protein in a variety of organs; it has major cardiac sequelae, including restrictive cardiomyopathy, abnormalities of cardiac impulse formation and conduction, systolic dysfunction, and orthostatic hypotension. In general, patients will exhibit at least one and often several of these cardiac manifestations. There are a host of dermatological findings in amyloid disease. Perhaps the most common of these are lesions consisting of small papules that are especially likely to be seen on the face, scalp, neck folds, or intertriginous folds. In addition, small, smooth and yellowish papules may be seen in the areas around the eyes and mistaken for xanthomata. While they are characteristically rounded, they frequently exhibit a hemorrhagic component, as in Figure B, which is an important point in the differential diagnosis. In some patients, nodules of a larger size may appear.

Fabry's disease is an X-linked disorder of glycosphingolipid metabolism, which is due to a deficiency of the enzyme ceramide trihexosidase. The disorder is characterized by the accumulation of glycolipids within the myocardium, skin, and kidneys. Systemic hypertension, mitral valve prolapse, renovascular hypotension, and congestive heart failure are all common clinical manifestations of the disease. Fabry's disease may also be associated with a restrictive cardiomyopathy that may be difficult to distinguish from cardiac amyloidosis. Ocular signs in the disorder are common. Approximately 90 per cent of patients have corneal opacities, while two-thirds of patients have conjunctival vessel tortuosity as illustrated in Figure C. Hypertensive cardiovascular disease, renal failure, and cerebrovascular disease are the major causes of death in this disorder.

Progressive systemic sclerosis, or scleroderma, presents as a progressive tightening and thickening of the skin, with Raynaud's phenomenon occurring at some time in almost all patients. Cardiac involvement is extremely common in this disorder and is a frequent cause of death, second only to involvement of the kidneys as a factor shortening survival. Scleroderma heart disease is primarily a myocardial process, leading to vascular insufficiency and fibrosis in the small vessels of the heart, which produces cardiomyopathy with both congestive heart failure and conduction system abnormalities. Pericarditis is also extremely common. The CREST variant of this syndrome includes patients with calcinosis, Raynaud's phenomenon, esophageal dyskinesia, sclerodactyly, and telangiectasia. Recurrent painful ulcerations of the fingertips, which may become infected, are a common problem in this disorder, and are illustrated in Figure D. These are believed to result from the vascular disorder that produces Raynaud's phenomenon in these patients. They must be cared for in a careful and meticulous manner to avoid serious infection and even digital loss.

594-D, 595-C, 596-B, 597-E *(Braunwald, pp. 1800–1814)*

While there are many effects of endocrine abnormalities on the cardiovascular system, alterations in blood pressure occur most commonly. Adrenal insufficiency, or Addison's disease, is characterized classically by significant hypotension, while excessive production of adrenal steroids (hyperaldosteronism) is often accompanied by hypertension. Cushing's syndrome, the most common syndrome of glucocorticoid excess, leads to hypertension by an unknown mechanism. Acromegaly, hyperthyroidism, and pheochromocytoma all cause hypertension.

Adrenal insufficiency in association with hypoaldosteronism and hyperkalemia may also present with conduction defects. An increasingly common form of hypoaldosteronism is that associated with hyporeninism. This syndrome is most commonly observed in older diabetic patients with mild degrees of renal impairment and hypertension. Usually, these patients present with unexplained hyperkalemia, which may be secondary to damage to the juxtaglomerular apparatus. This syndrome may be exacerbated in diabetic patients with mild hypertension by administration of beta blockers, which further compromise aldosterone release, leading to the appearance of hyperkalemia.[1]

Perhaps the most common endocrine diseases affecting the cardiac system involve abnormalities of the thyroid gland. The clinical features of hyperthyroidism are well known, including an increase in resting heart rate, palpitations, and atrial fibrillation. The addition of thyroid hormone to cultured heart cells results in dramatic increases in heart rate and myocardial contractility. These increases have been suggested to be due to primary changes in protein synthesis with increases in the activity of the sodium pump and alterations in myosin isoenzymes. In severe hyperthyroidism, there may be generalized cardiac enlargement accompanied by signs and symptoms of heart failure. In patients with coronary artery disease the frequency of angina pectoris is usually increased. Hyperthyroid patients with cardiovascular disease are often resistant to therapy. In particular, both congestive heart failure and cardiac arrhythmias are resistant to conventional doses of cardiac glycosides. The mechanism underlying this resistance may involve increases in the volume of distribution of the cardiac glycosides as well as an increase in sodium-potassium ATPase activity.

Hypothyroidism, or myxedema, results in a pale, flabby, and grossly dilated heart, with myocardial cell swelling and interstitial fibrosis. Frequently, pericardial effusions occur, especially in overt myxedema. The diagnosis is suggested by cardiomegaly and low voltage on the ECG. There appear to be direct effects on cardiac contractility associated with hypothyroidism. These may be due to a reduction in the normal number of myocardial beta receptors as well as alterations in catecholamine-induced calcium mobilization.

Pheochromocytoma is a dramatic endocrine/cardiac illness, with a classic presentation of labile hypertension, diaphoresis, and orthostatic hypotension associated with left ventricular hypertrophy and sinus tachycardia. In many of these patients there may be myocarditis consisting of focal necrosis with infiltration of inflammatory cells and occasionally contraction band necrosis.[2] In some studies, 50 per cent of patients who died from pheochromocytoma had myocarditis at autopsy. It is possible that this may reflect a catecholamine-mediated cardiomyopathy, perhaps due to sustained coronary vasoconstriction.

Growth hormone is one of a family of proteins whose overall function is to regulate growth of the organism. An excess of growth hormone produces the classic clinical picture of acromegaly. Cardiac manifestations of acromegaly include cardiac enlargement that is greater than would be anticipated for the generalized organomegaly, as well as hypertension, premature coronary artery disease, congestive heart failure, and cardiac arrhythmias.[3] Since there is no direct relationship between the degree of cardiac enlargement and the level of circulating growth hormone, other factors such as the insulin-like growth factors IGF_1 and IGF_2 have been suggested to play a role in cardiomegaly. Cardiomegaly is actually the most common cardiovascular manifestation of acromegaly, occurring in 15 to 50 per cent of patients. Hypertension in acromegaly is usually mild, uncomplicated, and readily responsive to drugs. Patients without significant hypertension or atherosclerosis may develop significant cardiac dysfunction due to acromegalic cardiomyopathy.

REFERENCES

1. Lee, T.H., Salomon, D.R., Rayment, C.M., and Antman, E.M.: Hypotension and sinus arrest with exercise-induced hyperkalemia and combined verapamil/propranolol therapy. Am. J. Med. *80*:1203, 1986.
2. McManus, B.M., Fleury, T.A., and Roberts, W.C.: Fatal catecholamine crisis in pheochromocytoma: Curable form of cardiac arrest. Am. Heart J. *102*:930, 1981.
3. McGuffin, W.L., Sherman, B.M., Roth, J., Gorden, P., Kahn, C.R., Roberts, W.C., and Frommer, P.L.: Acromegaly and cardiovascular disorders. Ann. Intern. Med. *81*:11, 1974.

598-A, 599-B, 600-A, 601-A, 602-B *(Braunwald, pp. 1725–1728; see also Answers 586–589 above)*

The *Marfan syndrome* is a generalized disorder of connective tissue which is characterized by abnormal cross-linked elastin in the aorta.[1] Characteristic clinical findings include involvement of the eye, the skeletal system, and the cardiovascular system. Affected individuals have ocular manifestations that include a defective suspensory ligament of the lens and thus *ectopia lentis*. In addition, involvement of the retinal connective tissue and an excessive length of the eyeball itself lead to retinal detachment and severe myopia. Skeletal manifestations of Marfan syndrome include excessive limb length, arachnodactyly, kyphoscoliosis, and anterior chest deformity. The cardiovascular system becomes involved in a variety of ways. Aortic aneurysm with subsequent dissection due to the abnormal elastin in the ascending aorta is frequently documented. In addition, aortic regurgitation from dilatation of both the aortic root and the aortic annulus or from myxomatous involvement of the valve leaflets is also noted. Myxomatous degeneration of the mitral valve and its apparatus may lead to mitral regurgitation (see Braunwald, Fig. 54–14, p. 1726).

The Marfan syndrome is inherited in an autosomal dominant fashion, with variable phenotypic expression. Cardiovascular complications occur in between 30 and 60 per cent of patients, depending upon the series reported. In one series the average age at death was 32 years. Of this group, the majority died secondary to cardiovascular complications, with aortic dilatation, rupture, and/or dissection accounting for 80 per cent of the cardiovascular fatalities.[2] Another series noted a similar cardiovascular cause of death in 50 per cent of patients by the age of 32.[3] Management of the Marfan syndrome includes the use of beta-adrenoreceptor blocking agents to attempt to decrease hemodynamic stress upon the weakened vascular tissues and appropriate surgical intervention on the aorta in selected cases. Attempts to replace aortic and/or mitral valves and reconstruct the ascending aorta in patients with Marfan syndrome are often complicated by the underlying connective tissue defect.

Pseudoxanthoma elasticum is an inherited disorder of connective tissue which leads to involvement of the skin, eyes, and gastrointestinal and cardiovascular systems. The disease actually seems to be a heterogeneous group of disorders with a basic defect noted in elastic tissue but without any specific basic biochemical lesion yet appreciated.[4] Pathological examination of cardiovascular components reveals disruption of the elastic membrane in affected blood vessels with abnormal and frequently calcified elastic fibers. Pathological studies of the heart may reveal changes similar to those noted in the vessels.[5] The valve leaflets may be involved, as may be the endocardium of both atria and ventricles. The physical appearance of patients affected with pseudoxanthoma elasticum is characterized by a thickened, coarse, and grooved skin with a leathery and "crepe-like" appearance. Involvement is most common in the areas of the face, neck, axillae, and inguinal folds. Small papular lesions resembling xanthomas may be noted in these areas, leading to the characteristic for which the syndrome is named. Ocular involvement is marked by angioid streaking and chorioretinitis, with subsequent visual impairment.

As might be predicted from the pathological changes noted, the clinical cardiovascular manifestations of pseudoxanthoma elasticum include peripheral vascular disease, hypertension, coronary artery disease, and restriction to filling of the ventricular cavities due to subendocardial fibrosis, with subsequent (diastolic) heart failure. In addition, prolapse of the mitral valve may be noted. There appears to be a predilection for involvement of the arteries of the upper extremities in this disorder, which may help distinguish it from typical atherosclerosis. Roentgenography may demonstrate calcification of limb arteries. The most likely cause of hypertension in pseudoxanthoma elasticum is involvement of the renal arteries with compromised renal blood flow and subsequent renal vascular hypertension. In one study of 200 cases of pseudoxanthoma elasticum, angina was present in 29 per cent.[6] Myocardial infarction and sudden death are not seen commonly but are well-documented complications during the second and third decades. There is no specific management for the disorder. Angina, congestive heart failure, hypertension, and their sequelae are managed in the conventional manner.

REFERENCES

1. Abraham, P.A., Perejda, A.J., Carnes, W.H., and Vitto, J.: Marfan syndrome. Demonstration of abnormal elastin in aorta. J. Clin. Invest. *70*:1245, 1982.
2. Murdoch, J.L., Walker, B.A., Halpern, B.I., Kuzma, J.W., and McKusick, V.A.: Life expectancy and causes of death in the Marfan syndrome. N. Engl. J. Med. *286*:804, 1972.
3. Gott, V.L., Pyeritz, R.E., Magovern, G.J., Jr., Cameron, D.E., and McKusick, V.A.: Surgical treatment of aneurysms of the ascending aorta in the Marfan syndrome. Results of composite graft repair in 50 patients. N. Engl. J. Med. *314*:1070, 1986.
4. Rowe, D.W., and Shapiro, J.R.: Diseases associated with abnormalities of structural proteins. *In* Kelly, W.N., Harris, E.D., Jr., Ruddy, S., and Sledge, C.B. (eds.): Textbook of Rheumatology. Philadelphia, W.B. Saunders Company, 1985.
5. Akhlar, M., and Brody, H.: Elastic tissue in pseudoxanthoma elasticum: Ultrastructural study of endocardial lesions. Arch. Pathol. *99*:667, 1975.
6. Eddy, D.D., and Farber, E.M.: Pseudoxanthoma elasticum: Internal manifestations. A report of cases and a statistical review of the literature. Arch. Dermatol. *86*:729, 1962.

603-A, 604-B, 605-B, 606-C (Braunwald, pp. 1624–1626)

The *Turner* and *Noonan* syndromes share several superficial features, including shortness of stature, webbing of the neck, skeletal anomalies, renal abnormalities, and congenital heart disease. Because of these clinical similarities, Noonan syndrome is frequently referred to as "male Turner syndrome" or Turner phenotype with normal chromosomes. However, there are several striking genetic and clinical differences that can readily distinguish these two disorders. The Turner syndrome occurs exclusively in females due to the fact that in about 60 per cent of patients all cells are deficient in one of the two chromosomes (45,X). The remaining 40 per cent of patients are mosaics and contain (45,X/46,XX). Most fetuses with the (45,X) form of Turner syndrome die in utero and are aborted spontaneously. Of those that survive, cardiovascular abnormalities occur in 35 to 50 per cent.[1] Coarctation of the aorta is by far the most common abnormality that is encountered, accounting for 70 per cent of all cardiac anomalies. Other abnormalities include bicuspid aortic valve, hypertrophic obstructive cardiomyopathy, atrial septal defect, mitral valve prolapse, and dextrocardia. Stenosis of the pulmonic valve is rarely if ever seen in Turner syndrome in contrast to Noonan syndrome. Patients with Turner syndrome also frequently develop hypertension, which is independent of the coarctation.

Noonan syndrome appears similar to Turner syndrome, although there is a unique facial appearance, with hypertelorism, strabismus, small chin, and low-set ears in patients with Noonan syndrome. In contrast to Turner syndrome, in Noonan syndrome both males and females are affected and the karyotype in both sexes is normal. Noonan syndrome is inherited as an autosomal dominant trait. Approximately 50 per cent of patients have congenital heart disease, with the most common lesion being valvular pulmonary stenosis, occurring in about 60 per cent of patients. Characteristically, the annulus of the pulmonary valve is normal, but the valves are thickened and immobile. Other findings include atrial septal defect and hypertrophic cardiomyopathy. Although diagnosis is difficult, the presence of ocular abnormalities (ptosis, hypertelorism, and epicanthus) in association with pulmonary artery stenosis should suggest Noonan disease.[2]

REFERENCES

1. Nora, J.J., Torres, F.G., Sinha, A.K., and McNamara, D.G.: Characteristic cardiovascular anomalies of XO Turner syndrome, XX and XY phenotype and XO/XX Turner mosaic. Am. J. Cardiol. 25:639, 1970.
2. Mendez, H.M.M., and Opitz, J.M.: Noonan syndrome: A review. Am. J. Med. Genet. 21:493, 1985.

607-C, 608-A, 609-B, 610-A, 611-A *(Braunwald, pp. 946–950; 1664–1668)*

The two-dimensional echocardiogram illustrated in Figure A displays an apical, four-chamber view of *tricuspid atresia*, demonstrating a dense band in the tricuspid annulus and a large left ventricle. This anomaly is marked by the absence of the tricuspid orifice and the presence of an intraatrial communication and hypoplasia of the right ventricle, with a communication between the systemic and pulmonary circulations that is usually a ventricular septal defect. In approximately 60 to 70 per cent of patients with this disease the great arteries have normal relationship, and the remainder have D-transposition of these vessels. In addition, pulmonic stenosis or atresia may be present and other cardiac abnormalities may coexist, especially in patients with transposition. Clinically, the marked diminution in pulmonary blood flow usually leads to severe cyanosis (see Braunwald, Fig. 30–53, p. 949). In those infants in whom transposition coexists with a ventricular septal defect and an unobstructed pulmonary outflow tract, torrential pulmonary blood flow will occur, leading to heart failure rather than cyanosis as the predominant problem. The majority of infants with tricuspid atresia have pulmonary hypoperfusion and the clinical picture of cyanosis with electrocardiographic findings of LV hypertrophy, left axis deviation, and RA enlargement.[1]

Echocardiographic examination in this disorder is usually diagnostic. At cardiac catheterization the RV cannot be entered from the RA. When the great arteries are normally related, pulmonary blood flow is found to be maintained via a ventricular septal defect or a patent ductus arteriosus. However, in complete transposition, the pulmonary artery blood flow is derived directly from the LV. Functional correction of tricuspid atresia has been accomplished by the Fontan procedure, which consists of construction of a prosthetic conduit between the RA and pulmonary artery and closure of the intraatrial comunication (see Braunwald, Fig. 30–56, p. 950).[2]

The two-dimensional echocardiogram in Figure B is a parasternal long-axis view of *tetralogy of Fallot*, which demonstrates both overriding of the aorta and the presence of a ventricular septal defect. The two other components of this malformation are obstruction to RV outflow and RV hypertrophy. The clinical presentation in tetralogy of Fallot is determined principally by the degree of obstruction to pulmonary blood flow which exists in each patient. In general, infants with tetralogy of Fallot become symptomatic and cyanotic before the age of 1 year. There is a direct correlation between the time of onset of symptoms and the severity of pulmonary outflow tract obstruction that exists. Intense cyanotic spells related to sudden increases in venoarterial shunting and simultaneous decreases in pulmonary blood flow occur between 2 and 9 months of age and may be life-threatening. Physical examination of infants with tetralogy of Fallot usually reveals varying degrees of underdevelopment and cyanosis, with clubbing of the terminal digits not uncommonly obvious within the first year of life. A RV impulse and systolic thrill may often be appreciated along the left sternal border. A systolic flow murmur across the pulmonic valve is often present, and the intensity and duration of this murmur vary inversely with the severity of the pulmonic outflow tract obstruction. The ECG usually shows RVH, and is occasionally accompanied by RA hypertrophy as well. A normal-size but boot-shaped heart ("couer en sabot") with prominence of the RV and a concavity in the region of the underdeveloped RV outflow tract may be seen on roentgenographic examination (see Braunwald, Fig. 6–37, p. 162). Echocardiographic examination is often diagnostic in this disorder. Cardiac catheterization with angiography is necessary to confirm the diagnosis, to quantitate the magnitude of shunting, to evaluate the architecture of the right-sided cardiac chambers, and to document the coronary artery anatomy prior to surgical repair. Coronary artery anatomy may have surgically important variations in this disorder, including origin of the anterior descending artery from the right coronary artery, or a single right or left coronary artery giving rise to the coronary vessels.[3]

The management of tetralogy of Fallot consists of total correction of the anomaly with early definitive repair being advocated in most centers once infants are medically prepared for intracardiac surgery. Pulmonary arterial size is the single most important determinant in evaluating a patient for primary repair of the anomaly. In patients in whom marked hypoplasia of the pulmonary arteries is present, a systemic-pulmonary arterial anastomosis may be used in a palliative manner to allow the infant to survive until childhood or adolescence, at which time total correction may be carried out at a lower risk.

REFERENCES

1. Bharati, S., and Lev, M.: Conduction system in tricuspid atresia with and without regular D-transposition. Circulation 56:423, 1977.
2. Fontan, F., Deville, C., Quaegebeur, J., Ottenkamp, J., Sourdille, N., Choussat, A., and Brom, G.A.: Repair of tricuspid atresia in 100 patients. J. Thorac. Cardiovasc. Surg. 85:647, 1983.
3. Fellows, K.E., Freed, M.D., Keane, J.F., Van Praagh, R., Bernard, W.R., and Castaneda, A.C.: Results of routine preoperative coronary angiography and tetralogy of Fallot. Circulation 51:561, 1977.

612-B, 613-A, 614-B, 615-C, 616-D *(Braunwald, pp. 1736–1741)*

Chronic hemolytic anemias, such as sickle cell anemia and thalassemia, have a variety of accompanying cardiovascular problems, including cardiomegaly, congestive heart failure, and sudden death. In addition, the specific diseases in question may have characteristic cardiopulmonary complications. In sickle cell disease, frank cardiac decompensation usually occurs in patients who have coexisting complications of the disease such as renal failure, pulmonary thrombosis and infarction, and systemic infections, or underlying cardiovascular abnormalities that are independent of the sickle cell process. Pulmonary infarction is a common complication of sickle cell anemia, and is thought to be due to thrombosis in situ rather than to embolization. Acute myocardial infarction may rarely complicate sickle cell disease, and this may involve the papillary muscle because of its susceptibility to hypoxia, since it is at the terminal portion of the coronary circulation. Cardiomegaly occurs in almost all patients with sickle cell anemia, despite the absence of other common causes of cardiomegaly. Multiple blood transfusions given as treatment for the underlying anemia may lead to myocardial iron deposition or hemosiderosis, which can contribute to the impairment of cardiac function that is noted in sickle cell disease. However, this complication occurs much more frequently in homozygous thalassemia (see below). In sickle cell disease there are no specific eletrocardiographic abnormalities, but approximately 80 per cent of patients have an abnormal ECG. Arrhythmias, on the other hand, occur only rarely with sickle cell anemia, although they may be more prevalent during acute, painful crises.[1]

The thalassemias are a group of inherited disorders that result from an imbalance in the production of hemoglobin chains and therefore a decreased production of hemoglobin A, leading to a hypochromic, microcytic anemia. Cardiac complications are the major cause of death in patients with thalassemia. Iron overload due to frequent transfusions is a common problem in thalassemia and often causes cardiomegaly. In addition, the iron deposition may lead to electrocardiographic abnormalities including arrhythmias and higher grades of heart block due to deposition of iron in the AV node and conduction system. Approximately half of all patients with thalassemia have episodes of pericarditis which may be recurrent and present in a classic manner. Roentgenographic evidence of cardiac enlargement in children regresses when hemoglobin is maintained above 10 g/dl in this disorder, and supportive therapy with an adequate transfusion program, splenectomy, and early treatment of infections has prolonged the lives of patients with thalassemia.[2] Calcification of chordae tendineae is not seen in either sickle cell anemia or thalassemia.

REFERENCES

1. Maisel, A., Friedman, H., Flint, L., Koshy, M., and Prabhu, R.: Continuous electrocardiographic monitoring in patients with sickle cell anemia during pain crisis. Clin. Cardiol. 6:339, 1983.
2. Yee, H., Mra, R., and Nyunt, K.M.: Cardiac abnormalities in the

thalassemia syndromes. Southeast Asian J. Trop. Med. Public Health 15:414, 1984.

617-A, 618-D, 619-B *(Braunwald, pp. 1717–1720)*

A group of arthritic syndromes including ankylosing spondylitis, Reiter's disease, psoriatic arthritis, and several intestinal arthropathies has been classified as *seronegative spondyloarthropathies* because they share common clinical features, including predilection of arthritis for the sacroiliac and lumbosacral joints and predominance of the disease in men as opposed to women. They are distinguished from rheumatoid arthritis by the absence of increased rheumatoid factor. These diseases are associated with the histocompatibility antigen HLA B-27.

Ankylosing spondylitis is the most common of these syndromes to involve the heart, and classically causes dilatation of the aortic valve ring with fibrous thickening, scarring, and inflammation of the aortic valve. There is also dilatation of the sinuses of Valsalva so that the lesions resemble those of syphilis, although in ankylosing spondylitis the lesions are confined to the valve ring and do not affect the rest of the aorta. Mitral regurgitation is infrequent and usually insignificant in these diseases, although over many years, dilation of the left ventricle can lead to some mitral regurgitation.[1] AV block and conduction defects are common because of extension of fibrosis into the muscular septum and destruction of the proximal bundle branches. Pericardial rubs may occur during severe acute episodes but are rare in the chronic syndrome. The prevalence of the aortic lesion is related to the duration of spondylitis and peripheral joint involvement, reaching an incidence of 10 per cent in those with spondylitis for 30 years or more, and 18 per cent if peripheral joint involvement is also present.

Rheumatoid arthritis is a much more common disease than ankylosing spondylitis but less frequently involves the heart. The most characteristic pathological lesion of rheumatoid arthritis, the nodular granuloma, may involve the myocardium, endocardium, and valves of the heart. The extent of this involvement is proportional to the severity of the disease and is usually associated with rheumatoid nodules present subcutaneously and elsewhere. The most common clinical finding is pericarditis. Pericardial effusions may be demonstrated by echocardiography in 30 per cent of all patients studied and 50 per cent of those with subcutaneous nodules.[2] It is thought that this is an autoimmune phenomenon, since immunohistochemical staining of the pericardium reveals plasma cell infiltration and deposits of immunoglobulin. It is rare that cardiac function or valve function is impaired in rheumatoid arthritis, although in severe forms, granulomas may appear on the valves, leading to regurgitation. The most common cardiac finding in rheumatoid arthritis is first-degree AV block.[3]

REFERENCES

1. Roberts, W.C., Hollingsworth, J.F., Bulkley, B.H., Jaffee, R.B., Epstein, S.E., and Stinson, E.B.: Combined mitral and aortic regurgitation in ankylosing spondylitis. Angiographic and anatomic features. Am. J. Med. 56:237, 1984.

2. MacDonald, W.J., Jr., Crawford, M.H., Klippel, J.H., Zvaifler, N.J., and O'Rourke, R.A.: Echocardiographic assessment of cardiac structure and function in patients with rheumatoid arthritis. Am. J. Med. 63:890, 1977.
3. Cathcart, E.S., and Spodick, D.H.: Rheumatoid heart disease. A study of the incidence and nature of cardiac lesions in rheumatoid arthritis. N. Engl. J. Med. 266:959, 1962.

620-A, 621-D, 622-B, 623-A (Braunwald, pp. 1765–1767; 1778–1779)

Tissue plasminogen activator (tPA) is the major physiological activator of plasminogen and is synthesized predominantly in endothelial cells. The protein is synthesized in a single-chain form, which is subsequently converted to a two-chain form by proteolytic cleavage of a single plasmin-sensitive site. Both the single-chain and the two-chain forms have endogenous proteolytic activity. The α chain of tPA is derived from the amino terminal portion of single-chain tPA and contains a pair of finger-like structures referred to as "kringle" domains. The lysine binding sites located on these kringle domains confer binding specificity for fibrin. Thus, tPA is a relatively fibrin-specific activator, which converts plasminogen to plasmin two to three times more efficiently in the presence of fibrin. The protease domain of tPA contains a proteolytic site that converts plasminogen to plasmin. This portion of the protein is homologous to other serine proteases, such as urokinase and trypsin.[1] Urokinase is a two-chain serine protease with a molecular weight of 33,000 daltons, which is synthesized both in renal tubular epithelial cells and in endothelial cells. While urokinase converts plasminogen to plasmin by hydrolyzing the same bond as that acted on by tPA, the proteolytic activity of urokinase is not enhanced by the presence of fibrin and therefore it may activate circulating plasminogen as effectively as plasminogen absorbed onto fibrin thrombi.

Both platelets and endothelial cells secrete a plasminogen activator inhibitor (PAI) that participates in the careful endogenous regulation of the fibrinolytic system. Alpha$_2$-plasmin inhibitor is structurally homologous to other serine protease inhibitors such as antithrombin III and circulates in plasma so that it is available to neutralize free plasmin.[2] However, the kringle domains and the active-site serine of plasmin must be accessible for binding and neutralization by alpha$_2$-plasmin inhibitor. Therefore, when plasmin is bound to fibrin, it is "protected" from the neutralizing effect of alpha$_2$-plasmin inhibitor. This mechanism helps to maintain the fibrinolytic activity of plasmin within a particular thrombus while minimizing systemic fibrinolysis.

Thus, the fibrin clot itself plays a central role in the regulation of fibrinolysis. Fibrin binds plasminogen and thus concentrates it within the clot. The presence of fibrin also simultaneously enhances the activity of tPA while inhibiting the activity of alpha$_2$-plasmin inhibitor. These mechanisms help to make the endogenous fibrinolytic system relatively clot-specific and protect against systemic fibrolysis.

REFERENCES

1. Loscalzo, J., and Braunwald, E.: Tissue plasminogen activator. N. Engl. J. Med. 319:925, 1988.
2. Moroi, M., and Aoki, N.: Isolation and characterization of alpha$_2$-plasmin inhibitor from human plasma. A novel proteinase inhibitor which inhibits activator-induced lysis. J. Biol. Chem. 251:5956, 1976.